I0060964

Cancer

Cares, Treatments and Preventions

Cancer – Cares, Treatments and Preventions

Publisher: iConcept Press Ltd.
Cover design: Pineapple Design Ltd.
Interior design: iConcept Press Ltd.
Typesetting and copy editing: iConcept Press Ltd. and Pineapple Design Ltd.

ISBN: 978-1-922227-492

This work is subjected to copyright. All rights are reserved, whether the whole or part of the materials is concerned, specifically the rights of translation, reprinting, re-use of illustrations, recitation, broadcasting, reproduction on microfilms or in other ways, and storage in data banks. Duplication of this publication or parts thereof is only permitted under the provisions of the authors, editors and/or iConcept Press Ltd.

Printed in the United States of America

Copyright © iConcept Press 2014

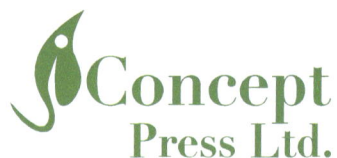

iConcept
Press Ltd.

www.iconceptpress.com

Contents

Preface

Cancer is a broad group of diseases involving unregulated cell growth, in which cells divide and grow uncontrollably, forming malignant tumors, and invade nearby parts of the body. Cancer may also spread to different parts of the body through the lymphatic system or the bloodstream. *Cancer – Cares, Treatments and Preventions* discusses some recent advances in cancer research.

There are totally 12 chapters in this book. Chapter 1 discusses the epidemiology of smoking and tobacco prevention efforts globally with emphasis on anti-tobacco education at the Elementary School level. Chapter 2 considers both the protection and inclusion of pregnant women in clinical trials. Guidance and an algorithm for determining which is appropriate for studies is included. Chapter 3 describes a method called Multiple reaction monitoring (MRM), which is a a targeted MS-based technology that provides the specificity, throughput, and multiplexing capabilities required for candidate biomarker quantitation in patient samples. It enables reliable and accurate quantitation of putative cancer biomarkers. This general approach will help to "credential" candidate markers and will help bridge the gap between discovery and pre-clinical validation. Chapter 4 discusses monoclonal antibodies (mAbs). mAbs and their derivatives, continue to be the focus of the biopharmaceutical industry for many diagnostic and therapeutic applications. In spite of vast improvements in our capability to deal with mAbs, they still pose many challenges.

Chapter 5 reviews four currently distinguished strategies to achieve tumor-specific infection and presents a transductional targeting strategies to specifically redirect viruses towards surface receptors on tumor cells. Chapter 6 reviews past and present treatment philosophies and regimens for treating Ewing's sarcoma. The authors also highlights how the identification of new therapeutic targets can be exploited through the use of tumor-specific agents. Chapter 7 examines what can be expected from using animal models to learn about cancers that affect humans. As humans and animals are examples of evolved, complex systems extrapolating outcomes from perturbations that occur at or effect higher levels of organization will be unlikely. This in part explains the profound lack of progress in finding treatments to human cancers. Chapter 8 provides a comprehensive overview of mitochondrial energy metabolism and cancer, analyzes mitochondrial protection and energy metabolic improvement of Astragalus Polysaccharides (APS), proposes a novel cancer-preventive mechanism from the perspective of effects of APS on mitochondrial oxidative phosphorylation and intracellular adenylates levels, and provides a new way of perspective, thinking and hope for the prevention and treatment of cancer.

Chapter 9 discusses clinically applied radiopharmaceuticals studied and used in Oncology. Constructive summary tables and up-to-date references provide the student and clinician with a working knowledge and understanding of different Nuclear Medicine techniques. Chapter 10 identifies indications for DT technique for chest imaging. Moreover, the authors performed experiments to measure the artificial pulmonary nodules detection capabilities of the DT imaging system for use as an effective screening method and compared the results with those of radiography and CT imaging. Chapter 11 presents a study to understand the behaviours of normal and diseased breast images from the Digital Database for Screening Mammography (DDSM), considering measures of lacunarity and fractal dimension with the corresponding texture signatures. The malignant nodules with the respective adjacent structures (partial pixels) also were quantified applying a multilevel segmentation method based on maximum entropy. All obtained results provide important information about the studied structures and may contribute with the developments of CAD systems. Chapter 12 presents recent advances in the field of Raman-based optical-biopy for cancer detection. A revision concerned applications to breast, oral, cervical cancers, technological challenges and perspectives is discussed.

Editing and publishing a book is never an easy task. Each chapter in this book has gone through a peer review, a selection and an editing process so as to guarantee its quality. Without the supports and contributions of the authors and reviewers, this book can never be able to complete. We would like to thank all of the authors in this book and all of the reviewers who participated in the reviewing process: Erin J. Aiello Bowles, Leandro Alves Neves, Myron Arlen, M. A. Azam, Anna Rita Bizzarri, Donald J Buchsbaum, Eline M Bunnik, Helena R. Chang, Bor-Sen Chen, Yu Chen, Liu Cheng, Zongbin Cui, AS Fathinul Fikri, José Alberto Fonseca-Moutinho, Nicolaas AP Franken, Simone Fulda, Stacie E. Geller, Amir H. Golnabi, T.F. Heston, Jeff Holst, Agnes Hotz-Wagenblatt, J. A. M. J. L. Janssen, Rainer J Klement, Leighton Ku, Sanghun Lee, Kirsten A. Leiss, Derek LeRoith, Annabelle Lewis, Yan Li, M. Liedlgruber, E. Maioli, Philippe Marchetti, Steven E Massey, Edward F. Miles, Marco Montillo, Kotsedi D Monyeki, Takeshi Morii, Christopher T Naugler, Dorte Lisbet Nielsen, Robin J. Parks, Maikel P. Peppelenbosch, Eugenio Picano, Keerthana Prasad, Wei-Jun Qian, Prithi Rajan, Jae Y. Ro, Franklin David Rumjanek, C. Haris Saslis-Lagoudakis, J. Fah Sathirapongsasuti, Bernhard Schaller, Emad A Shalaby, David W. Speicher, Amere Subbarao Sreedhar, Vivek Subbiah, Aladar A. Szalay, Mark Tangney, Martin Trepel, Koji Ueda, Felipe Vadillo-Ortega, Hongsheng Wang, Yitao Wang, Bang-Wen Xie, Dongzi Yang, Shozo Yokoyama and Hyun Jo Youn. We hope that you, the reader, will find this book interesting and useful. Any advices please feel free and are always welcome to tell us.

iConcept Press Ltd
March 2014

Smoking and Cancer:
Anti-Tobacco Advertisement &
Education Programs in Elementary Schools

Sara Surani
Pulmonary Associates, Corpus Christi, Texas USA

Salim Surani
Texas A&M University, USA

1   Introduction

Every 6 seconds, a person dies of a tobacco related illness. Every 24 hours, > 14,000 people die of a tobacco related cause. When these statistics are combined, tobacco will kills 6 million individuals per year internationally. 1.25 billion People worldwide are smoker, if action is not taken, 650 million smokers alive today will eventually die of tobacco related diseases. Nine out of 10 of these deaths resulting in lung cancer are attributed to smoking, and 3 of 10 cancer related deaths can be attributed to smoking. If no action is taken, tobacco will take the lives of 8 million people every year, and the lives of 250 million adolescents within the upcoming decades. Tobacco users have significant health care cost due to tobacco related illness. It is estimated to cost $500 billion worldwide. In addition, to the health care cost smoking results in significant productivity loss due to illness (Tobacco Free Kids, 2012).

Since 6,000 BC, tobacco and nicotine have been utilized and cultivated in the American civilization. Tobacco was not only merely consumed, but also symbolized vital roles in religious rites and ceremonies from the Indian to Mayan civilizations. While the Mayans exploited tobacco as a solar incense to bring rain during the dry seasons, the Aztecs used it for ceremonial purposes. Aside from the Eastern Hemisphere, the early usage of tobacco also has roots in the Western Hemisphere. In 1492, Christopher Columbus and company witnessed the American Indians igniting tobacco leaves. From that point onwards, the utilization and consumption of tobacco dispersed worldwide, ranging from its introduction to Middle East in 1500's, to China, Japan, and India in 1600's and to New Zealand in 1700s (Hymowitz, 2011).

The understanding of tobacco has taken a 360 degree turn over the past centuries. The ancient physicians of the 16th to 19th century believed on the medicinal values of tobacco. For example, the Cohilia Indians of California used tobacco as an agent to ward off evils. Indians from other tribes believed the properties of tobacco to be a remedy for biliary colic's, frost bites and burns. Additionally, in 1597, John Gerard published a book on therapeutics and illustrated the qualities of tobacco for the treatment of headaches, rheumatism, and protection against infections. As a result, in 1665, during the Great Plague of London, many individuals found the chewing of tobacco prophylactic and preventative. As was the case with the Yellow Fever epidemic in Philadelphia during 1973. The evidence of tobacco hazards emerged in 1670 when Dutch anatomist Theodor Keckring described a black tongue and copious soot in the trachea of a smoker's autopsy. Later, there was evidence of cancer in the noses among those who inhaled tobacco (Hymowitz, 2008).

2   Health Hazards of Tobacco Use

Over the years, extensive literature has linked smoking to various types of cancer, including cancer of the lung, head, neck, breast, and oral organs (Carbone, 1992; White, 1990). Conclusions from the Surgeon General's report have linked cigarette smoking during childhood and adolescence to a raging epidemic the young population. Moreover, passive smoking has resulted in chronic respiratory disease, fertility issues among men and women, an increased incidence of spontaneous abortion, abruptio placenta, preeclampsia, eclampsia, fetal growth retardation (especially if the mother was smoking during pregnancy), lower respiratory tract illness, an increase in middle ear disease, asthma, and atrophy. (Preventing Tobacco Use Among Youth and Young Adults: A report of the Surgeon General, 2012)

There are > 7,000 chemicals in the tobacco smoke, 69 of them can cause cancer (Guntupalli, 2010). Of those polycyclic aromatic hydrocarbons (PAH) and the tobacco specific nitrosamine 4-(methylnitrosamine)-1-(3-pyridyl)-1-butanone (NNK) are strongly linked to lung cancer. Nicotine, though not listed as carcinogen, is the most addictive substance in the tobacco smoke. The smoking of the cigarette leads to inhalation of several harmful substances. Polycyclic aromatic hydrocarbons (PAHs), nicotine-derived nitrosamine ketone (NNK) and other carcinogens undergo metabolic activation, leading to the formation of DNA adducts, which are the carcinogen metabolites bound covalently to DNA, mainly at guanine or adenosine site. This in turn leads to mutation and other changes as RAS, MYC, p53, p16, RB, FHIT and other critical genomic changes, leading to lung cancer. Similarly, the carcinogens leading to mutations in the DNA also lead to cancers in other organs (Hecht, 1999).

In addition to cancer, cigarette smoking has also been attributed to 80 million cases of COPD worldwide, with approximately 3 million deaths due to COPD. This comprises of approximately 5% of adult deaths globally (Halbert et al., 2006). The cigarette smoke contains highly noxious oxidants, which induces inflammation in the lung and the airways and has been confirmed by the bronchial biopsies. The increases in airway inflammation, and the structural changes in the airway, are worsened by persistence of smoking (Laniado-Laborin, 2009; Saetta et al., 1993). Significant progress has been made in understanding the relationship between smoking and lung cancer, but is yet to be determined why a person may get cancer after smoking, whereas another person who smokes may not get it. Future studies addressing the genetic markers of the individual person may help to shed some light addressing the individual genes response to the carcinogens.

The correlation of smoking and cancer has been widely accepted for the past several decades. In comparison to non-smokers, smokers were found to have a 10-fold higher risk of death from lung cancer, and heavy smoking were found to have an even higher risk (Carbone, 1992; Ockene et al., 1990). Additionally, Ockene and Shaten (1991) reported that among the 12,000 males who were studied for 10 years during the Multiple Risk Factor Intervention Trial (MRFIT), smoking was attributed to lung cancer in all 12,000 cases. The mortality ratio also increases with the number of cigarettes smoked per day, in addition to the degree of inhalation. During a 26 year follow-up study consisting of approximately 250,000 people, McLaughlin et al. (1990) reported a 47% excess risk rate of mortality from renal cancer among smokers, and among heavy smokers the relative risk was 2.1-fold higher than the risk among nonsmokers. In addition, another study confirmed that smokers were found to have a 2-fold higher risk of leukemia, the risk was even higher for myeloid leukemia (Mills et al., 1990).

3   Epidemiology of Smoking

Eighty-one and a half percent of the adult smokers smoked their 1st cigarette before the age of 18, and the remaining 16.5% took their "first puff" before they were 26. In addition, one-third of the adult smoker population have smoked their 1st cigarette before the age of 14 (Preventing Tobacco Use Among Youth and Young Adults: A report of the Surgeon General, 2012). According to the 2009 National Youth Tobacco Survey report (NYTS), 23.2% of high school seniors are current smokers and an additional 11.6% are smokeless tobacco users (Institute of Medicine. Keeping patients safe: Transforming the work environment of nurses, 2004).

The use of tobacco at an early age is associated with significant health hazards starting from an early age, as well as later in the individual's life. Eventually, this leads to a national economic impact, often resulting in financial instability. In addition, sufficient data suggests that smoking tobacco provokes lower grades, and supports the notion that a consequential decrease in academic performance leads to smoking (Bergen *et al.*, 2005; Bryant *et al.*, 2000; Hu *et al.*, 1998; Young & Rogers, 1986). However, several studies have also shown no correlation between smoking and academic grades (Azevedo *et al.*, 1999; Leatherdale *et al.*, 2008).

4   Cigarette Advertisements

In recent years, tobacco companies have spent billions of dollars in cause marketing, focusing on specific target groups. These techniques have taken into consideration the behavioral aspect of the clientèle. More importantly, they have focused on product design, product messaging, pricing, distribution, mass media, movies, and advertisements; however, tobacco companies have long argued that their marketing efforts have not been directed at certain groups, nor their marketing efforts have led to an increase in tobacco consumption among the younger population. The tobacco industry spent 12.4 billion dollars in 2002 in comparison to 13.11 billion dollars for commercial marketing in 2005, which has abated to 9.9 billion dollars in 2008 as per the Federal Trade Commission filling (FTC) (Baldwin & Daugherty, 2004). In addition, explicit efforts have been initiated branding cigarette packages for different age groups. Marlboro, Newport, and Camel were the top 3 brands for varying age groups, as "Joe Camel" was to lure the children towards smoking. The tobacco companies also recruited new smokers and aesthetically appealing advertisements in order to inspire the adolescents to start (Lovato *et al.*, 2003; Perry, 1999). Earlier studies in 1990's from Fisher *et al.* (1991) showed that children were familiar with different tobacco brands. It was ascertained that 91% of 6-year-old children were able to correctly match the picture of Joe Camel with the cigarette, in comparison to a picture of Walt Disney's Mickey Mouse. An additional study by Chapman *et al.* (1982; 2009) from Australia also pointed out that 11-14 year old adolescents who smoked cigarettes were more likely to identify the cigarette advertisement with a missing word and were able to complete the marketing cigarette slogans as compared to non-smoking adolescents. Cigarette brand recognition among smokers was found to be significantly higher than non-smokers in other studies as well (Botvin *et al.*, 1993; Hanewinkel *et al.*, 2010). In 1998, a study by Arnett *et al.* (2001) also demonstrated that 95% of students in grades 6 – 12 had seen at least 1 advertisement featuring "Joe Camel" or Marlboro, and 50% had seen related advertisements > 5 times. More than 50% of those students believed that "Joe Camel" made smoking more appealing, and 40% of them felt the same way about Marlboro. Other studies have shown that students were also receptive to the smoking advertisement and also they showed the tendency to favor magazines that contained tobacco advertisements (Feighery *et al.*, 2001).

A study by Pierce *et al.* (1998) showed that residents from California who had never smoked, but had a favorite cigarette advertisement, were more likely to commence smoking then those who were not aesthetically pleased by tobacco advertisements. It was also estimated that 34% of experimentation by children was attributed to tobacco marketing and advertisement. The same group also assessed the cigarette advertisement campaign conducted after the 1998 settlement. Longitudinal cohorts who were 10-13 years when they were enrolled in 2003 were surveyed about their favorite cigarette brand., At the 5th interview in 2007, the boys' ad preference remained stable over 5 years, whereas for females, it remained stable for 4 years. However, when "Joe Camel's" advertisement appeared, the percentage of females who reported a favorite ad increased from 10% to 44%. Researcher have found the "Joe Camel" brand accounts for favorite tobacco ad among the adolescent population (Pierce *et al.*, 2010). In addition to commercials, movies have also been an avenue for the tobacco marketing industry to convey a "cool image" when portraying celebrities with cigarettes. With the recent efforts, the utilization of tobacco in general audience movies has gradually declined.

Additionally, the tobacco industry also used the interplay between cigarette marketing and peer pressure. Peer and parental influence was associated with both the decisions of the children and adolescent to take up tobacco. To look cool and to appear popular was an inherent behavior among teens as well. Tobacco industries systematically exploited these common adolescent desires, using imagery to create a sense of popularity, coolness, and individuality. Pechmann (2002) and Kelder *et al.* (2002) showed that an exposure to both cigarette ads and peers who smoke tend to have paramount influence on the future risk of smoking. The tobacco industry has also been able to match the prices of other competitors in the industry and kept and maintained the cost in an affordable range. The data from Walker (2011) precisely demonstrated that an increase in the tobacco price constricted the consumption rate. This strategy was adopted by the law makers as an effort to increase the tobacco tax, henceforth increasing the tobacco price which resulted in the decrease of tobacco use.

Recently, tobacco industries entered web based marketing and have spent more than $13.2 million in 2008 in U.S. alone (Baldwin & Daugherty, 2004). In 2004, Brown and Williamson launched their KOOL MIXX hip-hop campaign, but voluntarily withdrew the campaign due to alleged law suits from several states' attorneys general. In addition, RJ Reynolds has established a website where smokers can participate in an online survey to be entered for sweepstakes (Lewis *et al.*, 2004). In 2011, web sites with the tobacco brands advertising surfaced across various the internet sites. This practice could increase with the increasing availability of alternate products such as smokeless tobaccos and electric cigarettes that may serve as a challenge due to the current generation's complete dependence on the internet. Surprisingly, when the phrase "discount tobacco" was searched on Google on 8/18/2012 it yielded 2.2 million search results.

Several studies have examined the augmentation of the online buying of tobacco products. Unger and colleagues (Unger *et al.*, 2001) reported that in 1999 – 2000, 2% of children < 18 reported buying cigarettes online in California, whereas a study by Fix and coworkers showed that 6.5% of 9[th]graders purchased cigarettes online (Fix *et al.*, 2006). Because of the current legislations, a vast majority of the current corporate web sites now have tobacco legislation updates, educational, and corporate information. Between 1982 – 1987, the tobacco companies influenced the Japanese government through US Trade Representatives to eliminate advertisement restrictions, resulting in 10-fold increase in export between 1985 – 1996. They also use popular Hollywood movie stars to influence the cool image of smoking (Lambert *et al.*, 2004).

5   Tobacco Prevention Globally

Tobacco has become a global challenge. To counter the global smoking, in May 2003 the World Health Organization (WHO) adopted the WHO framework on tobacco control. This was embraced by United Nations in order to take the action against tobacco prevention globally. This framework was signed by 115 countries to do a comprehensive ban on tobacco advertisement, promotion and sponsorship. This treaty was designed to help galvanize the preventive effort to combat the use of tobacco globally, and to help countries develop their policy for tobacco control. WHO came up with 6 policies which a now universally known as "MPOWER", which stands for:

- Monitor tobacco use and prevention policies,
- Protect people from tobacco smoke,
- Often help to quit smoke,
- Warn about the dangers of tobacco,
- Enforce bans on tobacco advertising, promotion and sponsorship, and
- Raise taxes on tobacco." (WHO, 2008)

Raising the taxes as a part of the governmental regulations and policies has been 1 of the most powerful tools to curtail the rate of tobacco smoking. In addition to getting higher tax revenue, the government has been spending less health care dollars on tobacco related illness due to declines in smoking. The public policies have also been garnered to ban smoking in public places and prevent hazards of second hand smoke. Ireland, on implementation of their smoke-free environment policies, demonstrated a decline of 83% in ambient air nicotine content. In addition second hand smoke among bar workers plunged to 0hours exposure per week from 30 hours per week, a significant decline in second hand smoking (WHO, 2008). In addition, supports for smoke free area are becoming popular with > 60% of population in New Zealand, New York City, California, Ireland, and Uruguay are supporting that. The tobacco industries have been advocating that smoke free bars and restaurants may hurt small business', but conversely a survey by Zagat (restaurant survey), showed that the smoke free environment actually is more beneficial for the business (WHO, 2008).

6   Anti-Tobacco education Program in School

So far we have discussed briefly the ill effect of smoking, health related issues related to smoking as well as smoking and cancer. We also briefly discussed tobacco marketing and the different avenues tobacco industries have utilized in order to improve their market share of smokers. These industries particularly focused on the child and adolescent populations, as the data indubitably asserted that > 80% of current smokers started smoking before age 18.

Governments, advocates against smoking, and several organizations have started educating the public, as well as children, regarding the perilous effects of smoking. From media campaigns to legislation, from community education outreach activities to raising taxes on tobacco products, also in addition to numerous law suits against the tobacco industry have all vigorously attempted to curtail the smoking and utilization of tobacco products. So far, regulations, smoke-free environments, raising taxes on tobacco products, and the banning of advertisements directed towards smoking have all worked in the United States and several countries to some extent; however, the tobacco industry has expanded their horizon to developing countries where the use of tobacco is on rise. Extensive efforts have been directed towards school based education, in an attempt to prevent the "first puff." We will look at several studies, methods, and means in further detail alongside discussing the school based education programs which our group has undertaken.

Over the past 3 decades, several school based programs have been initiated, ranging from curriculum based programs, movies, and educational material to coaching by teachers and school nurses. Additional studies on informational, affective/motivational and psychological approaches to prevent smoking have been deemed ineffective (Beattie, 1984; Thompson, 1978), though, a study by McGuire (1964) has shown moderate effectiveness. In 1994, the Surgeon General report revealed that school based programs that taught resistance skills exhibited momentous reductions among youth smoking. Several studies, reviews, and meta-analysis' have shown that school based programs, when accompanied with interactive programs offering interaction, role playing, and the practice of social skills have been quite effective (Flay, 2007; Hwang et al., 2004; Park, 2006; Tingle et al., 2003). In addition, the Center of Disease Control (CDC) continues to recommend school based prevention programs and suggests offering the tobacco education curriculum from kindergarten to 12th grade, with more emphasis in the high school (Addressing Tobacco Use and Addiction, 2007).

Hurd et al. (1980) reported improvement in the self reported smoking among 7th grade students at the end of 6 months, when the results of control students were compared with the results of students who received the curriculum and monitoring. Denson and Stretch (1981) from Canada reported a 6.5% reduction in student self reported tobacco use at the 2-year follow-up period. School based programs were conducted for 6th and 7th grade students: consisting of 4 sessions, an animated film, lectures, and an interactive group discussion. Evans (1981) showed a 5.1% point decrease in self reported regular or frequent tobacco use. The program was school based, comprising of 1,852 participants. The educational information was delivered during physical education time by multiple graduate or undergraduate coordinators. Studies from San Jose, California done by Telch et al. (1982) found an 11% reduction in an intervention group at 33 months among 9th graders on self reported smoking. In addition, several other studies have shown reduction in the self reported smoking post intervention (Aveyard et al., 2001; Botvin et al., 1990; Dielman et al., 1985; Killen et al., 1988; Perry et al., 1992).

Hwang et al. (2004) looked at the social influence, cognitive behavioral influence, and life skills among adolescents. They discovered that social influence approaches had effect size (ESs) of 0.12 at a short term follow up, and drop down to 0.07 at an interval > 3 years. Cognitive behavioral and life skills approach showed an effect at short term interval, but effectiveness dropped on long term interval. Morehouse and Tobler (2000) and Tobler (1997) summarized the results of a series of their meta-analyses, concluding that school based programs that utilize interactive learning approaches among similar age group peers as their leaders were deemed the most effective. Additionally, Walter et al. (1989) studied school based education among 4th grade students, recording an indicative effectiveness in their prediction of students not smoking when they grow older. This teacher based curriculum was conducted 2 hours per week and continued from 4th grade through 9th grade.

The Cochrane Review published a summary concerning preventative smoking school based programs in 2006. Their main challenge consisted of the program's inability to meet the randomization control trials criteria. Of the 94 randomized control trials, only 23 were classified as valid (category 1). There was a single category 1 trial that focused on information giving, and 2 category 1 studies focused on teaching social competence. Additionally, there were 13 category 1 studies which focused on social influence interventions. Among the pool of studies, Hutchinson smoking prevention was projected to be the largest study. It was conducted from September 1984 to August 1999 and was designed in order to attain the most rigorous randomized trial to see the long term impact of theory based social influence among children from grade 3rd to 12th on smoking prevalence among youth. The trials consisted of 8,388 participating children and achieved the implementation fidelity and a 94% follow up rate. They found no significant differences in the prevalence of daily smoking between the control and intervention group (Peterson et al., 2000). After thorough review, the Cochrane Review felt that there were only 3 high quality randomized control trials that studied the effectiveness of combining social influences and social competence interventions, and 4 that tested the multi-modal interventions, half of which showed substantial positive results (Thomas & Perera, 2006).

Numerous school base programs have shown to have a short term effect, but the efficacy of the intervention fails to merit on a long term horizon; however, when the intervention was conducted with interactive sessions, long term positive results sprouted among the students (Wiehe *et al.*, 2005). Additionally, Skara and Sussman (2003) reviewed multiple studies of 25 programs for tobacco prevention with ≥ 2 years follow-up. It was found that 18 studies reported significant short-term effects, 15 of which reported the long-term effects. Of the studies with significant short-term effects, 72% had significant long-term effects. Zaza *et al.* (2005) and colleagues, in their book, identified 17 studies suitable for their analysis. They ascertained that over time, school based education in coalescence with mass media campaigns and community education have resulted in a consistent reduction in adolescent smoking. Dobbins *et al.* (2008) examined reviews and meta-analyses from 1985 – 2007. It was concluded that school based program were effective on a short term basis in effort to reduce smoking intention, onset and prevalence. Flay and colleagues showed that school based programs can have the long-term effect if they have ≥ 15 sessions and an interactive lessons based on social skills and influence (BR, 2007; Preventing Tobacco Use Among Youth and Young Adults: A report of the Surgeon General, 2012). Home smoking environment plays also an important role among childhood smoking. Home smoking ban can influence smoking behavior, smoking believes and motivation to quit smoking. This is more important among African American and Hispanic ethnicities, where smoking is more prevalent at homes (Muilenburg Legge *et al.*, 2009). In addition to an increase in prevalence of smoke free homes can decrease the incidence of sudden infant death syndrome (Behm *et al.*, 2012). The infants do get significant second hand smoke exposure if parents are smoking. In a study, 27% of infants were found to have detectable level of cotinine (Daly *et al.*, 2010). Efforts must be directed towards parental involvement in combating smoking behavior among children.

7   Anti-Tobacco Education at the Elementary School Level

Most intervention programs have been designed for high school students, or students entering 7th or 8th grade. However, according to a report by the University of Michigan, Monitoring the Future, they reported that 6.1% of 8th graders and 11.8% of 10th graders are current smokers (Pietroiusti *et al.*, 2009). The authors of this chapter have designed a program in order to prevent the "first puff" at a very early age. McAlister and coworkers also discovered that the combination of intensive media and community campaigns can result in a significant reduction in adult tobacco usage (Murray *et al.*, 1989). Due to this, the anti-smoking education shown has only a diminutive effect when the program is initiated after the individual starts smoking. Additionally, it has been recorded that the tools and methods utilized in the delivery of the message are vitally important. Videos and age appropriate material can be an substantial factor in the success rate (Glynn, 1985). Since tobacco industries have utilized movies, films, and other avenues to lure and attract children, it is only logical for the anti-tobacco programs to utilize the same media and social network to counter those effects. Studies have shown that a single component approach seems to be ineffective on most instances, whereas using a multi-prong approach involving movies, story books, coloring books, and stickers along with the presenter may help to create a more memorable approach.

The authors' group targeted school children from 1st – 3rd grade with the main goal to educate children in order to prevent the "first puff" (Surani *et al.*, 2011). A program entitled "*AntE Tobacco*" was designed for elementary level students and was developed using a collaboration of movies, storybooks and coloring books, which were all replicas of the movie presented. The movie educated the children on the harmful effects of smoking, whereas the storybooks and coloring books served as a reinforcer that the children took home, read, and worked on. The vibrantly colored stickers and other attractants were also distributed in order to give students the "cool effect" and a sense of pride. The movie attempted to deliver 2 key messages: "Say no to smoking the first time and every time" and "stop using tobacco before it kills you" (Surani, *et al.*, 2011).

The programs were conducted by trained physicians, nurses, allied health professionals, and trained volunteers. Each program lasted 50 minutes. The program was initiated with a brief question-and-answer session, along with pre-test questions to assess the baseline status of the student's knowledge. This was followed by a 13 minutes "*AntETobacco*" video presentation and concluded with a post-test questionnaire and a second question and answer session. The "*AntE Tobacco*" message in the movie was conveyed through a colony of ants. "In the story, a young ant is lured by the excitement of tobacco, succumbs to temptations, is caught with tobacco by the grandpa ant, taught the dangers of tobacco and then vows never to try it again. He then learns that the reason grandpa ant is tired all of the time is because he uses tobacco. The family convinces the grandpa that, with their help, that they can all "*say no to tobacco*". The cartoon addresses both smokeless tobacco usage and cigarettes in a way children can understand with a storyline centered around family, pictures with bright colors, and loveable characters with whom they can relate." (*Foundation*) The presenter spent approximately 30 minutes, total, in addressing basic information about hazards of smoking, the myths about smoking, and clarifying any issues which children may have.

Overall, a total of 6,595 children were educated. The child's baseline knowledge of smoking, its' addictive nature and the effects of passive smoking were assessed. Children in 3rd grade were better informed on the pre-test compared to children in 1st grade. Results showed that approximately 6% of the participating child's siblings and 23% of the participating child's parents smoked. Interestingly, 83% knew it was tough to quit once they started smoking and 3% believed that they could smoke in a school environment (all the schools in the USA are smoke free facilities) (Surani, *et al.*, 2011). Post video, the children were given a post-test in order to assess the understanding of the message. The effectiveness of the movie and storybook was also assessed by performing a random survey to see if the children remembered the message delivered to them in the form of a storybook. The survey of the randomly selected school showed significant improvement in the retention at the 6-weekinterval. This was felt to be secondary to children reading the story book at home which was complete replica of the movie; that may be serving as reinforce towards their knowledge and improvement in a 6 week post test score (Surani, *et al.*, 2011). This study, observed in Galveston, Texas, USA, was limited by survey instrument being not validated, and a sample size gathered from single geographical area. The same group recorded that approximately 80% of the children do not consider children who smoke to be "popular and cool" on the post-intervention.

8   Conclusion

Considering the tremendous amount of public health education, mass media campaigns, and school based education programs, community education activities, and several reports by Surgeon Generals, smoking among children remains prevalent and at rise in the developing countries. Since 90% of the adult smokers start smoking before the age of 18 serves as an impetus of destruction for the health of the future generations. In addition, > 3.6 million kids < 18 are current smokers, 20% of which are smokers when they leave high school. More than 6.3 million children who are 18 years old today will die as a result of a smoking-related illness (Institute of Medicine. Keeping patients safe:Transforming the work environment of nurses, 2004; Pietroiusti *et al.*, 2009). A significant effort in the developed countries has assisted to some degree in order to decrease the rate of smoking, but more efforts are needed in the developing countries if the preventable risk of cancer desires to be extirpated. According to Surgeon General's report conclusion, "The evidence is sufficient to conclude that mass media campaigns, comprehensive community programs, and comprehensive statewide tobacco control program can prevent the initiation of tobacco use and reduces its prevalence among health". (Institute of Medicine. Keeping patients safe:Transforming the work environment of nurses, 2004) In summation, school based programs can produce at least short-term effects and reduce the prevalence of smoking among the youth of the current and future generations. Still, studies need to focus on the effectiveness of comprehensive school based and mass media programs directed towards children at very early age in order to prevent the "first puff." If this task is achieved, it can lead to the prevention of the health hazards of smoking and smoking related cancers.

References

Addressing Tobacco Use and Addiction. (2007) (Vol. a). Atlanta (GA): Centers for Disease Control and Prevention. U.S. Department of Health and Human Services, Centers for Disease Control and Prevention, Division of Adolescent and School Health.

Arnett, J. (2001). Adolescents' responses to cigarette advertisements for five "youth brands" and one "adult brand". Journal of Research on Adolescence, 11(4), 19.

Aveyard, P., Sherratt, E., Almond, J., Lawrence, T., Lancashire, R., Griffin, C., & Cheng, K. K. (2001). The change-in-stage and updated smoking status results from a cluster-randomized trial of smoking prevention and cessation using the transtheoretical model among British adolescents. Prev Med, 33(4), 313-324. doi: 10.1006/pmed.2001.0889S0091-7435(01)90889-8 (pii)

Azevedo, A., Machado, A. P., & Barros, H. (1999). Tobacco smoking among Portuguese high-school students. Bull World Health Organ, 77(6), 509-514.

Baldwin, D. C., Jr., & Daugherty, S. R. (2004). Sleep deprivation and fatigue in residency training: results of a national survey of first- and second-year residents. Sleep, 27(2), 217-223.

Beattie, A. (1984). Health education and the science teacher: invitation to a debate. Education and Health, 7(2), 15.

Behm, I., Kabir, Z., Connolly, G. N., & Alpert, H. R. (2012). Increasing prevalence of smoke-free homes and decreasing rates of sudden infant death syndrome in the United States: an ecological association study. Tob Control, 21(1), 6-11. doi: tc.2010.041376 (pii)10.1136/tc.2010.041376

Bergen, H. A., Martin, G., Roeger, L., & Allison, S. (2005). Perceived academic performance and alcohol, tobacco and marijuana use: longitudinal relationships in young community adolescents. Addict Behav, 30(8), 1563-1573. doi: S0306-4603(05)00040-7 (pii)10.1016/j.addbeh.2005.02.012

Botvin, G. J., Baker, E., Dusenbury, L., Tortu, S., & Botvin, E. M. (1990). Preventing adolescent drug abuse through a multimodal cognitive-behavioral approach: results of a 3-year study. J Consult Clin Psychol, 58(4), 437-446.

Botvin, G. J., Goldberg, C. J., Botvin, E. M., & Dusenbury, L. (1993). Smoking behavior of adolescents exposed to cigarette advertising. Public Health Rep, 108(2), 217-224.

BR, F. (Ed.). (2007). The long term promise of effective school-based smoking prevention programs.: Washington Academy Press.

Bryant, A. L., Schulenberg, J., Bachman, J. G., O'Malley, P. M., & Johnston, L. D. (2000). Understanding the links among school misbehavior, academic achievement, and cigarette use: a national panel study of adolescents. Prev Sci, 1(2), 71-87.

C Pechmann, S. K. (2002). An experimental investigation of the joint effects of advertising and peers on adolescents' beliefs and intentions about cigarette consumption. Journal of Consumer Research, 29(1), 15.

Carbone, D. (1992). Smoking and cancer. Am J Med, 93(1A), 13S-17S.

Chapman, S., & Fitzgerald, B. (1982). Brand preference and advertising recall in adolescent smokers: some implications for health promotion. Am J Public Health, 72(5), 491-494.

Chapman, S., & Freeman, B. (2009). Regulating the tobacco retail environment: beyond reducing sales to minors. Tob Control, 18(6), 496-501. doi: tc.2009.031724 (pii)10.1136/tc.2009.031724

Daly, J. B., Wiggers, J. H., Burrows, S., & Freund, M. (2010). Household smoking behaviours and exposure to environmental tobacco smoke among infants: are current strategies effectively protecting our young? Aust N Z J Public Health, 34(3), 269-273. doi: AZPH525 (pii)10.1111/j.1753-6405.2010.00525.x

Denson, R., & Stretch, S. (1981). Prevention of smoking in elementary schools. Can J Public Health, 72(4), 259-263.

Dielman, T. E., Lorenger, A. T., Leech, S. L., Lyons, A. L., Klos, D. M., & Horvath, W. J. (1985). Fifteen-month follow-up results of an elementary school based smoking prevention project. Resisting pressures to smoke. Hygie, 4(4), 28-35.

Dobbins, M., DeCorby, K., Manske, S., & Goldblatt, E. (2008). Effective practices for school-based tobacco use prevention. Prev Med, 46(4), 289-297. doi: S0091-7435(07)00454-9 (pii)10.1016/j.ypmed.2007.10.003

Feighery, E. C., Ribisl, K. M., Schleicher, N., Lee, R. E., & Halvorson, S. (2001). Cigarette advertising and promotional strategies in retail outlets: results of a statewide survey in California. Tob Control, 10(2), 184-188.

Fischer, P. M., Schwartz, M. P., Richards, J. W., Jr., Goldstein, A. O., & Rojas, T. H. (1991). Brand logo recognition by children aged 3 to 6 years. Mickey Mouse and Old Joe the Camel. Jama, 266(22), 3145-3148.

Fix, B. V., Zambon, M., Higbee, C., Cummings, K. M., Alford, T., & Hyland, A. (2006). Internet cigarette purchasing among 9th grade students in western New York: 2000-2001 vs. 2004-2005. Prev Med, 43(3), 191-195. doi: S0091-7435(06)00197-6 (pii)10.1016/j.ypmed.2006.04.022

Flay, B. R. (Ed.). (2007). The long term promise of effective school-based smoking prevention programs. Washington: National academies Press.

Foundation, I. s. Y. L.   Retrieved 8/22/2012, from http://www.itsyourlifefoundation.org/?page_id=17

Guntupalli K., Surani S., Shastri S., Laxmipathi G. and Casturi L. (2010). Evils of Tobacco: It's Your Life Foundation.

Halbert, R. J., Natoli, J. L., Gano, A., Badamgarav, E., Buist, A. S., & Mannino, D. M. (2006). Global burden of COPD: systematic review and meta-analysis. Eur Respir J, 28(3), 523-532. doi: 09031936.06.00124605 (pii)10.1183/09031936.06.00124605

Hanewinkel, R., Isensee, B., Sargent, J. D., & Morgenstern, M. (2010). Effect of an antismoking advertisement on cinema patrons' perception of smoking and intention to smoke: a quasi-experimental study. Addiction, 105(7), 1269-277. doi: ADD2973 (pii)10.1111/j.1360-0443.2010.02973.x

Hecht, S. S. (1999). Tobacco smoke carcinogens and lung cancer. J Natl Cancer Inst, 91(14), 1194-1210.

Hu, T. W., Lin, Z., & Keeler, T. E. (1998). Teenage smoking, attempts to quit, and school performance. Am J Public Health, 88(6), 940-943.

Hurd, P. D., Johnson, C. A., Pechacek, T., Bast, L. P., Jacobs, D. R., & Luepker, R. V. (1980). Prevention of cigarette smoking in seventh grade students. J Behav Med, 3(1), 15-28.

Hwang, M. S., Yeagley, K. L., & Petosa, R. (2004). A meta-analysis of adolescent psychosocial smoking prevention programs published between 1978 and 1997 in the United States. Health Educ Behav, 31(6), 702-719. doi: 31/6/702 (pii)10.1177/1090198104263361

Hymowitz, N. (2011). Smoking and cancer: a review of public health and clinical implications. J Natl Med Assoc, 103(8), 695-700.

Hymowitz, N. (Ed.). (2008). Physician intervention for smoking cessation. New York: Nova Science Publishers Inc.

Institute, N. c. Harms of Smoking and Health Benefits of quitting Retrieved 10/14/2012, 2012, from www.cancer.gov/cancertopics/factsheet/Tobacco/cessation

Institute of Medicine. Keeping patients safe:Transforming the work environment of nurses. (2004). Washington DC: National Academic Press.

Kelder, S. H., Pechmann, C., Slater, M. D., Worden, J. K., & Levitt, A. (2002). The National Youth Anti-Drug Media Campaign. Am J Public Health, 92(8), 1211-1212.

Killen, J. D., Telch, M. J., Robinson, T. N., Maccoby, N., Taylor, C. B., & Farquhar, J. W. (1988). Cardiovascular disease risk reduction for tenth graders. A multiple-factor school-based approach. Jama, 260(12), 1728-1733.

Lambert, A., Sargent, J. D., Glantz, S. A., & Ling, P. M. (2004). How Philip Morris unlocked the Japanese cigarette market: lessons for global tobacco control. Tob Control, 13(4), 379-387. doi: 13/4/379 (pii)10.1136/tc.2004.008441

Laniado-Laborin, R. (2009). Smoking and chronic obstructive pulmonary disease (COPD). Parallel epidemics of the 21 century. Int J Environ Res Public Health, 6(1), 209-224. doi: 10.3390/ijerph6010209

Leatherdale, S. T., Hammond, D., & Ahmed, R. (2008). Alcohol, marijuana, and tobacco use patterns among youth in Canada. Cancer Causes Control, 19(4), 361-369. doi: 10.1007/s10552-007-9095-4

Lewis, M. J., Yulis, S. G., Delnevo, C., & Hrywna, M. (2004). Tobacco industry direct marketing after the Master Settlement Agreement. Health Promot Pract, 5(3 Suppl), 75S-83S. doi: 10.1177/1524839904264596

Lovato, C., Linn, G., Stead, L. F., & Best, A. (2003). Impact of tobacco advertising and promotion on increasing adolescent smoking behaviours. Cochrane Database Syst Rev(4), CD003439. doi: 10.1002/14651858.CD003439

McGuire, W. (1964). Some Contemporary approaches. Afdvances in Experimental Social Psychology, 1, 39.

McLaughlin, J. K., Hrubec, Z., Heineman, E. F., Blot, W. J., & Fraumeni, J. F., Jr. (1990). Renal cancer and cigarette smoking in a 26-year followup of U.S. veterans. Public Health Rep, 105(5), 535-537.

Mills, P. K., Newell, G. R., Beeson, W. L., Fraser, G. E., & Phillips, R. L. (1990). History of cigarette smoking and risk of leukemia and myeloma: results from the Adventist health study. J Natl Cancer Inst, 82(23), 1832-1836.

Morehouse, E., & Tobler, N. S. (2000). Preventing and reducing substance use among institutionalized adolescents. Adolescence, 35(137), 1-28.

Muilenburg Legge, J., Latham, T., Annang, L., Johnson, W. D., Burdell, A. C., West, S. J., & Clayton, D. L. (2009). The home smoking environment: influence on behaviors and attitudes in a racially diverse adolescent population. Health Educ Behav, 36(4), 777-793. doi: 36/4/777 (pii)10.1177/1090198109339461

Murray, D. M., Pirie, P., Leupker, R. V., & Pallonen, U. (1989). Five- and six-year follow-up results from four seventh-grade smoking prevention strategies. J Behav Med, 12(2), 207-218.

Ockene, J. K., Kuller, L. H., Svendsen, K. H., & Meilahn, E. (1990). The relationship of smoking cessation to coronary heart disease and lung cancer in the Multiple Risk Factor Intervention Trial (MRFIT). Am J Public Health, 80(8), 954-958.

Ockene, J. K., & Shaten, B. J. (1991). Cigarette smoking in the Multiple Risk Factor Intervention Trial (MRFIT). Introduction, overview, method, and conclusions. Prev Med, 20(5), 552-563.

Park, E. (2006). School-based smoking prevention programs for adolescents in South Korea: a systematic review. (Review). Health Educ Res, 21(3), 407-415. doi: 10.1093/her/cyl038

Perry, C. L. (1999). The tobacco industry and underage youth smoking: tobacco industry documents from the Minnesota litigation. Arch Pediatr Adolesc Med, 153(9), 935-941.

Perry, C. L., Kelder, S. H., Murray, D. M., & Klepp, K. I. (1992). Communitywide smoking prevention: long-term outcomes of the Minnesota Heart Health Program and the Class of 1989 Study. Am J Public Health, 82(9), 1210-1216.

Peterson, A. V., Jr., Kealey, K. A., Mann, S. L., Marek, P. M., & Sarason, I. G. (2000). Hutchinson Smoking Prevention Project: long-term randomized trial in school-based tobacco use prevention--results on smoking. J Natl Cancer Inst, 92(24), 1979-1991.

Pierce, J. P., Choi, W. S., Gilpin, E. A., Farkas, A. J., & Berry, C. C. (1998). Tobacco industry promotion of cigarettes and adolescent smoking. Jama, 279(7), 511-515. doi: joc71624 (pii)

Pierce, J. P., Messer, K., James, L. E., White, M. M., Kealey, S., Vallone, D. M., & Healton, C. G. (2010). Camel No. 9 cigarette-marketing campaign targeted young teenage girls. Pediatrics, 125(4), 619-626. doi: peds.2009-0607 (pii)10.1542/peds.2009-0607

Pietroiusti, A., Neri, A., Somma, G., Coppeta, L., Iavicoli, I., Bergamaschi, A., & Magrini, A. (2009). Incidence of metabolic syndrome among night-shift healthcare workers. Occup Environ Med, 67(1), 54-57.

Preventing Tobacco Use Among Youth and Young Adults: A report of the Surgeon General. (2012) (pp. 16-19). Atlanta, GA: U.S. Department of Health and Human Services, Centers for Disease Control and prevention, National Center for Chronic Disease Prevention and Health Promotion, Office on smoking and Health.

Evans, R.I., Rozelle, R.M., Maxwell, S.E., Raines, B.E., Dills, C.A., et al. (1981). Social modelling films to deter smoking in adolescents: results of a three-year field investigation. Journal of Applied Psuchology, 66(4), 16.

Surani, S., Hesselbach, S. and Guntupalli, K. (2011). Intervention affecting perception and attitude towards tobacco use among elementary students in Galveston. Chest, 11(1), 140.

Saetta, M., Di Stefano, A., Maestrelli, P., Ferraresso, A., Drigo, R., Potena, A., . . . Fabbri, L. M. (1993). Activated T-lymphocytes and macrophages in bronchial mucosa of subjects with chronic bronchitis. Am Rev Respir Dis, 147(2), 301-306.

Skara, S., & Sussman, S. (2003). A review of 25 long-term adolescent tobacco and other drug use prevention program evaluations. Prev Med, 37(5), 451-474. doi: S009174350300166X (pii)

Surani, S., Reddy, R., Houlihan, A. E., Parrish, B., Evans-Hudnall, G. L., & Guntupalli, K. (2011). Ill Effects of Smoking: Baseline Knowledge among School Children and Implementation of the "AntE Tobacco" Project. Int J Pediatr, 2011, 584589. doi: 10.1155/2011/584589

Telch, M. J., Killen, J. D., McAlister, A. L., Perry, C. L., & Maccoby, N. (1982). Long-term follow-up of a pilot project on smoking prevention with adolescents. J Behav Med, 5(1), 1-8.

Thomas, R., & Perera, R. (2006). School-based programmes for preventing smoking. Cochrane Database Syst Rev(3), CD001293. doi: 10.1002/14651858.CD001293.pub2

Thompson, E. L. (1978). Smoking education programs 1960-1976. Am J Public Health, 68(3), 250-257.

Tingle, L. R., DeSimone, M., & Covington, B. (2003). A meta-evaluation of 11 school-based smoking prevention programs. J Sch Health, 73(2), 64-67.

Glynn, T.J., et al. (1985). Community intervention trial for smoking cessation (COMMIT): I. Cohort results from a four year community intervention. American Journal of Public Health, 85(2), 10.

Tobacco Overview. (2012) Retrieved 8/24, 2012, from www.tobaccofreekids.org/facts_issues/tobacco_101

Tobler, N. S. (1997). Meta-analysis of adolescent drug prevention programs: results of the 1993 meta-analysis. NIDA Res Monogr, 170, 5-68.

Unger, J. B., Rohrbach, L. A., & Ribisl, K. M. (2001). Are adolescents attempting to buy cigarettes on the internet? Tob Control, 10(4), 360-363.

Walker, O. a. (Ed.). (2011). The Tax Burden of Tobacco: Historic Compilation 2010. Arlington VA: Orzechowski and Walker.

Walter, H. J. (1989). Primary prevention of chronic disease among children: the school-based "Know Your Body" intervention trials. Health Educ Q, 16(2), 201-214.

White, C. (1990). Research on smoking and lung cancer: a landmark in the history of chronic disease epidemiology. Yale J Biol Med, 63(1), 29-46.

WHO. (2008). MPOWER: Six policies to reverse the tobacco epidemic Retrieved 10/13/2012, 2012, from www.who.int/tobacco/mpower/mpower_report_six_policies_2008.pdf

Wiehe, S. E., Garrison, M. M., Christakis, D. A., Ebel, B. E., & Rivara, F. P. (2005). A systematic review of school-based smoking prevention trials with long-term follow-up. J Adolesc Health, 36(3), 162-169. doi: S1054-139X(04)00460-4 (pii)10.1016/j.jadohealth.2004.12.003

Young, T. L., & Rogers, K. D. (1986). School performance characteristics preceding onset of smoking in high school students. Am J Dis Child, 140(3), 257-259.

Zaza, S., Briss, P. A., & Harris, K. W. (Eds.). (2005). Tobacco. Atlanta (GA): Oxforg University Press.

Including and Protecting Pregnant Women in Clinical Trials

Lori Allesee

Section of Integrated Ethics, Department of Critical Care
The University of Texas MD Anderson Cancer Center, USA

Colleen M. Gallagher

Section of Integrated Ethics, Department of Critical Care
The University of Texas MD Anderson Cancer Center, USA

1   Introduction

Not too long ago, a cancer diagnosis put a mother and a fetus in an adversarial battle for survival. Physicians would offer their pregnant patients two possible plans of care: 1) Delay treatment until the baby was born, or 2) Begin cancer treatment and abort the pregnancy. Often oncologists viewed treating the expectant patient as a liability – not only could the cancer treatment harm the fetus, doctors thought being pregnant might worsen the cancer prognosis.

By the 1990s, clinical researchers had collected information on pregnant women with breast cancer that challenged the traditional plans of care for pregnant women. Meanwhile, federal regulations were undergoing significant changes. Specifically, laws were being amended to adopt a policy of inclusion of pregnant women in clinical trials.

Today, although there is more scientific literature addressing the relationship between cancer and pregnancy than there was 30 years ago, research is still limited. And, despite changes in the research environment, investigators and their sponsors are still reticent to include pregnant women in research. Needless to say, there is a gap in the science of cancer research. Cancer is diagnosed in only 1 in 1,000 pregnancies, making it a relatively uncommon diagnosis. However, the incidence of cancer in pregnant women appears to be on the rise. This trend likely correlates with the growing number of women who are postponing motherhood. Between 1990 and 2004 cancers complicated by pregnancy increased from 1 in 1,560 to 1 in 1,180 pregnancies (McKain *et al.*, Results section, para. 1).

Even with the growing numbers, many pregnant women face cancer unsure of the best or even adequate treatment options for themselves or their fetus. The Food and Drug Administration has approved only a handful of medications for use during pregnancy and those medications relate to pregnancy issues. Consequently, medications that are designed to treated chronic illnesses, like cancer, are used without approval (Lyerly *et al.*, 2008, pp. 5-22).

So the question then becomes, "Should I include pregnant women in my clinical trial?" The answer is, it depends. There are still legal and ethical obstacles for the pregnant woman, investigators and institutional review members to study. This chapter outlines the ethical principles to consider when deciding whether to include a pregnant woman in clinical trials. Further, this chapter draws on the advice and experience of ethicists, federal regulators, case law, and researchers who have pioneered practices to safeguard the inclusion of pregnant women in clinical trials.

2   History of the Inclusion and Exclusion of Pregnant Women in Clinical Trials

Abuses in medical research, drug tragedies, and the subsequent, and often, reactionary federal regulations have greatly shaped a pregnant woman's participation in clinical trials. Two historical events largely define the history of exclusion –the Diethylstilbestrol (DES) and thalidomide tragedies. Diethylstilbestrol (DES) was manufactured in 1938 to prevent miscarriage. Five to 10 million pregnant women and their children were exposed to the drug (Center for Disease Control, 2012, DES history section, para. 1). Later, it was realized that the drug did not prevent miscarriage, and over time, it was linked to cancer in the daughters of the treated women. By 1971, DES was no longer prescribed (DES history section, para. 1 –

4). The resulting and continuing DES litigation has had widespread financial impact on the pharmaceutical industry chilling many companies from being receptive to pregnant women in their clinical trials.

Meanwhile, in Europe, the thalidomide disaster (1950s – 1960s) also contributed to an expansion of exclusionary policies of pregnant women in clinical trials. Thalidomide was being prescribed to treat morning sickness in pregnant women and was later linked to birth defects in thousands of newborns (Macklin, 2010, p. 632). The United States escaped a similar disaster as the Food and Drug Administration never authorized its sale. The drug, however, was distributed to United States physicians during its clinical testing.

The United States history of exclusion continued through 1993. In that year, Congress established the National Institute of Health Revitalization Act, which recognized that the systematic exclusion of pregnant women from clinical trials was failing women. Pregnant women and their physicians literally had no evidence-based information on which to base their decisions for maternal and fetal care. Consequently, Congress reversed its policy of exclusion in favor of inclusion. In 1993, the federal regulations were amended to include pregnant women (National Institute of Health Revitalization Act of 1993). And, in the following year, 1994, the Institute of Medicine issued a report declaring that pregnant women be "presumed eligible" as research subjects (Lyerly *et al.*, 2009, p. 5-22). Notwithstanding these policy changes, it is widely observed that researchers and institutional review boards continue the practice of conservationism and exclusion. This reticence largely stems from the unknown and potential unknown dangers to the fetus and the subsequent liability.

3   Ethics of Inclusion for Pregnant Women

Since the adoption of the revised regulations, the call for the inclusion of pregnant women in clinical trials has garnered heightened attention from medical, legal and ethics scholars as well as the mainstream media. The arguments for the inclusion of pregnant woman largely rest on a number of autonomy-based and social justice-based principles. Proponents for inclusion believe that the addition will reduce the effects of medical discrimination against pregnant woman by building a better base of evidenced-based medical knowledge with an eye toward improving health care.

In developing this ethical framework for this argument, ethicists have employed the accepted principles of clinical medicine and clinical research, specifically: 1) Autonomy, 2) Beneficence and Nonmaleficence, and 3) Justice (Belmont Report, 1979, Part B; Beauchamp & Childress, 1994, p. 12-13). These principles are examined within the context of the inclusion of pregnant woman and their fetuses below.

3.1 Autonomy

Autonomous decision-making is a fundamental concept in both law and ethics. The principle of autonomy recognizes respect for the individual and acknowledges a person's right to self-determination. In the context of pregnancy, the principle of autonomy is inherently problematic. For instance, there are situations where maternal autonomy challenges fetal autonomy and vice versa.

The competing questions arise, "Does participating in this clinical trial empower the fetus or pose an unanticipated risk to autonomy?" and "Does participating in this clinical trial empower the woman or pose threats to her autonomy?

Consider the case of Angela Carder. At 13, Angela Carder was diagnosed with Ewing's sarcoma. During her adolescent years, she sought aggressive and experimental treatment in the form of chemotherapy and radiation that put her cancer into remission. Years later, a secondary form of cancer developed and she pursued chemotherapy, radiation and surgery. Aggressive treatment again resulted in remission. During this period of remission, Angela Carder married and became pregnant.

Now, 27 years-old and 25 weeks pregnant, Angela Carder was once again diagnosed with the same disease that she had battled with during her adolescence. Surgery and experimental therapies were ruled out as treatment options. Her condition was terminal. Consequently, she and her physician agreed to course of action that would prolong her own life while also helping the fetus reach 28 weeks gestation until the fetus reached 28-weeks gestation, however, Angela Carder refused to accept interventions for her fetus. At 26 weeks, both mother and fetus began experienced rapid deterioration. Angela Carder had lost consciousness and was ventilator dependent. The family was then asked to consent to a Cesarean section with the goal of saving the fetus. Medically, it was believed that this intervention would shorten Angela Carder's life, but would increase the fetus' chance of survival. In line with Angela Carder's wishes, the family decided against the Cesarean section (Steinbock, 2011, 190 – 192, In re A.C., 573 A.2d 1235, 1990).

Given the facts of this case, should the physician follow Angela Carder's wish? Did Angela Carder possess the capacity to refuse the intervention? These ethical questions are framed in terms of protecting autonomy through maternal decision-making. But, reflect on the competing questions: If the physician followed Angela Carder's wish was he undermining the fetus' autonomy? Do the physician's obligations to the fetus ever override the obligations to a pregnant patient?

The hospital was also considering these questions. Eventually, fearing legal liability, the hospital sought judicial intervention to perform a cesarean section to deliver the fetus. Among other issues, her physicians and the hospital were concerned about the effects of her decisions on her fetus and her ability to make competent decisions (in re A.C., 573 A.2d 1235, 1990).

Meanwhile, Angela Carder regained consciousness and appeared to have mouthed words expressing her refusal for a surgical intervention. Nonetheless, the trial court, granted the petition applying a justice based argument -- the state's interest in protecting a viable fetus. A Caesarean section was ordered. Although, Angela Carder's representative appealed, the operation was performed. The baby died 2.5 hours later, and Angela Carder succumbed to the cancer two days after the surgery.

Eventually, a higher court overturned the trial court's decision arguing that the substituted judgment of the mother trumps a decision based on viability. Using an autonomy-based argument, the appellate ruled: courts do not compel one person to permit a significant intrusion upon his or her bodily integrity for the benefit of another person's health…It has been suggested that fetal cases are different because a woman who "has chosen to lend her body to bring a child into the world" has an enhanced duty to assure the welfare of the fetus, sufficient even to require her to undergo Cesarean surgery. Surely, however, a fetus cannot have rights in this respect superior to those of a person who has already been born (in re A.C., 573 A.2d 1235, 1990).

Not all agree with the ethical or legal framework in the In re A.C. decision. Those who advocate for greater fetal protections argue that maternal autonomy is not without its limits, and place pregnant woman and the fetus in a special class of persons. In short, those who lobby for fetal rights argue that a pregnant woman has a greater moral responsibility to protect the fetus from harm.

If the facts in the Angela Carder case are manipulated and placed in the clinical research scenario, the same ethical conclusion as that in the In re A.C. decision can be reached. For instance, if Angela Carder had been involved in a clinical trial where her 26-week-old fetus was benefitting from treatment, but was jeopardizing her own health, would it be ethically appropriate for her to opt out of the research? Conversely, could researchers compel her to remain in the trial?

In this scenario, there is greater consensus that the principle of autonomy permits a research subject to voluntarily withdraw provided that the consequences of that action are discussed (Grady, 2012, p.43 – 44). Drawing on the same reasoning, the federal regulations echo this sentiment (U.S. Department of Health and Human Services. Protection of Human Subjects, 45 C.F.R. § 46, 2012).

Managing the ethical maternal/fetal conflict in clinical research requires building a strong informed consent process. Informed consent takes on different meanings in the courts and in clinical research. In the law, informed consent is generally a duty imposed on the physician to properly disclose significant risks inherent to treatment. Consider for example the holding in Shack v. Holland: Conditioned prospective liability to the fetus is created when an unborn child's mother is not sufficiently informed of risks, hazards and alternatives of delivery procedures administered, and such liability attaches upon birth and insures to benefit of child as cause of action for lack of informed consent (Shack v. Holland, 389 N.Y.S. 2d 988 (Sup. Ct., 1976)).

On the other hand, in ethics, the scope of informed consent consists of a two-part process: 1) The investigator-subject dialogue of informed consent, and 2) The formal documentation requirement (Beauchamp and Childress, 2009, p. 120 – 121). A more robust discussion of this process is described in Section 4. Clearly, the fetus cannot participate in the informed consent process. It is generally recognized, however, that parents have the right and responsibility to make health care decisions for their children (Canesi ex rel. Canesi v. Wilson, 730 A2d. 805 (N.J. 1999)). Further, the rationale for developing an informed consent process is that the best way to protect the fetus is by educating the pregnant women in making informed choices. Through informed consent, investigators can realize respect for a woman's autonomy and recognize the freedom of women to exercise their judgment in order to act in their best interest.

3.2 Beneficence and Nonmaleficence

The relationship between a pregnant woman and her fetus is complex and gives rise to many ethical dilemmas facing researchers and clinicians. In clinical medicine, beneficence and nonmaleficence duties require physicians to objectively assess therapeutic options that offer the pregnant woman and the fetus the greatest balance of benefit over risk for the patient whereas in clinical research these principles require a weighted analysis of the minimization of risks and enhancement of benefits to the subjects and society (Beauchamp & Childress, 2009, pp. 197 – 198).

Assessing harm and benefit in the research including the pregnant woman is difficult because there are many unknown variables. The American Congress of Obstetrics and Gynecologists (ACOG) (2007) provides for a pregnant woman to benefit from a clinical trial the research must be designed to provide a valid analysis as to whether women are affected differently than men. This type of differential analysis is basic to benefiting women and preventing harm during pregnancy (Ethical Principles Supporting the Inclusion of Women, para. 1).

Investigators must also weigh the competing interests of the risks and benefits to the woman with the harms and benefits to the fetus. This conflict lurks in the minds of many investigators largely because the issue of fetal rights continues to be on-going philosophical debate.

However, some ethicists point out that concern for fetal well-being is paradoxical. Investigators exercising concern out of fear for the fetal safety are forming this judgment with little empirical data on the safety of the therapy on the fetus or the pregnant woman. "If research is important to tell us when medications are unsafe, it is also important to reassure us when drugs *are* safe." (Lyerly *et al.*, 2009, p. 5-22).

To better ensure beneficence and nonmaleficence based-decisions, ACOG (2005) recommends that investigators address decisions about maternal or fetal well-being within the framework of scientific evidence and understood within the context of the pregnant woman's value system (Recommendations, para. 1 – 2). Some ethicists advance a beneficence-centered position based on fetal rights. This argument holds that because of the medical needs presented during pregnancy, approximately two-thirds of pregnant women are prescribed drugs during their pregnancy (National Institute of Child Health and Human Development, 2003). Caused in part by the history of exclusion and by reticence of investigators and sponsors, these drugs, for the most part, have been prescribed without information about fetal safety. The inadequate research poses serious risks of harm to fetuses (Lyerly *et al.*, 2008, p. 5 – 22).

The idea that investigators and institutional review boards are better positioned than a pregnant woman to assess the risks and benefits is overly paternalistic. Policies of this kind stereotype women and vulnerable and unable to determine when the potential benefits to them or their fetus are outweighed by the harm (Kass *et al.*, 1996, 37). Turning back to the case of Angela Carder, the court supported the concept that harm and benefit should be viewed from the lens of the patient. The following beneficence-based structure was used to determine how health care decision should be made when harm is involved to a patient: Courts in substituted judgment cases have also acknowledged the importance of probing the patient's value system as an aid in discerning what the patient would choose. We agree with this approach. Most people do not foresee what calamities may befall them; much less do they consider, or even think about, treatment alternatives in varying situations. The court in a substituted judgment case, therefore, should pay special attention to the known values and goals of the incapacitated patient, and should strive, if possible, to extrapolate from those values and goals what the patient's decision would be. Although treating physicians may be an invaluable source of such information about a patient, the family will often be the best source. Family members or other loved ones will usually be in the best position to say what the patient would do if competent (In re A.C., 573 A.2d 1235, 1990).

As such, balancing these two ethical principles with autonomy and justice compel investigators to utilize solid research designs, develop monitoring systems and employ highly competent researchers (Jonsen *et al.*, 2010, p. 203 – 210). Optimal cancer treatment requires sound research to enable pregnant women to make educated and informed decisions about maternal harm (Lyerly *et al.*, 2009, p. 5 – 22).

3.3   Justice

Distributive justice requires a fair distribution of goods and services, including fair access to clinical trials. Injustice results when a person is arbitrarily denied a benefit for which he was entitled or when some excessive burdens are undeservedly imposed. The most common way of understanding this principle is that equals should be treated equally. But who is equal? Are all women equal? Are all pregnant women equal? Are all fetuses equal?

Experience, age, competence, merit, and position are common criteria employed to justify disparate treatment. Treating people equally, however, requires application of a widely accepted formula that equalizes benefits and burdens. A fair distribution should consider the following: 1) To each person an equal share, 2) To each person according to need, 3) To each person according to effort, 4) To each person according to contribution, 5) To each person according to merit, and 6) To each person according to free-market exchanges (Beauchamp and Childress, 2009, p. 243). When considering inclusion of pregnant subjects in cancer research the first two aspects are often violated.

In this given context, when pregnant women do not have access to clinical research, it could be reasoned that they are denied the possibility of having the potential for benefit that is available to non-pregnant persons. Such policies would violate the principle of justice by denying then equal share. In fact, ACOG's Committee on Ethics (2007) maintains that the automatic exclusion of pregnant women from clinical trials constitutes a violation of justice. This argument is shaped by the consideration that women and their fetuses should be given what is due to them. To illustrate, pregnant women are currently being treated based on studies which have largely excluded women and, more pointedly, ignored pregnant women. Justice requires that pregnant women be included in trials to benefit from research as other groups do (p. 1 – 4).

Similarly, a woman with cancer is in need of treatment. Treatment delayed is often treatment denied. For many women treatment is provided through clinical trials. This lack of inclusion in the clinical trials violates justice in the second aspect. At the same time the violation of aspects three, four and five happens because a pregnant woman may be willing to contribute to the knowledge, accept the risk, and therefore be giving the same effort and contribution as a woman who is not pregnant.

This argument can also be expanded to say that that the lack of research on pregnant women reaches beyond maternal health. It is not sufficient to merely investigate the therapeutic benefits and risks of care during pregnancy. Resolving the issue of underrepresentation also requires an examination of the long-term effects of treatment over the woman's lifetime (Faden, 2011, p. 21). Underrepresentation potentially violates the sixth aspect of justice. "The most compelling reason to justify the inclusion of pregnant women in a greater number of studies is the need for evidence gathered under rigorous scientific conditions that place fewer women and their fetuses at risk than the much larger number of pregnant women who will be exposed to the medications once they come to market." (Macklin, 2010, p. 632).

4   Ensuring Ethical Maternal and Fetal Protections in Clinical Trials

Law and ethics compel additional protections for investigators studying pregnant women and fetuses. Bioethicists largely accept the federal legal requirements, the United States Department of Health and Human Services and the Food and Drug Administration regulations, placed on institutional review boards.

Beyond the legal requirements, the ethical acceptability of inclusion rests on the medical or scientific necessity of the study and on the minimization of risks to the woman and the fetus (Goldkin *et al.*, 2010, 2241 – 2243). Ensuring ethical maternal and fetal protections therefore requires a properly designed study. Many investigators have established protocols that include informed consents that address the risk-benefit analysis with regard to fetal exposures and maternal health, and present therapeutic alternatives to clinical trial enrollment. Further, ethicists encourage adoption of study end-points and data collection systems to monitor maternal and fetal findings.

This section outlines the additional protections required by the United States Department of Health and Human Services (hereinafter referred to as Protection of Human Subjects, 45 C.F.R. 46), that must be provided to pregnant women and fetuses involved in research and highlights informed consent requirements. It also discusses the best ethical practices and provides practical guidance drawn from completed cancer studies.

It should be acknowledged that this chapter does not account for the costs connected with the implementation of the federal regulations or the ethical guidelines. The drivers for these standards are subject autonomy and patient safety. Justification for the costs in balance with the benefit to minorities provided is a matter of ongoing debate and is broader than the purpose of this chapter. That said, the burden of this oversight in time and money must be acknowledged. First, the regulations have contributed to the slowing pace of clinical research. It is estimated that the regulatory compliance process now accounts for 5 years of the 12 to 15-year drug approval process (Steard *et al.*, 2010, p. 2927 – 2928). In the 1960s, the process – from discovery to marketing – took an estimated 8 years (Steard *et al.*, 2010, p. 2927 – 2928). Second, the complex regulatory environment has added to the rising costs of clinical trials. The rate of increase has grown to 12.2 percent from 7.3 percent from 1970-1980 (Steard *et al.*, 2010, p. 2927 – 2928).

Despite these figures, NIH-funded studies do not permit cost as a factor in determining whether to include a pregnant woman (National Institute of Health Revitalization Act of 1993). It is the policy of NIH that funded research includes representative samples of subpopulations unless the inclusion would be inappropriate with respect to the health of the subjects or counter to the purpose of the trial. (National Institute of Health Revitalization Act of 1993).

4.1   Designing the Protocol: Research with Women Who Become Pregnant During a Clinical Trial

Although the special protections required by the federal regulation do not specifically apply when pregnancy is incidental to participation, a research protocol should consider additional safeguards when participation could pose risk to a potential mother and fetus. This is cautionary advice because almost half of pregnancies are unintended (Lyerly *et al.*, 2008, p. 5 – 22).

The World Health Organization's Council for International Organizations of Medical Sciences (CIOMS) (2002) has a broad policy of inclusion of women of reproductive age: "The potential for becoming pregnant during a study should not, in itself, be used as a reason for precluding or limiting participation" (Guideline 16: Women as Research Subjects, para. 1).

CIOMS (2002) does, however, advise investigators to initiate a thorough discussion on the risks of becoming pregnant while on the trial. This conversation should involve a weighted analysis of continued participation in the trial (Guideline 16: Women as research subjects, para. 5).

Guidance suggests when the following conditions are met, continued participation in research on the now pregnant participant may be appropriate: 1) When the potential benefits of ongoing fetal exposure outweigh the potential risks; 2) When prospect of beneficial treatment overshadows the risk of stopping the therapy, and 3) When the likely benefits of treatment offset the threat of fetal exposure to additional drugs (Feibus & Goldkin, 2011, p. 18).

4.1.1 Anticipate Risk of Pregnancy

Every clinical trial involving women of reproductive age should anticipate the risk of pregnancy. CIOMS (2002) identified the following ethical guidelines to assist investigators in the event of a pregnancy. First, in preparing for the risk of pregnancy investigators must draw up a disclosure about the potential risks that may be incurred by the subject and the fetus if the participant becomes pregnant. In some studies it may be appropriate to urge participants against becoming pregnant. Second, investigators should adopt a notification system whereby a pregnancy is immediately disclosed to the investigator. Third, a multi-disciplinary institutional review board should review an assessment of the risks on the woman and the fetus. Finally, the investigator should provide women with access to pregnancy tests and contraceptives (Guideline 16: Women as Research Subjects, para. 1 – 5).

It should be noted, however, that the risk of pregnancy should not authorize mandatory use of contraceptives. ACOG (2007) has concluded that such mandates are unethical. Mandatory contraceptive requirements violate women's autonomy, especially those who are not sexually active. Women should be allowed to choose a birth control method in accordance with her individual needs and beliefs (Research Related to Diagnosis and Therapy, para. 2 – 6).

4.1.2 Draft Special Informed Consents

Informed consent is the "practical embodiment of respect for persons and for individual autonomy" (del Carmen & Joffee, 2005, p. 636 – 637). Although informed consent will be obtained at the beginning of every clinical trial, a new and institutional review board-reviewed consent disclosure should be prepared in the event that a woman becomes pregnant and decides that she will continue t. This is because the informed consent process assumes greater significance in the context of a pregnant woman research subject. Here, ethics requires a careful balance between maternal and fetal interests and advancement of medical science.

The primary purpose of the new consent form is to protect the research subjects – now the pregnant woman and the fetus. This new disclosure should outline a plan for pregnancy management, clarify the risks and benefits of continued participation, and address the risks and benefits of alternative therapies (Moreno, 1999 p.30; Feibus & Goldkind, 2011 p. 19).

Especially in the area of oncology, it is critical that investigators minimize the risk of "therapeutic misconception." In a clinical trial, therapeutic misconception occurs when research participants do not understand that the overarching goal of clinical research is to produce generalizable knowledge regardless of the trial's ability to provide a direct therapeutic benefit to the research subject (Pentz et al., 2012, pp. 4571 – 4572).

Therapeutic misconception is likely to arise where the physician plays dual roles in a patient's care. That is, where the physician is also an investigator. Where the ethical duties overlap, the physician-investigator has protective responsibilities. The physician must protect the autonomy of a patient by offering truthful information about the trial while also shielding the research subject from unnecessary risks and exploitation (Litton & Miller, 2010, p. 1491 – 1492).

Resolving the therapeutic misconception begins by initiating a conversation with the patient. This communication should seek to clarify the difference between participation in a clinical trial and routine clinical care; explain a risk-benefit analysis regarding enrollment in a study trial versus clinical care outside of the trial; disclose the uncertainties within the trial; and balance any altruistic missions of advancing research (del Carmen and Joffe, 2005, p. 639).

Finally, there is controversy about whether substituted consent, that is, consent of the father, is required. ACOG (2007) maintains that the pregnant woman's consent alone is sufficient to most research, and does not recognize paternal rights before birth (Informed Consent, para. 5). CIOMS (2002), on the other hand, provides that the pregnant woman should determine the acceptability of risks. However, when research involves the fetus, the father's assent should be obtained (Guideline 17: Pregnant women as research participants para. 4 – 6). As outlined more thoroughly in Figure 2, the federal regulations do require paternal consent when the prospect of direct benefit is for the fetus alone. Figure 1 details the ethical and legal requirements of informed consent, and Figure 2 illustrates the consenting requirements of the federal legislation.

Legal and Ethical Requirements of Informed Consent.	
Ethical Elements of Informed Consent	Legal Requirements of Informed Consent
The basic elements of ethical informed consent and refusal involve: 1. Disclosure of material information, including purpose of the trial, potential risks and benefits; 2. Patient understanding of the information, risk and benefits 3. Capacity to make decisions, 4. Voluntary participation in the trial, and 5. Patient consentto participate in the trial. Source: Beauchamp and Childress, 2009, pp. 120-121.	The legal requirements of informed consent include: 1. A statement explaining the trial's purpose, the procedures to be followed, the duration of participation, and identification of experimental procedures; 2. A description of foreseeable risks and discomforts; 3. A description of benefits that the participant can reasonably expect; 4. Disclosure of alternative treatments or procedures that might be advantageous to the participant; 5. A statement about participant confidentiality, 6. An explanation of compensation and available medical treatments if injury occurs; 7. Contact information for trial-related questions and to help with research-related injuries; and 8. A statement that participation is voluntary and that there is no penalty and no loss of benefits for discontinuing participation. Further, the disclosure may require: 1. A statement that there may be unforeseeable risks to the participants if the participant is or may become pregnant, 2. Disclosure of circumstances under which the investigator may terminate a participant's enrollment, 3. Disclosure of costs to the participant, 4. Disclosure of the consequences and procedures of orderly termination of subject participation, 5. A statement that participants will be informed of significant new findings that might affect their willingness to participate, and 6. The approximate number of participants enrolled in the trial. Source: 45 C.F.R. § 46.116, General requirements of informed consent (2012).

Figure 1: This chart distinguishes the ethical elements with the legal requirements of informed consent. Obtaining informed consent is a process. It begins with a discussion between the investigator and the pregnant woman and concludes with formal documentation.

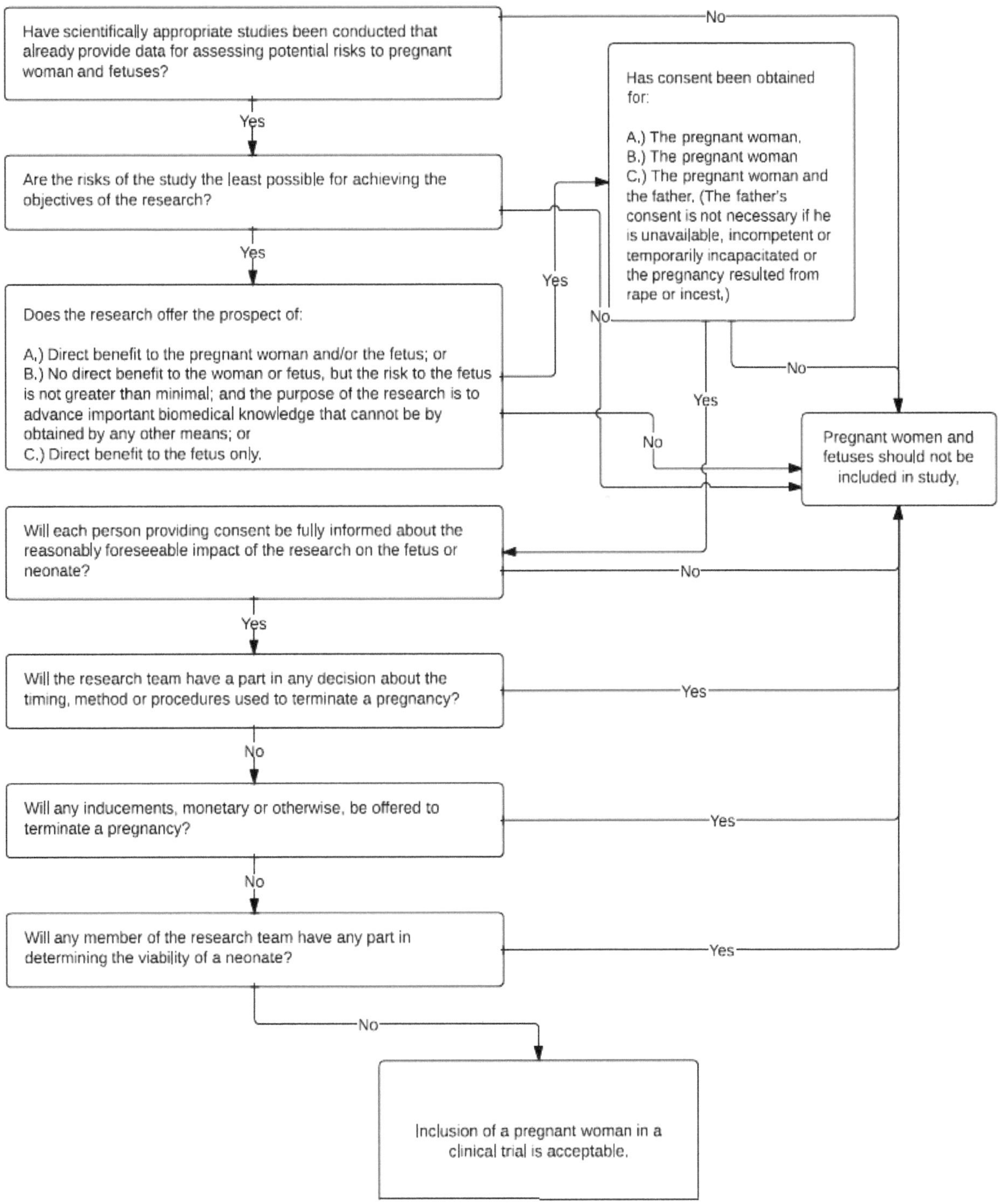

Figure 2: Algorithm outlining the federal regulation process. Source: 45 C.F.R. § 46.204 (a – j) (2012).

4.1.3 Offer Counseling

Prudent investigators provide pre-participation counseling to subjects considering pregnancy, interim counseling for those who become pregnant, as well as need-based counseling when appropriate. Some ethicists specifically propose establishing counseling services aimed to address contraceptive use and the risk fetal toxicity (Feibus & Goldkind, 2011, p. 19). Counseling needs to include the pregnant subject's desire for children and her knowledge of possible challenges to her future fertility. The management of each pregnant subject diagnosed with cancer has to be highly individualized and involves a multidisciplinary team of medical personnel. The patient and her family need counseling regarding the diagnosis, long-term prognosis, options of termination of pregnancy, choice of chemotherapeutic agents and radiation and their effects on the fetus and pregnancy.

4.1.4 Build in a Process for Institutional Review Boards or Ethics Committee Review

All research involving pregnant women should be reviewed and approved with a multidisciplinary team – either an institutional review board or an integrated ethics committee. It is essential that investigators have access to institutional review boards and ethics committees for oversight and assistance in resolving moral questions and for the purpose of ongoing education. Such access promotes the ethical standards of research protocols and improves the conduct of biomedical research (CIOMS, 2002, Introduction, para. 2).

4.2   Designing the Protocol: Cancer Research Including Pregnant Women

When designing a research protocol including pregnant women several preliminary issues will need to be addressed. These issues include determining the appropriate conditions for research; addressing the issues of informed consent to the mother and fetus in the informed consent; anticipating risks and identifying minimal risks to the mother and fetus; providing counseling; and monitoring care.

4.2.1   Determine Appropriate Conditions for Research

The federal regulations governing the additional protections for pregnant women in clinical trials are generally considered to be ethically sound. These ten strict guidelines are set out in the Protection of Human Subjects, 45 C.F.R. § 46.201 – 46.211. Because of the limitations of this chapter only 9 will be examined, Accordingly, pregnant woman and fetuses may be involved in research:

1. *Where scientifically appropriate*, preclinical studies (including studies on pregnant animals) and clinical studies (including studies on non-pregnant woman) have been conducted and provide data for assessing potential risks to pregnant women and fetuses;

2. When the risks to the fetus are no more than minimal, meaning either:

    a. The risk is solely by interventions or procedures that hold out the prospect for direct benefit for the woman or the fetus, or

    b. There is no such prospect of benefit, the risk to the fetus is not greater than minimal and the purpose of the research is the development of important biomedical knowledge, which cannot be obtained by any other means;

3. If the risk is the least possible for achieving the objectives of research;

4. Where the consent of the pregnant woman has been obtained, and the research holds out the prospect either:

   a. Direct benefit to the pregnant woman,

   b. Direct benefit to the pregnant woman and the fetus, <u>or</u>

   c. No benefit to the woman or the fetus and risk to the fetus is not greater than minimal <u>and</u> the purpose of the research is the development of important biomedical knowledge that cannot be obtained by any other means;

5. Where the consent of both the pregnant woman and the father has been obtained, and the research holds out the prospect of direct benefit solely to the fetus. The father's consent is not necessary:

   a. If he is unable to consent because of unavailability, incompetence or temporary incapacity; or

   b. If the pregnancy resulted from rape or incest;

6. Where all individuals providing consent are fully informed regarding the reasonably foreseeable impact of the research on the fetus or neonate;

7. If no inducements, monetary or otherwise to terminate the pregnancy are offered;

8. Where individuals engaged in the research will have no part in any decisions as to the timing, method, or procedures to terminate a pregnancy; and

9. Provided that individuals engaged in the research will have no part in determining the viability of a neonate (Protection of Human Subjects, 45 CFR, 2012, § 46. 204 (a – j), 2012).

Figure 2 provides the federal algorithm that institutional review board members are to use when determining whether to approve research involving pregnant woman and fetuses.

CIOMS (2002) has set forth similar, but less rigid guidelines: Research should be performed only if it is relevant to the particular health needs of pregnant woman or her fetus, or to the health needs of pregnant woman in general, and when appropriate, if it is supported by reliable evidence from animal experiments, particular as to risks of teratogenicity and mutagenicity (Guideline 17: Pregnant women as research participants, para. 2).

4.2.2   Draft Informed Consent

Informed consent is a requirement for all research. Drafting an informed consent that considers the inclusion of pregnant woman largely involves use of the same legal and ethical framework as is involved in drafting an informed consent for women who become pregnant during a clinical trial. To reiterate, such disclosures must address pregnancy management, analyze the potential risks and benefits of participation for both the pregnant and fetus, and examine the risks and benefits of alternative therapies (Moreno, 1999; Feibus & Goldkind, 2011).

The most significant difference in this analysis is that the pregnant woman is starting a therapy rather than continuing a therapy. From the outset, investigators should ensure that pregnant women have a fundamental understanding of the purpose, benefit, and risk of the study. To reduce the incidence of therapeutic misconception and increase realistic expectations, it is important for the researcher to address any belief that the trial will provide a direct benefit to her or the fetus. Some researchers advise that pregnant women discuss their participation in a clinical trial with an independent physician or a research advocate before making a decision (ACOG, 2005, Informed Consent, para. 1 – 7).

The National Cancer Institute (2011) aspires to have "research advocates" become a standard practice in cancer research. Research advocates offer a nonscientific, but experienced voice to the research process in order to support a collective patient perspective. NCI has outlined a recommended framework to help identify, involve and support advocates involved in cancer research, but at this time, the recommendations are limited to its own research activities (p. i – 1).

4.2.3   Anticipate Risks and Address Minimal Risks for the Pregnant Woman and Her Fetus

For research that does not hold the prospect for direct health benefit to pregnant woman or fetus, investigators must show "no more than minimal risk." Addressing the vague term of "minimal risk" in the protocol poses challenges for investigators, institutional review board members, ethicists and reviewing lawyers alike.

As defined in 45 C.F.R. § 46, minimal risk means: The probability and magnitude of harm or discomfort anticipated in the research are not greater in and of themselves than those ordinarily encountered in daily life or during the performance of routine physical or psychological examinations or tests.

The elusive definition creates the opportunity for inconsistent interpretation, and to date, there are no formal studies on how institutional review board members apply "minimal risk" to their review of research. Therefore, the institutional review board's interpretation of the definition is important to disclose, as it is significant to informing adequate maternal consent (Strong, 2011, p. 530 – 537; Levine, 2001, p. 41).

4.2.4   Provide Counseling

Pregnant woman with a cancer diagnosis may experience overwhelming emotional stressors. Participation in a clinical trial can exacerbate these feelings and necessitate access to counseling services. ACOG (2011) advocates that pregnant women should have access to ethics consultation services, social services, and counseling services to address concerns about the trials effects on her pregnancy (Other Necessary Support Services, para. 1).

Consistent with ACOG's (2011) recommendation for women who become pregnant during a clinical trial, the group also advances the concept of employing an independent advocate or physician for pregnant women. This safeguard may be particularly beneficial when the proposed protocol presents significant risk to either pregnant woman or fetus (The Decision-Making Process, para. 1 – 6).

4.2.5   Monitor Maternal and Fetal Health Outcomes

Research designs that incorporate short- and long-term maternal and fetal monitoring are endorsed by research and professional organizations (CIOMS, 2002, Guideline 17: Pregnant women as research participants, para. 6 and ACOG, 2007, The Ethical Context, para. 1). Such efforts should include high-risk obstetrical care; post-obstetrical care; regular fetal growth; ultrasonography and fetal heart monitoring; and pediatric educational development observations (Goldkin *et al.*, 2010, p. 2243).

4.2.6   Build in a Process for IRB Review or Ethics Committee Review

To ensure ethical design and conduct of research, investigators must adopt a multi-disciplinary review process. As discussed previously, these committees provide investigators with assistance in addressing ethical dilemmas, particularly as they relate to the fetus, and offer education to better the conduct of research (Presidential Commission for the Study of Bioethical Issues, 2011, pp. 93 – 98 and CIOMS, 2002, Introduction, para. 2).

5   Exclusions to Conducting Clinical Trials on Pregnant Women

There are many situations in which conducting clinical research trials on pregnant women would be unethical. One example of when exclusion is ethically acceptable is a Phase I trial offering no prospect of medical benefit to the pregnant woman or the fetus (Allesee & Gallagher, 2011, 1 – 4). Another instance is "where fetal abnormality is not recognized as an indication for abortion, pregnant women should not be recruited for research in which there is a realistic basis for concern that fetal abnormality may occur as a consequence of participation as a subject in research" (CIOMS, 2002, Guideline 17: Pregnant Women as Research Participants, para 5 – 6).

When a pregnant woman's participation is precluded there may be other methods of obtaining information, such as cohort studies, retrospective studies or pregnancy registries (Goldkin *et al.*, 2010, p. 2243.)

6   Limitations to Conducting Clinical Trials on Pregnant Minors

This chapter does not examine the ethics of including pregnant minors in clinical research. Researchers and institutional review board members must make additional considerations before including minors. Most critically, inclusion of pregnant minors requires researchers to be familiar with state laws governing eligibility for participation in research (Human Subjects Protection, 2012, § 46.402).

7   Conclusion

Considerable efforts of researchers, ethicists and federal regulators have helped to bridge a gap in the science of cancer research involving pregnant women. During the past three decades progress has been made to improve the lives of women and their fetuses with improved research. Research already completed has changed the way in which oncologists now practice medicine. But, much work remains.

Some argue that reticence for inclusion may be based on legal liability. Reaction to liability may be consequential and further perpetuate fears. As referenced previously, the DES litigation had a profound impact on clinical trials. In 1980, the California Supreme Court decided a landmark case, involving a plaintiff who alleged that she developed cancer as a result of a drug her mother took while pregnant. The Court ruled: "As between an innocent plaintiff and negligent defendants, the latter should bear the cost of the injury" (Sindell v. Abbott Laboratories, 1980).

But, anxiety over liability may be misplaced. Lawsuits have slowed in the past 20 years. An observational study conducted at an institutional review board (IRB) workshop on legal liability highlights this point. Within this workshop, there was not one participant that could point to a single example of a successful litigation against an institutional review board

There is also an irony to the IRB's fear of litigation. The failure to conduct research that yields understanding about fetal safety and maternal health may actually expose IRBs to greater liability than if they had supported the research (Wisner & Levine, 2011, pp. 44 – 45). Connecting investigators and researchers with pregnant women requires thorough understanding of the legal and ethical dilemmas posed because of the inextricable link between the woman and her fetus. The decision to include pregnant women in cancer research trials involves consideration of ethical principles and legal regulations. Weighing the decision of whether to include pregnant woman in clinical trials will require balancing the ethical principles of autonomy, beneficence, nonmaleficence and justice, and compliance with the law. Even when inclusion is acceptable, additional legal and ethical protections may be required. Those protections include designing protocols that detail the appropriate conditions for research, monitoring maternal and fetal outcomes, providing for a thorough informed consent process, offering counseling services and articulating a process for oversight.

Finally, although this chapter advocates for the inclusion of pregnant women in clinical trials, caution is advised. There are acceptable and ethically justifiable reasons to exclude pregnant women from clinical trials. When situations do not merit the inclusion of women it is recommended that other methods of gathering information be explored such as cohort studies, retrospective studies or pregnancy registries.

References

In re A.C., 573 A.2d 1235 (1990).

Allesee, L. & Gallagher, C.M. (2011). *Pregnancy and protection: the ethics of limiting a pregnant woman's participation in clinical trials, Journal of Clinical Research and Bioethics, 2(2), 1-5.*

American College of Obstetricians and Gynecologists (2011, August). *AGOG Committee Opinion: Maternal-Fetal Interventions and Fetal Care Centers, Number 501. Retrieved October 7, 2012 from http://www.acog.org/ Resources_And_Publications/Committee_Opinions/Committee_on_Ethics/Maternal-Fetal_Intervention_and_Fetal_Care_Centers.*

American College of Obstetricians and Gynecologists. (2005, November). *ACOG Committee Opinion: Maternal Decision Making, Ethics and the Law, Number 321. Retrieved October 7, 2012 from http://www.acog.org/ Rsources_And_Publications/Committee_Opinions/Committee_on_Ethics/Maternal_Decision_Making_Ethics_and_the_Law.*

The American Congress of Obstetricians and Gynecologists. (2007, September). *ACOG Committee Opinion: Research Involving Women, Number 377. Retrieved October 7, 2012 from http://www.acog.org/Resources_And_Publications/ Committee_Opinions/Committee_on_Ethics/Research_Involving_Women.*

Beauchamp, T. L. & Childress, J.F. (2009). *Principles of Bioethics. (6th edition). New York: Oxford University Press.*

Belmont Report (1979). *The Belmont Report: Ethical principles and guidelines for the protection of human subjects of research. Retrieved October 17, 2012 from http://www.hhs.gov/ohrp/humansubjects/guidance/belmont.html.*

Canesi ex rel. Canesi v. Wilson, 730 A2d. 805 (N.J. 1999).

The Center for Disease Control. (2012). *DES Update: Consumers. Retrieved October 17, 2012 from http://www.cdc.gov/des/consumers/about/history.html.*

Chervenak, F.A., McCullough, L.B. Skupski, D. & Chasen, S. T. (2003). Ethical Issues in the Management of Pregnancies Complicated by Fetal Anomalies, Obstetrical and Gynecological Survey, 58:7, 473-483.

del Carmen, M.G. & Joffee S. (2005). Informed consent for medical treatment and research: a review. The Oncologist, 10, 636–641.

Faden, R.R. (2011). Justice in Health Research. In U.S. Department of Health and Human Services, Public Health Service, National Institutes of Health, Office of Research on Women's Health, Pregnant Women: Issues in Clinical Research (pp. 20-23), Bethesda, Md. National Institute of Health.

Feibus, K. & Goldkind, S. F. (2011, May 17). Pregnant women &clinical trials: scientific, regulatory and ethical considerations, FDA Office of Women's Health Symposium.May 17, 2011, Silver Spring, M.D.

Grady, C. (2012). Ethical Principles in Clinical Research.In Gallin, J. I. & Ognibene, F.P. (Eds.). Principles and Practice of Clinical Research (3rded.) (pp. 43-44). Oxford, U.K.: Elsevier, Inc.

Goldkind, S. F., Sahin L. & Gallauresi, B. (2010, June 17). Enrolling Pregnant Women in Research – Lessons from the H1N1 Influenza Pandemic.The New England Journal of Medicine, 362(24) 2241-2243.

Hahn, K. M.E., Johnson P. J., Gordon, N., Kuerer, H., Middleton, L., Ramirez, M., Yang, W., Perkins, G., Hortobagyi G. N. &Theriault, R. (2006).Treatment of Pregnant Breast Cancer Patients and Outcomes in Children Exposed to Chemotherapy in Utero. Cancer. 107.

Jonsen, A. R., Siegler, M., & Winslade, W. J. (2010).Clinical Ethics: A Practical Approach to Ethical Decisions in Clinical Medicine.(7th edition).The McGraw-Hill Companies, Inc.

Kaposy, C. and Baylis, F. (2011). The common rule, pregnant women, and research: no need to "rescue" that which should be revised. American Journal of Bioethics. 11(5), 60-62.

Kass, N.E., Taylor, H.A., & King, P.A. (1996). Harms of Excluding Pregnant Women from Clinical Research: The Case of HIV-Infected Pregnant Women, The Journal of Law, Medicine & Ethics, 24(1), 36-46.

Levine, R. (2011). IRB Perspective. In U.S. Department of Health and Human Services, Public Health Service, National Institutes of Health, Office of Research on Women's Health, EnrollingPregnant Women: Issues in Clinical Research (p. 4437-43), Bethesda, Md.National Institute of Health.

Litton, J.K. & Theriault, R. L. (2010). Breast cancer and pregnancy: current concepts in diagnosis and treatment. The Oncologist.15(12).1238-1247.

Litton, P. & Miller, F. G. (2010). What physician-investigators owe patients who participate in research.Journal of the American Medical Association.304(13).1491-1492.

Lo, B. (2009). Ethical Issues in Obstetrics and Gynecology. In Resolving Ethical Dilemmas: A Guide for Clinicians (4thed.) (p. 286) Philadelphia, PA: Lippincott Williams & Wilkins.

Lyerly, A.D., Little, M.O., Faden R. (2008, November-December). Pregnancy and clinical research, Hastings Center Report, 38(6), inside back cover.

Lyerly, A. D., Little, M. O. &Faden, R. (2008). The second wave: toward responsible inclusion of pregnant women in research. International Journal of Feminist Approaches to Bioethics,1(2). 5-22.

Lyons, T. R., Schedin, P.J. & Borges, V. (2009). Pregnancy and breast cancer: when they collide. Journal of Mammary Gland Biology Neoplasia. 14(2), 87-98.

Macklin, R. (2010). The art of medicine: enrolling pregnant women in biomedical research. The Lancet. 375(9715), 632-633.

McKain L. F., Albano J.D & Desai M. (2009). Cancer in pregnancy: trends and research. Journal of Clinical Oncology.27 (Suppl; abstr e20720). There were no listed page numbers. Abstract can be found at http://www.asco.org/ ASCOv2/Meetings/Abstracts?&vmview=abst_detail_view&confID=65&abstractID=33278

Merkatz, R., Temple, R., Sobel, S., Feiden, K., & Kessler, D. (1993). Women in clinical trials of new drugs—a change in Food and Drug Administration policy. The New England Journal of Medicine. 329(4), 292-296.

Moreno, J.D. (1999). Ethical issues related to the inclusion of women of childbearing age in clinical trials. In Mastroianni, A.C., Faden, R. & Federman, D. (Eds.), Women and Health Research: Ethical and Legal Issues of Including Women in Clinical Studies, Volume 2. (pp. 29-34). Washington, DC: National Academy Press.

National Institute of Child Health and Human Development (2008, February 18). Obstetric-Fetal Pharmacology Research Units. Retrieved October 17, 2012 from http://grants.nih.gov/grants/guide/rfa-files/RFA-HD-03-017.html

National Institute of Health Revitalization Act of 1993, Pub. L. 103-146, § 131, 207 Stat. 122 (1993).

Pentz, R.D., White, M. Harvey, R. D., Farmer, Z.L., Liu, Y., Lewis, C. Dashevskaya, O., Owonikoko, T., Khuri, F. D., (2012). Therapeutic misconception, misestimation, and optimism in participants enrolled in phase I trials. Cancer, 118(18), 4571-4578. doi:10.1002.cncr.27397

Presidential Commission for the Study of Bioethical Issues.(2011, December).Moral Science: Protecting Participants in Human Subjects Research. Washington, D.C.

Robertson, J. (1999). Ethical issues related to the inclusion of pregnant women in clinical trials (II). In Women and Health Research: Ethical and Legal Issues of Including Women in Clinical Studies, Volume 2, Mastroianni, A. C., Faden, R.,&Federman, D. (Ed.) Washington, DC: National Academy Press.

Sandstand, N.C. (2008). Pregnant women and the fourteenth amendment: a feminist examination of the trend to eliminate women's rights during pregnancy. Law and Inequity.26(1), 171-202

Shack v. Holland, 389 N.Y.S. 2d 988 (Sup. Ct. 1976).

Sindell v. Abbott Laboratories, 607 P.2d. 924 (1980).

Steinbock, B. (1999). Ethical issues related to the inclusion of pregnant women in clinical trials (II). In Mastroianni, A.C., Faden, R. & Daniel Federman (Eds.), Women and Health Research: Ethical and Legal Issues of Including Women in Clinical Studies, Volume 2. (pp. 23-28). Washington, DC, National Academy Press.

Steinbock, B. (2011). The Moral and Legal Status of Embryos and Fetuses, 2nd Edition, New York, NY: Oxford University Press.

Stewart, D., Whitney, S., Kurzrock, R. (2010) Equipoise Lost: Ethics Costs, and the Regulation of Cancer Clinical Trials, Journal of Clinical Oncology, 29 (17) 2925-2935, doi 10.1200.JCO2009.27.5404.

Strong, C. (2011, Fall). Minimal risk in research involving pregnant women and fetuses.Journal of Law, Medicine and Ethics.39(3), 529-538.

U.S. Department of Health and Human Services, National Institutes of Health, National Cancer Institute (2011). Advocates in Research Working Group, NIH Publication 11-7687.

U.S. Department of Health and Human Services.Protection of Human Subjects, 45 C.F.R. § 46 (2012).

Wisner, K. & Levine, R. (2011). Discussion. In U.S. Department of Health and Human Services, Public Health Service, National Institutes of Health, Office of Research on Women's Health, EnrollingPregnant Women: Issues in Clinical Research (p. 44-49), Bethesda, Md. National Institute of Health.

World Health Organization (2002). Handbook for Good Clinical Research Guidance for Implementation, Geneva, Switzerland.

World Health Organizations, Council for International Organizations of Medical Sciences. (2002). Council for International Organizations of Medical Sciences: International Ethical Guidelines for Biomedical Sciences. Geneva, Switzerland.Retrieved October 17, 2012 from http://www.cioms.ch/publications/guidelines/guidelines_nov_2002_blurb. htm

A Targeted Mass Spectrometric Approach for Quantitating Candidate Cancer Biomarker Proteins in Undepleted and Non-Enriched Human Plasma

Andrew J. Percy, Andrew G. Chambers, Carol E. Parker
University of Victoria - Genome British Columbia Proteomics Centre
University of Victoria, Canada

Christoph H. Borchers
University of Victoria - Genome British Columbia Proteomics Centre /
Department of Biochemistry and Microbiology
University of Victoria, Canada

1   Introduction

According to recent global statistics, cancer has become the primary cause of mortality in economically developed countries and the second leading cause of death in developing countries (Jemal *et al.*, 2011). Lung cancer is the most frequent cancer and the leading cause of death in males worldwide, while breast cancer is the equivalent for females. Unfortunately, the incidence of new cancer cases is projected to increase from the current estimate of 12.7 million to 22.2 million by 2030 (Bray *et al.*, 2012), which will place a significant burden on global economic and health care systems. The heightened prevalence accentuates the need for accurate diagnostic tools for improving personalized medicine and extending patient survival.

Proteins, which are the structural and functional workhorses of the human body, are carried in the cardiovascular and lymphatic systems after being released, secreted, or leaked from surrounding cells, organs, and tissues. These biomolecules reflect the physiological state of a patient and can therefore serve as molecular indicators of disease and its progression. While proteins can be monitored for disease management in a variety of bodily fluids (e.g., cerebrospinal fluid, pancreatic juice), readily-accessible biofluids such as blood and urine are the preferred sample sources for patient monitoring. Despite its complexity and the wide dynamic range of its component proteins (Anderson *et al.*, 2002), plasma is one of the most commonly used biological samples for biomarker screening of human cancer (Aebersold *etal.*, 2005), as well as other non-communicable forms of disease (Addona *et al.*, 2011). The dominant clinical technology for targeted proteomics utilizes antibodies in an enzyme-linked immunosorbent assay (ELISA) methodology.

While ELISA remains the "gold-standard" in the clinic due to their relatively high-throughput and exceptional sensitivity, the exorbitant development time and cost makes this technique impractical for verifying and validating the large numbers of putative cancer-related biomarker proteins that currently exist (Anderson, 2010; Polanski *et al.*, 2006). Verification and validation of candidate biomarkers before clinical use is necessary to help guard against the false positives and negatives that can arise in disease diagnosis (Neagu *et al.*, 2011). For instance, plasma-based prostate-specific antigen (PSA) screening tests for prostate cancer in men have low specificity (Schröder *et al.*, 2008), which makes diagnostic confirmation through additional tests, such as a prostatic biopsy (Paulovich *et al.*, 2008), a necessity. If additional plasma proteins were FDA-approved for *in vitro* diagnostics, they could be screened along with PSA in a routine blood test, providing added diagnostic accuracy; thus, potentially avoiding the invasive biopsy procedure and the potential complications (e.g., inflammation, infection, metastasis) that can arise. Since ELISAs also have limited multiplexing capabilities and suffer from low analyte specificity, alternative quantitative proteomic approaches are necessary for the verification and validation of candidate cancer biomarkers, which were initially discovered through transcriptional profiling or untargeted and unbiased mass spectrometry (MS) (Rifai *et al.*, 2006).

Multiple reaction monitoring (MRM), a targeted MS-based technology, provides the specificity, throughput, and multiplexing capabilities required for candidate biomarker quantitation in patient samples. In this MS/MS technique, peptides in the chromatographic eluate are first volatized and ionized by electrospray ionization (ESI) processes. This enables their transfer into the vacuum chamber of the mass spectrometer where specific precursor ions (corresponding to intact peptides) are selected according to their mass-to-charge (*m/z*) ratio in the first mass analyser, subjected to collision-based fragmentation in the collision cell, and then transmitted into a second mass analyser where specific product ions (i.e., peptide fragments) are selected for detection (again by their *m/z* ratio). By combining the MRM technique with stable isotope-labeled standard (SIS) peptides (a heavy version of its natural form that causes a 6-10 Da mass shift), the absolute concentration of the peptides in the injected sample, and by inference their corresponding proteins, can be accurately and precisely determined. This MRM with SIS peptide approach is being used by other research groups to quantitate putative disease biomarkers in blood plasma (Anderson *et al.,* 2006; Hüttenhain *et al.*, 2012; Keshishian *et al.*, 2007). These research groups employ upfront depletion or enrichment to extend the depth of protein quantitation in the complex biological sample. Such pre-fractionation, however, is undesirable as it can diminish throughput, increase costs, and cause target analytes to be lost through non-specific or non-covalent interactions.

Recently, we have developed several bottom-up proteomic liquid chromatography (LC)/MRM-MS methods with internal SIS peptides to accurately quantitate disease biomarker proteins in undepleted and non-enriched human plasma (Chen *et al.*, 2012; Domanski *et al.*, 2012; Kuzyk *et al.*, 2009). Using a similar analytical approach and an alternative data analysis strategy, a method was developed to quantitate 27 high-to-moderate abundance proteins that have been reported to be differentially expressed in a variety of human cancers. The method demonstrated high robustness, accuracy, and throughput, which are essential requirements for its utilization in verifying and validating these proposed protein biomarkers for future clinical applications. The present chapter describes and discusses this developed method, which enables reliable and accurate protein quantitation of putative cancer biomarkers. We believe that this general approach will help to "credential" a fraction of the candidate markers (Paulovich *et al.*, 2008) and help bridge the gap between discovery and pre-clinical validation.

2   Materials and Methods

2.1   Chemicals and Reagents

All chemicals and reagents were of the highest analytical grade available and purchased from Sigma-Aldrich (St. Louis, MO, USA), Thermo Scientific (Rockford, Il, USA), or Promega (Madison, WI, USA). Human plasma, containing K_2-EDTA as the anticoagulant, was purchased from Bioreclamation (HMPLEDTA2; Westbury, NY, USA) and kept at -20°C until use. The plasma samples represent pooled whole blood donations collected from 30 healthy, gender- and race-matched donors between the ages of 18 and 50. Mobile phases and solutions were prepared with LC/MS grade solvents from Sigma-Aldrich.

2.2   Bioinformatics

Proteotypic peptides for 33 putative cancer-related biomarker proteins of high-to-moderate abundance were selected for chemical synthesis in their isotopically labeled form. Peptide selection adhered to the following criteria that were guided by proteomic database search tools (e.g., human PeptideAtlas (Deutsch *et al.*, 2008), Global Proteome Machine (Beavis, 2006)):

    i.   routinely observed in tryptic protein digests,

    ii. sequence unique to the protein within the target plasma proteome,

    iii. lack internal missed tryptic cleavage sites,

    iv. devoid of modifiable amino acid residues,

v. contain no sequential proline residues, and

vi. less than 20 residues in length.

Candidate peptides were then further filtered based on theoretical tryptic cleavage efficiency specified in the Peptide Cutter tool provided by ExPASy(ExPASy_Bioinformatics_Portal, 2005; Gasteiger *et al.*, 2005). The 82 peptides selected represent the most suitable candidates for precise protein MRM-based quantitation.

2.3   SIS peptide Synthesis, Purification, and Characterization

The isotopically labeled target peptides were prepared in-house as described elsewhere (Kuzyk *et al.*, 2012, in press; Kuzyk *et al.*, 2009). Briefly, tryptic SIS peptides were synthesized using Fmoc chemistry techniques that were performed on a Prelude peptide synthesizer (Protein Technology; Tucson, AZ, USA). Peptide purification was performed by reversed-phase high-performance liquid chromatography (RP-HPLC), with their elution monitored by UV absorbance (at 230 nm) on an Ultimate 3000 (Dionex; Sunnyvale, CA, USA). Collected fractions were measured by matrix-assisted laser desorption/ionization time-of-flight mass spectrometry (MALDI-TOF-MS), with the fractions containing the target peptide being pooled, lyophilized, and stored at –80°C until use. Lyophilized peptides were solubilized before characterization in 30% acetonitrile (ACN) containing 0.1% formic acid (FA). Peptide purity was further assessed by capillary zone electrophoresis, while amino acid analysis was used to confirm the peptide sequence and determine its concentration. These absolute concentrations were then adjusted by the percent purity of each synthetic peptide in the quantitative MRM analyses.

2.4   Transition Optimization

The optimal MRM precursor/product ion pairs (i.e., "transitions") for the target peptides, and their corresponding collision energies, were empirically optimized as described previously (Domanski *et al.*, 2012; Percy *et al.*, 2012). Briefly, the transition list to be optimized consisted of doubly- and triply-charged precursor ions (spanning the m/z 300 to 1400 range) and their corresponding b- and y-product ions generated by collision-induced dissociation. Once assembled, equimolar SIS peptide mixtures (at 1 µM in 30% ACN and 0.1% FA) were infused directly into the Agilent 6490 triple quadrupole mass spectrometer and analyzed *via* standard-flow ESI. Each MRM transition was scanned for 20 ms, while the collision energies were ramped in 4 V increments, from 5 to 53 V. Based on the results of this optimization, the 3 most intense transitions were selected, regardless of peptide charge, but with a preference for y-series product ions.

2.5   Detection of Endogenous Peptides

For the detection of endogenous peptides, biological samples were prepared for LC/MRM-MS using a conventional bottom-up proteomic workflow (Domanski *et al.*, 2012; Percy *et al.*, 2012). Briefly, aliquots of the 10X diluted biological sample were denatured with sodium deoxycholate (1% (w/v)), reduced with tris(2-carboxyethyl)phosphine hydrochloride (5 mM (w/v)), alkylated with iodoacetamide (10 mM iodoacetamide), and quenched with dithiothreitol (10 mM dithiothreitol). Thereafter, digestion was initiated with sequencing grade modified trypsin (Promega; Madison, WI, USA) spiked in at a 50:1 substrate:enzyme ratio. This reaction was allowed to proceeded for 16 h at 37 °C before being quenched with the chilled, acidified SIS peptide mixture (0.5% FA, pH <3). The SIS peptide mixture used was equimolar for the optimizations and concentration-balanced to reflect the endogenous plasma protein concentrations in the reproducibility and quantitation experiments. The acid-insoluble surfactant was pelleted by centrifugation (12,000 x g, 10 min) and the supernatant was removed for solid phase extraction (10 mg Oasis HLB cartridge; Waters; Milford, MA, USA). The eluted samples were then frozen for lyophilization, and were rehydrated prior to LC/MRM-MS analyses. The final concentration of all samples was 1 $\mu g/\mu L$, which assumes that the protein concentration in the initial plasma was 70 mg/mL.

All experiments were performed on a standard-flow ultra-high performance liquid chromatography (UHPLC)/MRM-MS platform that utilizes Agilent's latest technology (Agilent Technologies; Palo Alto, CA, USA). A standard-flow LC system rather than a nano-flow platform was employed for the MRM-based quantitative proteomic analyses, because we had previously demonstrated that the standard-flow platform yielded fewer chemical interferences and superior assay metrics (in terms of robustness, limit of quantitation, and dynamic range), when interfaced to the same mass spectrometer, if a ten-fold increase in sample loading was used (Percy et al., 2012). In all experiments, an optimal amount of plasma digest (10 μg), spiked with a SIS peptide mixture (100 fmol of SIS peptides in the optimizations or 0.01 to 1000 fmol of the balanced SIS mix in the experiments), was loaded onto the RP-UHPLC column (150 × 2.1 mm i.d., 1.8 μm particles) that was maintained at 50°C with a Peltier thermostat for precise temperature control and enhanced chromatographic separations. High-throughput peptide separations were achieved at a flow rate of 0.4 mL/min with a UHPLC solvent gradient program from 3 to 90% mobile phase B (0.1% FA in 90% ACN) over a 30 min run time. ESI was performed in the positive ion mode, using the optimal MRM acquisition parameters, as described previously (Domanski et al., 2012; Percy et al., 2012), as well as peptide-specific collision energies (5 – 41 V) and retention times (2.4 – 22.6 min). The final dynamic MRM method contained 120 transitions, which represented 60 interference-free peptide targets that corresponded to 27 cancer-associated plasma biomarker proteins. Each peptide was monitored by a single transition, with each transition integrated for a minimum of 13 ms to give a total cycle time of 370 ms. The total number of samples processed in each experiment is as follows: 2 in the interference assessment (n = 2), 3 in the reproducibility evaluation (n = 20), and 8 in the quantitative analysis (n = 5).

2.6   Interference Screening

The optimal MRM transitions were screened for chemical interference in the proteinaceous biological sample, as described previously (Domanski et al., 2012; Percy et al., 2012). Briefly, the peptide transitions for the SIS and endogenous (NAT) isoforms were monitored under matrix-free conditions (i.e., in mobile phase A: 0.1% FA) and in the biological matrix (i.e., tryptic-digested plasma) using the optimized LC gradient. The average relative ratios and %CVs between these ratios for the SIS peptide in buffer, the SIS peptide in plasma, and the NAT peptide in plasma were calculated from duplicate LC/MRM-MS analyses of each solution. The top 3 transitions for a given peptide were then ranked if two of the three transitions had a coefficient of variation (CV) below 20%, displayed identical SIS and NAT chromatographic behaviors, and were free from co-eluting ions. The transition that produced the highest average ratio was used as the quantifier in the quantitation experiments, unless otherwise specified.

2.7   Accurate and Precise Quantitation

Quantitative information on the interference-free target peptides, and thus by inference the corresponding proteins, was determined as described previously (Domanski et al., 2012; Percy et al., 2012). All MRM data was processed with Agilent's MassHunter Quantitative Analysis software (version B.04.00). Peaks were first evaluated for correct selection and integration accuracy before responses (i.e., NAT or SIS peak area) and relative responses (i.e., NAT:SIS or SIS:NAT peak area ratios) were determined. The lower limit of quantitation (LLOQ), the dynamic range, and the concentration of each target protein was extracted from an 8-point calibration curve (relative response as a function of the relative concentration, which spanned a 100,000-fold concentration range), with the curve for each peptide having been constructed with $1/x^2$ (x = concentration) weighting. The standard samples for the curve contained a variable amount of SIS and an identical amount of NAT, as detailed in section 2.5. In order to qualify, the 5 replicates for a given level must be both precise (< 20% CV) and accurate (80 – 120%), as per the recommendations of the US FDA ("US Food and Drug Administration. Draft Guidance for Industry: Bioanalytical Method Validation. US Food and Drug Administration, Rockville, MD, USA," 1999). The LLOQs were defined as the lowest point on the curve that obeyed the two-tailed precision and accuracy requirement, whereas the dynamic range was the quotient of the upper and lower LOQ. The concentration calculation utilized the relative response (NAT:SIS) of the peptide and its synthetic peptide concentration (corrected with percent purity) for each "qualified" concentration level. For proteins that had multiple target peptides, the peptide that provided the highest plasma protein concentration was used for the accuracy determinations. Quantitation accuracies were determined by comparing the calculated protein concentrations to their mean reported values from the literature.

3   Results and Discussion

Of the approximately 100 FDA-approved protein analytes in human plasma (Anderson, 2010), only 9 are currently used in diagnostic cancer screening and at least one (PSA) lacks the sensitivity and specificity required for definitive cancer assignments. Over the past decade, much effort has been directed toward protein biomarker discovery. By 2006, 1252 additional potential plasma protein markers for human cancer had been reported (Polanski et al., 2006). These proteins, however, have still not been verified or validated as true clinical markers of cancer. To meet this goal, analytical methods must be developed that are robust, sensitive, and accurate in order to have clinical utility. Furthermore, they must enable the multiplexed analysis of a panel of target analytes in a single high-throughput assay with the lowest possible cost. A targeted proteomics approach involving bottom-up UHPLC/MRM-MS with SIS peptides satisfies these requirements and is therefore ideally suited for the verification and validation phases of the protein biomarker pipeline. Described herein is the use of this approach for detecting and quantitating a panel of 27 candidate cancer protein biomarkers in undepleted and non-enriched human plasma.

3.1   Investigated Protein Panel

Using the 2006 list of candidate cancer protein biomarkers as a reference (Polanski et al., 2006) and the 10 ng/mL protein concentration lower limit previously found on this Agilent MS platform as a threshold (Domanski et al., 2012), a shorter list of 33 putative markers were selected for method development. These proteins span 5 orders of magnitude in concentration, from albumin (reported plasma protein concentration: 41 mg/mL) to insulin-like growth factor 1 (reported plasma protein concentration: 144 ng/mL), and have been linked to a variety of human cancers (see Figure 1 for a breakdown).

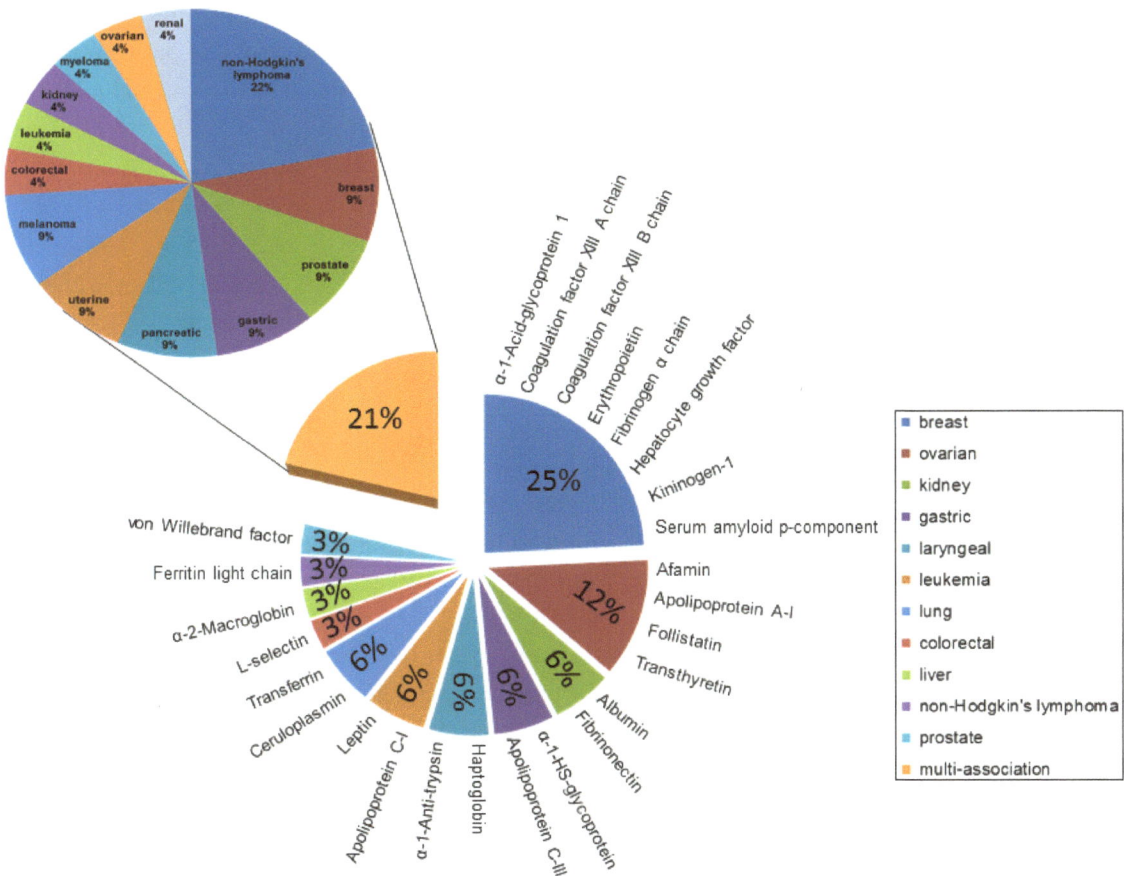

Figure 1: The correlation of candidate human cancer biomarker proteins with the cancer sub-type. The pie chart consists of 33 high-to-moderate abundance plasma proteins that comprise the initial target protein panel. The proteins with multiple associations include: β-2 microglobu-lin, C-reactive protein, intercellular adhesion molecule 1, insulin-like growth factor 1, insulin-like growth factor-binding protein 3, serum paraoxonase/arylesterase 1, and vitronectin.

Breast cancer has the highest association with 8 of the target proteins being reported as candidate markers (Polanski *et al.*, 2006). For each target protein, an average of 3 proteotypic tryptic peptides were selected for directed protein quantitation. The 82 peptides were chosen based on a set of selection criteria, described in detail by Kuzyk *et al.* (2012) and briefly described in the experimental section above, that were guided by web-accessible databases (e.g., PeptideAtlas (Deutsch *et al.*, 2008), Global Proteome Machine (Beavis, 2006)). Since peptides act as molecular surrogates for the proteins of interest, the criteria for peptide selection is necessarily strict. This enables increased accuracy and specificity in the MRM assay, which is required if a peptide is to be monitored in biomarker screening studies. The databases that proteotypic peptides are selected from are publicly available and contain lists of enzymatically-derived peptides which have been observed in tandem MS proteomics studies, along with other useful information, such as frequency of observation and sequence uniqueness. The information contained in the databases is compiled from a multitude of experiments that were performed on different MS platforms in diverse laboratories. For our MRM-based studies, only the most suitable candidates from the databases were chemically synthesized as SIS peptides. After synthesis, the concentration and purity were determined for each SIS peptide (average purity: 96%), which enables accurate and precise quantitation of the endogenous proteins by MRM.

3.2   Preliminary Optimizations

To develop a sensitive and accurate MRM assay, the precursor/product ion pairs for each peptide, along with their optimal collision energies, must first be empirically tuned. As previously demonstrated by Kuzyk *et al.* (Kuzyk *et al.*, 2009), this can improve the detection sensitivity by a factor of 11.4. This optimization is readily performed by direct infusion of the SIS peptides in solvent, as described above. Since the standards have identical chemical and physical properties to their endogenous (natural, NAT) counterparts (except for molecular weight), identical behaviors (in terms of chromatographic separation, electrospray ionization, and gas-phase fragmentation) are exhibited. This allows the collision energies obtained for the SIS peptides to also be used for the NAT peptide targets. The top 3 most-abundant transitions (predominantly y-ions), along with their corresponding collision energies (15 V on average), were used in further optimization experiments (see Table 1 for a list of the optimized parameters for the 82 peptides).

Using the curated list of top 3 transitions for each peptide, the optimal loading capacity for the standard-flow UHPLC/MRM-MS platform (10 μg protein digest on-column, (Domanski *et al.*, 2012)), and an optimal 30 min LC gradient for the target peptides, the MRM transitions were screened for chemical interference from the plasma matrix background. Interference screening is necessary due to the complexity of the digested plasma (Abbatiello *et al.*, 2010; Domanski *et al.*, 2012; Hüttenhain *et al.*, 2012; Keshishian *et al.*, 2007; Kuzyk *et al.*, 2009; Percy *et al.*, 2012; Sherman *et al.*, 2009), which involves thousands of proteins being converted to hundreds of thousands, if not, millions of peptides. In this project, screening was performed by monitoring the SIS and NAT peptide transitions under matrix-free and with-matrix conditions. From the resulting extracted ion chromatograms (XICs), the individual responses of SIS and NAT were obtained from each MRM transition. After calculating the ratios of the responses for the transitions of the SIS peptide in buffer, the SIS peptide in plasma, and the NAT peptide in plasma, relative to the most intense signal-producing transition in the set, the average relative ratio and the CVs for each peptides transition were determined. In general, for a transition to be considered interference-free, *both* forms of the peptide must be 1) free from co-eluting ions in the ion transmission windows, 2) be Gaussian in peak shape, 3) co-chromatograph with each other, and 4) have less than 20% CV in the average relative ratio (see Figure 2a,b for the XICs of a good peptide in plasma and buffer). Based on these constraints, 22 peptides were removed from the initial target panel, leaving 60 peptides (corresponding to 27 putative cancer plasma proteins) for inclusion in the final targeted MRM assay. Nine of these 22 peptides were removed because of interference, while 13 had an undetectable endogenous signal due to either low plasma protein concentration or poor tryptic digestion efficiency. For the remaining 60 peptides, the transition that exhibited the highest average relative ratio was usually selected as the transition on which the quantitation is based. Peptide SSPVVIDASTAIDAPSNLR from fibronectin (see Figure 2c,d for the XICs in plasma and buffer) and peptide GLIDEVNQDFTNR from fibrinogen α chain were the two exceptions in the panel. In this case, due to the detection of a non-specific signal that interfered with the y_5^+ ion pair on the SIS peptide in plasma, the y_7^+ MRM ion pair was instead selected for moni-

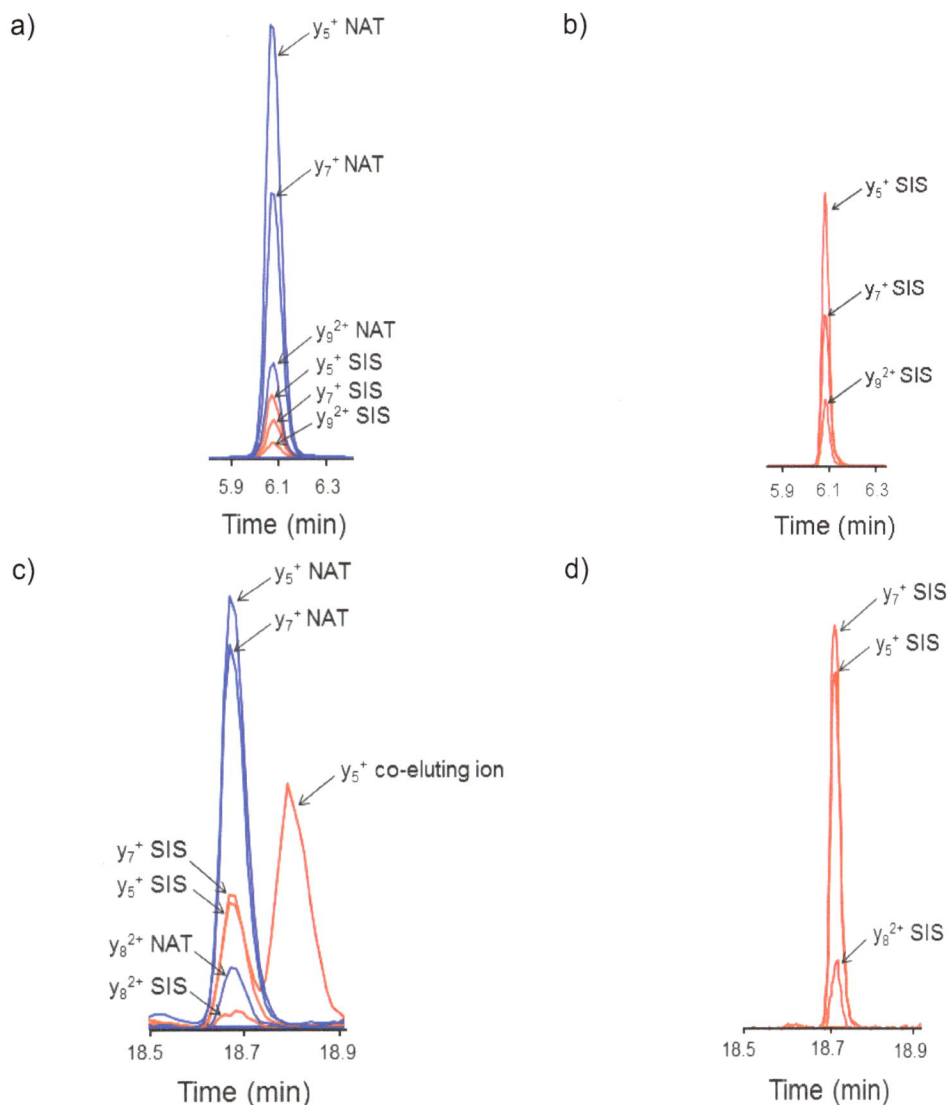

Figure 2: Extracted ion chromatograms for the three most abundant MRM ion pairs for two selected peptides from the interference test. Peptide GSESGIFTNTK from fibrinogen α chain in **a)** plasma and **b)** 0.1% FA. Peptide SSPVVIDASTAIDAPSNLR from fibrinonectin in **c)** plasma and **d)** 0.1% FA. The NAT ion pairs are displayed in blue, while the SIS ion pairs are in red.

toring (0.93, 7% CV vs. 0.99, 2% CV). This further stresses the importance of testing the MRM transitions for interference.

Since no patient samples were to be analyzed using this preliminary method, only a single transition for each interference-free peptide was targeted. If real patient samples were to be evaluated using this method, three transitions per peptide would be used, with the transition that yielded the highest average relative ratio serving as the quantifier ion pair, while the 2 lower-abundance ion pairs would act as qualifiers. The qualifiers would assist in determining possible peptide interferences that could potentially arise from other upregulated proteins in cancer patients. Nevertheless, the final MRM acquisition method developed used a concentration-balanced SIS peptide mixture, as opposed to the equimolar mixture that was utilized in the optimization experiments and employed previously in the literature (Hüttenhain *et al.*, 2012). The balanced ratios help improve the quantitative accuracy and minimize the analytical variation between analyses by providing SIS signals that are within an order of magnitude of their endogenous peptide counterparts (Kuzyk *et al.*, 2009). For the 60 peptides that comprised the final assay, the average NAT:SIS responses were 2.6 (see Figure 3 for the total ion chromatogram and XIC insets for two 1-min retention time windows). The balanced NAT:SIS ratios are in keeping with clinical guidelines for the creation of MS-based quantitative assays, as stated by Chance *et al.* (2006), and should enable precise MRM measurements.

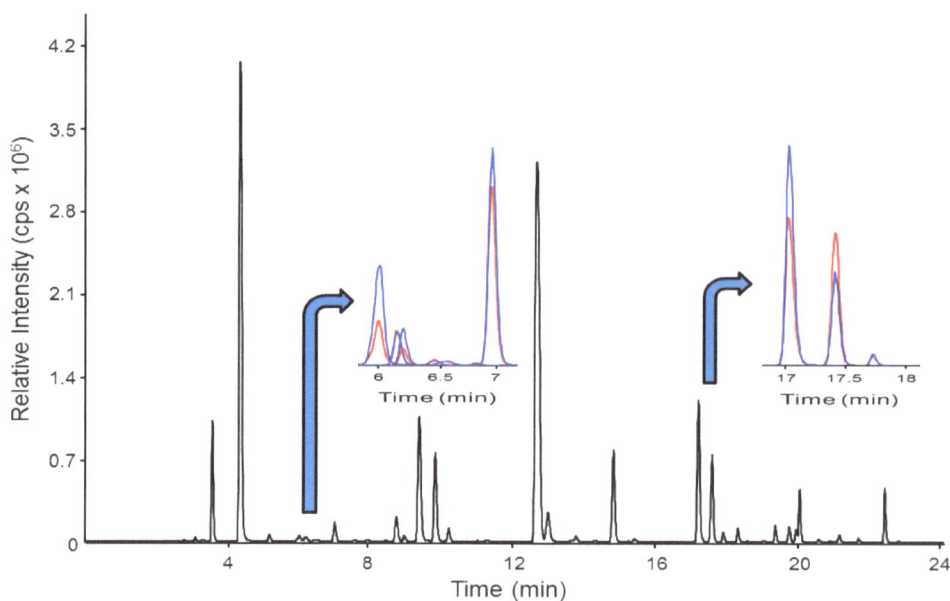

Figure 3: Representative total ion chromatogram for 60 interference-free tryptic peptides (representing 27 cancer-linked proteins), monitored in the final scheduled MRM assay on Agilent's standard-flow UHPLC/MRM-MS platform. The SIS peptide mixture was spiked into the plasma digest at concentrations that reflect their endogenous levels. The inset on the right illustrates the transitions for 3 high abundance peptides (SVLGQLGITK and VFSNGADLSGVTEEAPLK, α_1-anti-trypsin; GSPAINVAVHVFR, transthyretin) eluting between 17 and 18 min, while the inset on the left shows a collection of 7 lower-abundance peptides (2 from fibrinogen α chain and singles from apolipoprotein C-I, α_2-HS-glycoprotein, ceruloplasmin, fibrinonectin, and serum amyloid P-component) eluting between 6 and 7 min.

3.3   Robustness

A key performance requirement of any analytical method designed for use in multiple laboratories is that it be robust. Robustness is defined here in terms of retention time variability and signal stability. This ensures reliable and reproducible LC-MS performance during routine implementation, which is necessary if the method is to ultimately be used for biomarker screening. To evaluate the robustness of our developed method, 3 independent plasma digests were prepared and 20 analytical replicates were run for each sample on the standard-flow UHPLC/MRM-MS platform over the course of 3 consecutive days. The results from one day of analyses are displayed in Figure 4, with equivalent results being obtained for the other 2 days (data not shown). Plotted is the average retention time, the full-width at half maximum (FWHM), and the signal stability (measured as a relative response, NAT:SIS) for the 60-peptide MRM assay in each of the 20 replicates. As illustrated, highly reproducible RP-UHPLC separations (average CV: 0.08%) and narrow chromatographic peak widths (average FWHM: 4.4 s) were obtained, which supports the scheduling of a higher number of transitions, and therefore enables higher multiplexing. Stable relative-response measurements were also demonstrated (average CV: 4.08%), which are well below the 20% CV desired for clinical utility ("US Food and Drug Administration. Draft Guidance for Industry: Bioanalytical Method Validation. US Food and Drug Administration, Rockville, MD, USA," 1999). This supports the verification of a panel of high-to-moderate abundance candidate cancer biomarkers in a rapid and reliable manner.While proteins below the 100 ng/mL range were not investigated in this study, the probability of being able to accurately detect and quantify plasma proteins in the low ng/mL range using a similar method and an identical analytical platform is considered high, based on our previous findings (Domanski *et al.*, 2012). In that study, robust protein quantitation of undepleted and non-enriched plasma proteins was demonstrated with average CVs of 12% for the 7 target proteins that were in the 10 – 100 ng/mL range. Robustness for proteins in the pg/mL range is currently being investigated with novel analytical approaches using the MRM with SIS peptide approach and will be the subject of a future study.

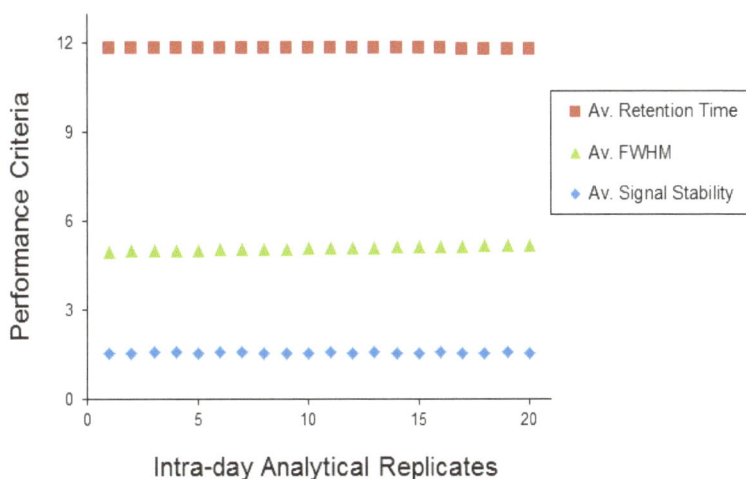

Figure 4: Performance criteria evaluation over one day of analytical replicate measurements. The average signal stabilities (NAT:SIS relative response; dimensionless), retention time (in min), and FWHM (in sec) of 57 interference-free peptides are plotted for 20 replicate measurements obtained on Agilent's standard-flow UHPLC/MRM-MS platform.

3.4   Accurate and Precise Quantitation

To further validate the developed MRM method, additional assay attributes (in terms of lower limit of quantitation, linear dynamic range, and protein concentration) must also be determined. These values can readily be extracted from calibration curves and further assessed with the aid of literature references. In our method, the curves were constructed with a maximum of 8 concentration levels for each interference-free peptide. Based on our precision and accuracy threshold for each level – and the requirement of a minimum of 3 qualified levels to generate a curve – 57 peptides were used to quantitate 27 cancer-related biomarker proteins (see Table 2 for a detailed list of the quantitative results). The corresponding curves displayed excellent linearity (average coefficient of determination: 0.99), with an average linear dynamic range of 10^3 and an average protein LLOQ of 78 µg/mL (see Figure 5a for the spread of the LLOQs for the 27 target proteins). As was the case with the intra-/inter-day reproducibility measurements, the quantitative assay also demonstrated high precision, with an average CV of 4.1% at the level where the endogenous and synthetic peptides were present at nearly equal concentrations. This further highlights the robustness of the standard-flow UHPLC-MS platform.

The determined protein concentrations ranged from 27 mg/mL (albumin) to 162 ng/mL (insulin-like growth-factor 1), which is close to their mean reported protein concentrations of 41 mg/mL and 144 ng/mL, respectively (see Figure 5b for the quantitative accuracy). Considering that albumin has the highest plasma protein abundance and has been classified as a rapidly digested protein (Proc *et al.*, 2010), the 1.5 fold discrepancy between the determined and reported plasma protein concentrations is surprising. This is probably attributable to insufficient denaturation, reduction, and alkylation, and may result from the large number of disulfide bonds (17 in total) and the fact that non-surface accessible peptides are being targeted (namely SLHTLFGDK, residues 89-97; AEFAEVSK, residues 250-257; FQNALLVR, residues 427-434). These 3 peptides, however, are reported to have high tryptic cleavage probability if albumin is completely unfolded and accessible (an average of 92%, based on the PeptideCutter predictor tool).

As illustrated in Figure 5b, plasma protein concentrations were underestimated for 3 proteins that were represented by single-peptide surrogates (apolipoprotein C-I, protein 20 in Figure 5b; β-2 microglobulin, protein 25 in Figure 5b; and α-1-acid glycoprotein 1, protein 26 in Figure 5b). This suggests that enzymatic cleavage at these particular sites was not efficient. The poor digestion observed for apolipoprotein C-I and α-1-acid glycoprotein 1 is not unexpected based on our findings from a previous quantitative study conducted under a similar set of denaturation and digestion conditions (Proc *et al.*, 2010). The resistance to digestion observed for α-1-acid glycoprotein 1, for instance, could possibly be explained by the effect of steric hindrance of the glycans (5 N-linked oligosaccharides) on the proteolytic digestion (Lee *et al.*, 2011). Glycosylation of β-2 microglobulin could also explain the poor tryptic digestion observed for peptide VNHVTLSQPK, despite having a 100% cleavage probability under completely unfolded conditions (as reported by the PeptideCutter tool). Alternatively, the literature reference to which our values were compared may have used a different sample source and/or a different sample collection protocol. This pre-analytical variability has been found to influence the protein concentration measured by MRM-MS, as demonstrated recently by Aguilar-Mahecha *et al.* (2012). When multiple peptide targets were present, the concentration of NAT in the plasma matrix was based on the peptide that provided the highest plasma protein concentration, since this peptide was considered to have been the most readily digested. Thus, this study confirmed the importance of monitoring multiple peptides per target protein in

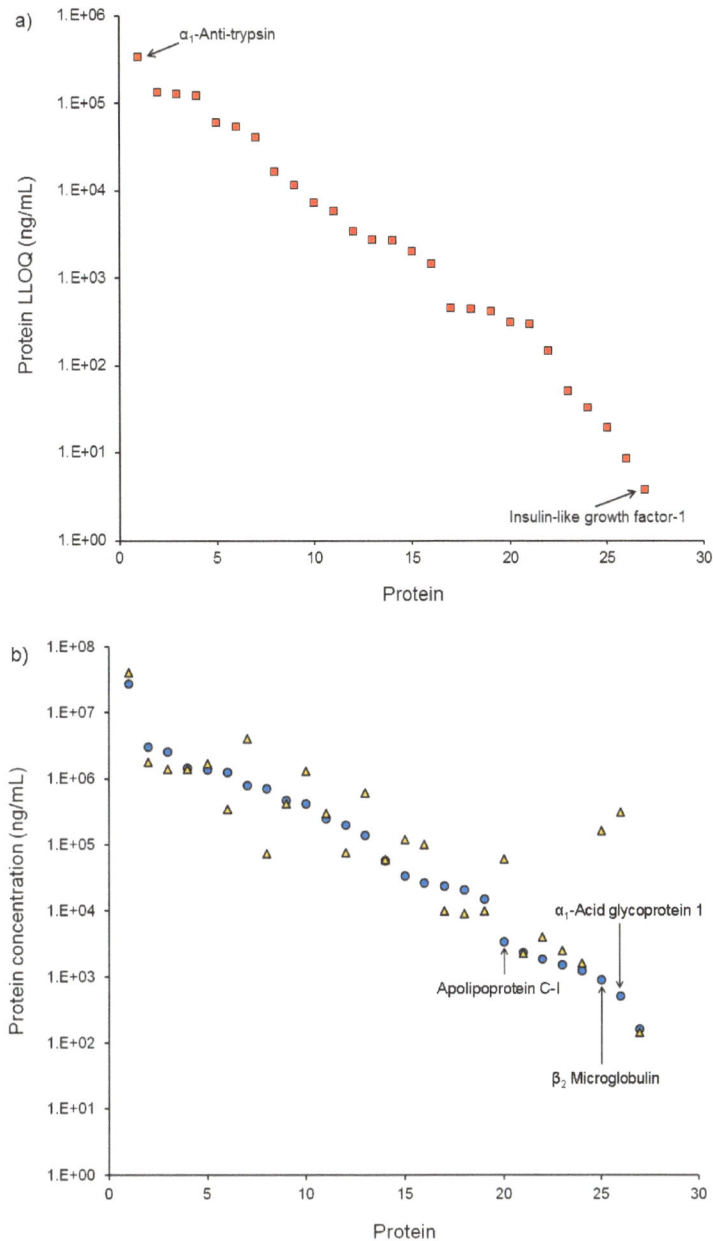

Figure 5: Determination of the sensitivity and accuracy of the protein quantitation. Plotted are **a)** the determined protein LLOQs (squares) in order of decreasing concentration, and **b)** the determined protein concentrations (circles), displayed in order of decreasing concentration, as well as the literature protein concentrations (triangles) for the 27 cancer-associated biomarker proteins. The plasma protein concentrations of the three indicated proteins were underestimated by this assay, possibly because their concentrations were based on single peptide surrogates that may have not been completely released during digestion.

order to help overcome the imperfect nature of tryptic digestion (Domanski *et al.*, 2012; Whiteaker *et al.*, 2010).

MRM-based protein quantitation, as presented in this chapter, demonstrates that plasma protein concentrations can be accurately and precisely measured using a robust analytical platform. Further development of this method is possible since MRM technology has the capacity to monitor hundreds to thousands of transitions in a single experiment, which enables the panel of target biomarker proteins to be dramatically increased. For instance, we have recently developed a method for quantitating 118 proteins in undepleted and non-enriched human plasma. These proteins cover a diverse array of clinically-relevant disease states that encompasses cancer, as well as cardiovascular disease and Alzheimer disease. Thus, a single highly-multiplexed analysis could be used to screen for many critical health problems, which would lead to improved patient outcomes while reducing costs.

4   Conclusions and Significance

Despite the tremendous success of protein biomarker discovery, the number of new FDA approved markers has remained relatively constant over a recent 15 year period from 1993 to 2008 (an average of 1 per year (Anderson, 2010)) due to the stringent requirements imposed for their verification and validation. Toward this end, we have developed a targeted MRM-based approach involving SIS peptides to enable the absolute quantitation of 27 proteins in undepleted and non-enriched human plasma. This example method demonstrates high reproducibility, accuracy, and specificity, while enabling proteins to be quantitated in a high-throughput and multiplexed manner with low sample consumption. We recognize that the successful verification and validation efforts require the analysis of large numbers of samples. We therefore hope that the described method will be adopted by plasma proteomic researchers in the field who will use it to test the utility of these, and other, candidate plasma protein biomarkers.

Acknowledgements

We wish to thank Genome Canada, Genome BC, and the Western Economic Diversification of Canada for providing platform funding. We also wish to recognize the fiscal, operational, and scientific support of the NCE CECR PROOF Centre of Excellence. We declare no financial or commercial conflicts of interest.

References

Abbatiello, S. E., Mani, D. R., Keshishian, H., & Carr, S. A. (2010). Automated Detection of Inaccurate and Imprecise Transitions in Peptide Quantification by Multiple Reaction Monitoring Mass Spectrometry. Clinical Chemistry, 56(2), 291–305.

Addona, T. A., Shi, X., Keshishian, H., Mani, D. R., Burgess, M., Gillette, M. A., Clauser, K. R., Shen, D., Lewis, G. D., Farrell, L. A., Fifer, M. A., Sabatine, M. S., Gerszten, R. E., & Carr, S. A. (2011). A pipeline that integrates the discovery and verification of plasma protein biomarkers reveals candidate markers for cardiovascular disease. Nature Biotechnology, 29(7), 635–643

Aebersold, R., Caprioli, R., Druker, B., Hartwell, L., & Smith, R. (2005). Perspective: a program to improve protein biomarker discovery for cancer. Journal of Proteome Research, 4(4), 1104-1109.

Aguilar-Mahecha, A., Kuzyk, M. A., Domanski, D., Borchers, C. H., & Basik, M. (2012).Comparison of blood collection tubes and processing protocols for plasma proteomics studies.PlosOne, 7(6), e38290. doi:38210.31371/journal.pone.0038290.

Anderson, L., & Hunter, C. L. (2006). Quantitative mass spectrometric multiple reaction monitoring assays for major plasma proteins. Molecular and Cellular Proteomics, 5(4), 573-588.

Anderson, N. L. (2010). The clinical plasma proteome: a survey of clinical assays for proteins in plasma and serum. Clin. Chem., 56(2), 177-185.

Anderson, N. L., & Anderson, N. G. (2002). The human plasma proteome:history, character, and diagnostic prospects. Molecular and Cellular Proteomics, 1(11), 845–867.

Beavis, R. C. (2006). Using the global proteome machine for protein identification.Methods in Molecular Biology, 328, 217-228.

Bray, F., Grey, N., Ferlay, J., & Forman, D. (2012). Global cancer transitions according to the Human Development Index (2008-2030): a population-based study. Lancet Oncology, 13(8), 790-801.

Chace, D. H., Barr, J. R., Duncan, M. W., Matern, D., Morris, M. R., Palmer-Toy, D. E., Rockwood, A. L., Siuzdak, G., Urbani, A., Yergey, A. L., & Chan, Y. M. (2006). Mass Spectrometry in the Clinical Laboratory: General Principles and Guidance; Approved Guideline, . Wayne, Pennsylvania, USA.

Chen, Y.-T., Chen, H.-W., Domanski, D., Smith, D. S., Liang, K.-H., Wu, C.-C., Chen, C.-L., Chung, T., Chen, M.-C., Chang, Y.-S., Parker, C. E., Borchers, C. H., & Yu, J.-S. (2012). Multiplexed Quantification of 63 proteins in Human Urine by Multiple Reaction Monitoring-based Mass Spectrometry for Discovery of Potential Bladder Cancer Biomarkers.Journal of Proteomics, 75(12), 3529-3545.

Deutsch, E. W., Lam, H., & Aebersold, R. (2008). PeptideAtlas: a resource for target selection for emerging targeted proteomics workflows. EMBO Reports, 9, 429–434.

Domanski, D., Percy, A. J., Yang, J., Chambers, A. G., Hill, J. S., Cohen Freue, G. V., & Borchers, C. H. (2012). MRM-based Multiplexed Quantitation of 67 Putative Cardiovascular Disease Biomarkers in Human Plasma. Proteomics, 12(8), 1222-1243.

ExPASy_Bioinformatics_Portal.(2005). Peptide Cutter. Retrieved July 2012

Gasteiger, E., Hoogland, C., Gattiker, A., Duvaud, S., Wilkins, M. R., Appel, R. D., & Bairoch, A. (Eds.).(2005). Protein Identification and Analysis Tools on the ExPASy Server. Totowa, NJ: Humana Press.

Hüttenhain, R., Soste, M., Selevsek, N., Röst, H., Sethi, A., Carapito, C., Farrah, T., Deutsch, E. W., Kusebauch, U., Moritz, R. L., Niméus-Malmström, E., Rinner, O., & Aebersold, R. (2012). Reproducible Quantification of Cancer-Associated Proteins in Body Fluids Using Targeted Proteomics. Science and Translational Medicine, 4(142), 1-13.

Jemal, A., Bray, F., Center, M. M., Ferlay, J., Ward, E., & Forman, D. (2011). Global cancer statistics.CA: A Cancer Journal for Clinicians, 61, 69-90.

Keshishian, H., Addona, T., Burgess, M., Kuhn, E., & Carr, S. A. (2007). Quantitative, multiplexed assays for low abundance proteins in plasma by targeted mass spectrometry and stable isotope dilution. Molecular and Cellular Proteomics, 6, 2212-2229.

Kuzyk, M. A., Parker, C. E., & Borchers, C. H. (2012, in press). Development of MRM based assays for plasma proteins. In H. Backvall (Ed.), Methods in Molecular Biology: Humana Press.

Kuzyk, M. A., Smith, D., Yang, J., Cross, T. J., Jackson, A. M., Hardie, D. B., Anderson, N. L., & Borchers, C. H. (2009). Multiple reaction monitoring-based, multiplexed, absolute quantitation of 45 proteins in human plasma. Molecular and Cellular Proteomics, 8(8), 1860-1877.

Lee, J. Y., Kim, J. Y., Park, G. W., Cheon, M. H., Kwon, K. H., Ahn, Y. H., Moon, M. H., Lee, H. J., Paik, Y. K., & Yoo, J. S. (2011). Targeted mass spectrometric approach for biomarker discovery and validation with nonglycosylated tryptic peptides from N-linked glycoproteins in human plasma.Molecular and Cellular Proteomics, 10(12), M111.009290.Epub 002011.

Neagu, M., Constantin, C., Tanase, C., & Boda, D. (2011).Patented Biomarker Panels in Early Detection of Cancer.Recent Patents on Biomarkers, 1, 10-24.

Paulovich, A. G., Whiteaker, J. R., Hoofnagle, A. N., & Wang, P. (2008). The interface between biomarker discovery and clinical validation: the tar pit of the protein biomarker pipeline. Proteomics: Clinical Applications, 2(10-11), 1386-1402.

Percy, A. J., Chambers, A. G., Yang, J., Domanski, D., & Borchers, C. H. (2012).Comparison of Standard-Flow and Nano-Flow Liquid Chromatography Systems for MRM-Based Quantitation of Putative Plasma Biomarker Proteins.Analytical and Bioanalytical Chemistry, 404(4), 1089-1101.

Polanski, M., & Anderson, N. L. (2006).A List of Candidate Cancer Biomarkers for Targeted Proteomics.Biomarker Insights, 1, 1–48.

Proc, J. L., Kuzyk, M. A., Hardie, D. B., Yang, J., Smith, D. S., Jackson, A. M., Parker, C. E., & Borchers, C. H. (2010). A Quantitative Study of the Effects of Chaotropic Agents, Surfactants, and Solvents on the Digestion Efficiency of Human Plasma Proteins by Trypsin.Journal of Proteome Research, 9(10), 5422-5437.

Rifai, N., Gillette, M. A., & Carr, S. A. (2006). Protein biomarker discovery and validation: the long and uncertain path to clinical utility. Nature Biotechnology, 24(8), 971-983.

Schröder, F. H., Carter, H. B., Wolters, T., van den Bergh, R. C., Gosselaar, C., Bangma, C. H., & Roobol, M. J. (2008). Early detection of prostate cancer in 2007. Part 1: PSA and PSA kinetics. European Urology, 53(3), 468-477.

Sherman, J., McKay, M. J., Ashman, K., & Molloy, M. P. (2009). How specific is my SRM?: The issue of precursor and product ion redundancy. Proteomics 9, 1120–1123.

US Food and Drug Administration. Draft Guidance for Industry: Bioanalytical Method Validation. US Food and Drug Administration, Rockville, MD, USA. (1999).

Whiteaker, J. R., Zhao, L., Anderson, L., & Paulovich, A. G. (2010).An Automated and Multiplexed Method for High Throughput Peptide Immunoaffinity Enrichment and Multiple Reaction Monitoring Mass Spectrometry-based Quantification of Protein Biomarkers.Molecular and Cellular Proteomics, 9, 184-196.

Monoclonal Antibodies as Targeted Therapies for Cancer

Bobby George
Reliance Life Sciences Pvt. Ltd, India

1   Introduction

It is well known that cancer arises through a multistep, mutagenic process whereby cancer cells acquire a common set of properties including unlimited proliferation potential, self-sufficiency in growth signals, and resistance to anti-proliferative and apoptotic cues. Furthermore, tumors evolve to garner support from surrounding stromal cells, attract new blood vessels to bring nutrients and oxygen, evade immune detection, and ultimately metastasize to distal organs (Hanahan & Weinberg, 2000). The complexity of alterations in cancer presents a daunting problem with respect to treatment. A key to successful therapy is the identification of critical, functional nodes in the oncogenic network whose inhibition will result in system failure, that is, the cessation of the tumorigenic state by apoptosis, necrosis, senescence, or differentiation. Furthermore, therapeutic agents attacking these nodes must display a sufficiently large therapeutic window with which to kill tumor cells while sparing normal cells. The two mainstay treatment options for cancer today - chemotherapy and radiation, are examples of agents that exploit the enhanced sensitivity of cancer cells to DNA damage.

Traditional cytotoxic chemotherapy works primarily through the inhibition of cell division. Over the last couple of decades with better understanding of mechanisms of oncogenesis, there has been a revolution with regards to the development of novel agents referred to as "targeted therapy". "Targeted" therapies, which aim to attack the underlying oncogenic context of tumors, when properly deployed, tend to be more effective relative to chemotherapy and radiation (Luo *et al.*, 2009). Targeted therapy blocks the proliferation of cancer cells by interfering with specific molecules required for tumor development and growth. The molecular pathways most often targeted in the treatment of solid tumors (e.g., breast, lung, and colorectal cancers) are those of the epidermal growth factor receptor (EGFR, also known as HER1), vascular endothelial growth factor (VEGF), and HER2/neu. Such pathways can be inhibited at multiple levels: by binding and neutralizing ligands (i.e., molecules that bind to specific receptor sites on cells); by occupying receptor-binding sites (thereby preventing ligand binding); by blocking receptor signaling within the cancer cell; or by interfering with downstream intracellular molecules (David, 2008). One of the ways in classifying the targeted therapies for cancer is given under Table 1. The fundamental basis of Ab-based therapy of tumors dates back to the original observations of antigen expression by tumor cells through serological techniques in the 1960s. The definition of cell surface antigens that are expressed by human cancers has revealed a broad array of targets that are over expressed, mutated or selectively expressed compared with normal tissues. Identification of antigens that are suitable for Ab-based therapeutics is important. The increasing knowledge in molecular oncology and the pathogenic mechanisms underlying malignant progression have identified numerous cell surface targets selectively overexpressed in tumors that form part of signaling pathways implicated in cell survival and growth. The advent of mAb technology has made it possible to raise Abs against specific antigens presented on the surfaces of tumors.

Abs are complex protein-based molecules produced by B-lymphocytes that bind to and help eliminate foreign and infectious agents in the body. Abs are grouped into five classes based on the sequence of their heavy chain constant regions: IgM, IgD, IgG, IgE and IgA (Louis *et al.*, 2010). Although there are several classes/subclasses of immunoglobulins in humans, current therapeutic Abs are mostly of the IgG1 isotype because of their long serum half-life and their capacity for strong effector functions as compared to those of other classes/subclasses (Tsuguo *et al.*, 2009). IgG is also the most frequently used subclass

No.	Group	Representative drugs
1	Angiogenesis inhibitors	Angiostatin, Bevacizumab, Endostatin
2	Biologic response modifier agents	Denileukin diftitox
3	Proteasome inhibitors	Bortezomib,
4	Multi-targeted kinase inhibitors	Imatinib mesylate, Nilotinib, Pazopanib, Sorafenib, Sunitinib
5	Therapeutic Abs	Alemtuzumab, Bevacizumab, Cetuximab, Gemtuzumab ozogamicin, Ofatumumab, Panitumumab, Pertuzumab, Rituximab, Transtuzumab, Ziv-aflibercept (a fusion protein)

Table 1: Targeted therapies for cancer.

for cancer immunotherapy. Abs are Y-shaped, having two sets of branches attached to a single stem (see Figure 1A). The arms of the Y (Fab) are the so-called variable regions, the tips of the arms contain antigen-binding regions (complementarity determining regions or CDRs) and the stem (Fc) is a constant region. The constant regions trigger effector functions (phagocytosis, cytolysis by cytotoxic lymphocytes or initiation of complement cascade followed by cell lysis) by linking the complex to other cells of the immune system. The mAbs are monospecific Abs that are produced by identical immune cells that are clones of a unique parent cell (see Figure 1B). They are structurally complex, having large molecular sizes (~150 kDa) and may have several functional domains within a single molecule.

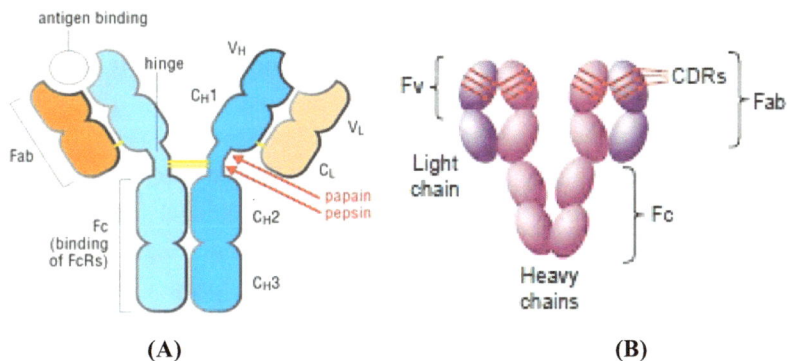

(A)   **(B)**

Figure 1: (A) IgG. Fc region is constituted by CH_2 and CH_3 domain of heavy (H) chain whereas Fab is made up of CH1 and variable domain formed by heavy (H) as well as light (L) chains. **(B)** Unmodified mAb. The mAbs have monovalent affinity, in that they bind to the same epitope. The heavy chains form a fused "Y" structure with 2 light chains running parallel to the open portion of the heavy chain. Modified from: Michael LL et al., 2002.

Today close to 30 mAbs are approved for human therapy and over 200 Abs currently in clinical development worldwide for a wide range of diseases, including cancer, autoimmunity and inflammation, organ transplantation, cardiovascular disease, infectious diseases and ophthalmological diseases (Bobby, 2012b). Commercial interest in mAbs is driven by increasing sales, many of them being blockbuster products generating over $1 billion (bn) in annual sales. In 2009, the global mAb market was worth an estimated $36 bn and between 2009 and 2015; the market is forecast to expand to $63 bn (Datamonitor, 2012).

Ab based therapeutics are being globally marketed as therapeutics for the treatment of various solid tumors and hematological malignancies. mAbs are also being used as disease-specific contrast agents for diagnostic imaging mainly for staging disease in patients suspected of recurrent or metastatic cancer (see Table 2). Aside from targeting antigens that are involved in cancer cell proliferation and survival, mAbs can also function to either activate or antagonize immunological pathways that are important in cancer immune surveillance. The mAbs due to their high affinity and specificity, with a differential expression of target antigen in tumor cells versus normal cells makes an ideal agent for cancer immunotherapy. Due to their protein structure, they can get denatured in the gastrointestinal tract, thus mAbs are administered intravenously. They do not undergo hepatic metabolism, so they are not subject to significant drug interactions. They have been used either as single agents; in combination therapy or as Ab drug conjugates (ADC) (Alejandro & Anthony, 2007). In this chapter we shall dwell on how mAbs are changing the face of cancer therapy.

2   Ab Evolution

2.1   Murine analogues

The modern era of targeted therapy for cancer came to limelight with the discovery of mAbs by Kohler and Milstein (Kohler & Milstein, 1975). This opened the door for the production of Abs of a single specificity (or mAb) in mice and later in rats. The first mAb to show reproducible anti-tumor activity were against GD3 ganglioside for melanoma (Houghton & Scheinberg, 2000). It was expected that, mAbs against tumor antigens would be of great therapeutic value in cancer patients. However these expectations were not met, as murine mAbs did not perform well in the human host. The first patient treated in the United States (US) with mAb therapy (a murine mAb, designated AB-89) was a patient with NHL (Nadler et al, 1980). Although treatment was not successful in inducing a significant clinical response, it did represent the first proof of principle in humans that a mAb could induce transient decreases in the number of circulating tumor cells, and form complexes with circulating antigen, all with minimal toxicity to the patient. Orthoclone OKT3®, was the first such commercially approved therapeutic mAb in 1986 for acute allograft rejection in heart, liver and renal transplantation. It was in Karolinska Institute that the first potential antitumor AbCa 17.1A was tested for activity in metastatic colon cancer (Mellstedt et al., 1989). The mAb was able to regress the metastatic lung lesions, but failed to prolong the survival. It was later discontinued in therapeutic trials.

Murine analogues became less effective with each injection in a clinical setting. This was because of the immunogenicity of murine proteins in humans and the rapid development of a human antimurine antibody (HAMA) response in the patients. This HAMA response neutralized the effectiveness of the murine mAbs and resulted in their rapid clearance from the body. Murine analogues, contributed to the early lack of success of mAbs as they had a short half-life in vivo (due to immune complex formation), limited penetration into tumor sites, inadequate host effector functions and the formation complexes after repeated administration, which resulted in mild allergic reactions and sometimes anaphylactic shock.

No.	Generic Name	Trade Name	Type / Format	First US Approval Year (Withdrawn)	Approved Clinical Indication(s)
A. Unconjugated Abs or Naked Abs					
1	Edrecolomab	Panorex®	Murine	1995* (2002)	CRC
2	Rituximab	Rituxan®/ MabThera®	Chimeric	26th Nov 1997	NHL, RA
3	Trastuzumab	Herceptin®	Humanized	25th Sep 1998	Breast Ca, Gastric Ca
4	Nimotuzumab	TheraCIM®	Humanized	1999*	HNC, Glioma, Lymphoma
5	Cetuximab	Erbitux®	Chimeric	12th Feb 2004	KRAS wild type CRC, HNC
6	Alemtuzumab	Campath-IH®	Humanized	7th May 2001	CLL
7	Bevacizumab	Avastin®	Humanized	26th Feb 2004	CRC, Ovarian & Lung Ca
8	Epratuzumab	Lymphacide	Humanized	2005	NHL
9	Mogamulizumab	Poteligeo®	Humanized	2012*	Lymphoma
10	Pertuzumab	Perjeta	Humanized	8th Jun 2012	Breast Ca
11	Panitumumab	Vectibix®	Human	27th Sep 2006	CRC
12	Zanolimumab	HuMaxCD4	Human	2008	T-cell Lymphoma
13	Ofatumumab	Arzerra®	Human	26th Oct 2009	CLL
14	Ipilimumab	Yervoy®	Human	25th Mar 2011	Melanoma
B. Immunoconjugates					
1√	111In-labeledSatumomab pende-tide	OncoScint™	Murine	29th Dec 1992	Ovarian and CRC
2√	99mTc-labeledAcritumomab	CEAScan™	Murine	28th Jun 1996	CRC
3√	99mTc-labeledNofetumomab merpentan	Verluma™ **	Murine	20th Aug 1996	SCLC, Breast, Ovary, Pancreas Ca
4√	Gemtuzumaboz ogamicin	Mylotarg®	Humanized	17th May 2000 (2010)	AML
5√	90Y-labeled IbritumomabTiuxe-tan	Zevalin®	Murine	19th Feb 2002	NHL
6√	131I -labeledTositumomab	Bexxar®	Murine	27th Jun 2003	NHL
7√	131I -labeled Metuximab	Licartin	Murine	2006*	Lung Ca
8	Brentuximab vedotin	Adcetris™	Chimeric	19th Aug 2011	Systemic anaplastic large cell lymphoma, HL

* Approval outside of EU/US

√ Approved as imaging agents

** No longer marketed by their sponsor for economic considerations

Table 2: Approved anticancer mAbs. AML: Acute myeloid leukemia; Ca: Cancer; CLL: Chronic lymphocytic leukemia; CRC: Colorectal carcinoma; HL: Hodgkin's Lymphoma; HNC: Head and neck cancer; In: Indium; KRAS: Kirsten rat sarcoma; MM: Multiple myeloma; NHL: Non-Hodgkin's lymphoma; RA: Rheumatoid arthritis; SCLC: Small cell lung Cancer; Tc: Technetium; Y: Yttrium (Modified from: Andrew *et al.*, 2012; Bobby 2012b; David 2008; Janice 2012a; Louis *et al.*, 2010).

3   Chimeric mAbs

To overcome the HAMA responses occurring from the usage of murine mAbs, efforts were made to make mAbs more human-like and less immunogenic wherein recombinant DNA technology was applied to Ab design to reduce the antigenicity of murine and other rodent-derived mAbs. In the early 1990s, using molecular biology techniques "chimeric" Abs were created by linking the murine genes encoding the antigen binding portion of the Ab (the variable region) to the genes encoding the constant region of human immunoglobulin light and heavy chains. By this approach, antigenicity could be reduced to permit multiple dosing, affinity could be maintained, the half-life of injected doses could be improved, and host immunologic effector function could be accessed (Morrison *et al.*, 1984). Many of the mAbs approved for commercialization in the 1990's and early 2000's were chimeric Abs with rituximab being first off the block. The use of chimeric Abs substantially reduced the HAMA responses but they still pose a moderate risk of immunogenicity to patients from their residual murine components.

3.1   Humanized mAbs

The technological advances paved the way for humanized mAb which is a mAb constructed with only antigen-binding regions (also called CDRs) derived from a mouse, and the remainder of the variable regions, and constant regions, derived from a human source (Jones *et al.*, 1986). The first humanized mAb to enter the clinic was Alemtuzumab (CamPath-1H) as first-line treatment for refractory B-cell CLL

3.2   Fully human mAbs

Further advancement in creating less immunogenic therapeutic Ab products was the ability to generate fully human mAbs using transgenic mice or phage display libraries (Lonberg, 2008). Human mAbs are produced by transferring human immunoglobulin genes into the murine genome, after which the transgenic mouse is vaccinated against the desired antigen, leading to the production of mAbs. Today, almost all mAb products currently in development are humanized or fully human.

3.3   Modified mAbs and Related Products

Molecular techniques that can alter Ab pharmacokinetics (PK), effector function, size and immunogenicity have emerged as key elements in the development of new Ab-based therapies. Evidence from clinical trials (CTs) of Abs in cancer patients has revealed the importance of iterative approaches for the selection of antigen targets and optimal Abs, including the affinity and avidity of Abs, the choice of Ab construct, the therapeutic approach (such as signaling abrogation or immune effector function) and the need to critically examine the PK and pharmacodynamic (PD) properties of Abs in early CTs (Andrew, 2012). The pathogenesis of many human diseases involves several mediators that function in distinct signaling pathways or that have redundant roles in the same pathway. Simultaneous blockade of several different disease mediators using bispecific Abs may lead to greater therapeutic efficacy and/or benefit more patients than targeting individual disease mediators. Bifunctional Abs are being engineered to effectively target tumor-associated antigens at low levels and then deliver a cytotoxic payload to tumor cells. Modified Abs such as antibody drug conjugates (ADCs), bispecific Abs, Fc or glyco-engineered Abs and Ab fragments/domains comprise 40% of the mAbs currently in Phase II or Phase III CTs (clinicaltrials.gov). Majority of these are undergoing evaluation as treatments for cancer or for immunological diseases (Janice, 2012a; 2012b). Catumaxomab (Removab®), is the first bispecific Ab to be approved by EMA (in 2009) for malignant ascites. Some of the mAbs which are in late phase of their clinical development in oncology setting have been enlisted in Table 3.

No.	INN	Indication in Phase III
1	Elotuzumab	MM
2	Girentuximab	Renal cell Ca
3	Inotuzumab ozogamicin	NHL
4	Obinutuzumab	CLL, NHL
5	Naptumomab estafenatox	Renal cell Ca
6	Necitumumab	Non Small Cell Lung Ca

Table 3: Antibody-based therapeutics in Phase III clinical trials in cancer. Modified from: Janice MR, 2012b.

4 Immunoconjugates

Conjugation procedures have been designed to improve the efficacy of Ab therapy. In these approaches, radioisotopes, natural toxins, chemotherapy agents, or other substances or cells are chemically linked or conjugated to mAbs to form an "immunoconjugate" (see Table 2). Several issues are critical for clinical success of any immunoconjugate. Conjugation must be successful for as many cytotoxic molecules as possible (high specific activity) in such a way that immunoreactivity of the Ab and cytotoxicity of the conjugated agent are retained. The immunoconjugate should also be specific, although this may be demonstrated more easily *in vivo* than *in vitro*, depending on the agent and the chemical linkage. The delivery of the highly toxic moiety to normal cells is undesirable and, therefore, substantial tumor-specific antigen expression is required for optimal delivery. The cytotoxicity of Abs and immunoconjugates is dose related and proportional to the amount of tumor antigen expressed. After systemic administration of the immunoconjugate, its efficacy is dependent upon the stoichiometric relationship of the delivered toxic payload to tumor cells. The number of antigen sites on target cells as well as the prevalence of antigen sites on normal tissues may significantly impact efficacy and toxicity of mAbs and immunoconjugate could help to overcome this weakness. Immunoconjugate stability within the plasma, and subsequent selective release of the payload within the cell cytoplasm, is critical to the success of immunoconjugates bearing toxin and cytotoxic agents. Cellular bioavailability is a key issue for the nonisotope immunoconjugates because they must be able to enter certain intracellular compartments in order to induce a cytotoxic effect.

4.1   Radiolabeled Abs

The immunoconjugates that are technically the easiest to make are radiolabeled Abs. Radiolabeled Abs are important clinically for both tumor imaging and therapy. Radiolabeled Abs have been able to detect tumors that are not detectable by conventional radiologic diagnostic techniques. The distribution of these radiopharmaceuticals depends on the mAb, human antimouse Ab, free antigen, tissue reactivity, tumor vascularity, the radioisotope, and the nature of any linker, such as a chelating agent that may be used in the creation of the immunoconjugate (Epenetos *et al.*, 1986). Radioimmunotherapy (RAIT) involves the administration of an Ab linked to a radioisotope. In RAIT, mAbs with selectivity for the target cells or tissues are linked to radioisotopes with high linear-energy transfer (LET), such as beta (^{131}iodine and ^{90}yttrium) or alpha (^{213}bismuth and ^{211}astatine) emitters that can cause DNA strand breaks and other effects, resulting in cell kill. The Abs themselves might contribute to tumor-cell kill through signaling effects. As radiation can also destroy normal cells, the targeting molecule must achieve a high target to non-target ratio. In general, beta particles, with a penetration range of millimeters, are suitable for therapy of bulk disease, whereas alpha particles, with a penetration range of a few cell diameters, are suitable for micro-metastases or circulating tumor cells (Theresa, 2002).

4.2   Immunotoxins

Immunotoxins are composed of internalizing mAbs or other ligands that are linked to extremely potent toxins, toxin subunits or ribosome-inactivating proteins that kill cells by inactivating protein synthesis or signal transduction. The toxins are derived from plants, fungi or bacteria. The basic principles that govern the choice of toxin are related to the potency of the agent and whether or not the Ab is internalized following binding to the target antigen. Plant and bacterial protein toxins including ricin, gelonin, diphtheria toxin or *Pseudomonas* exotoxin can be directly linked to Abs by gene fusion. Exotoxin A is the most commonly used toxin for targeted cancer therapy. Plant and bacterial immunotoxins traffic through endosomes or the Golgi and endoplasmic reticulum. Free toxin is then released to the cytoplasm where it inhibits protein synthesis and ultimately causes cell death.

4.3   Antibody–drug Conjugates (ADC)

The cytotoxic agent bound to the Ab needs to be highly potent so that the ADCs that do reach the target cell have the maximum killing potential. Other characteristics of the drug component of the ADC is that it must be non-immunogenic and non-toxic (dormant or inactive) when circulating in the blood. The binding of ADCs to specific tumor-associated antigens (TAAs) can trigger internalization of the binding complex and release the drugs inside the cancer cells for the intended cytotoxic action. Another development in this field has been in the linker that links the toxin molecule to the Ab. The linker has to be stable enough to ensure that the ADC remains intact until it reaches its target cell, so it has to be resistant to enzymes in the serum. Then, once the ADC is internalized, the linker and drug have to be released. As an example, "Gemtuzumab ozogamicin" (Mylotarg®, the ADC to be approved (under an accelerated approval mechanism)) which consists of calicheamicin conjugated to an anti-CD33 Ab by a stable bifunctional linker, undergoes hydrolysis in the acidic environment of the lysosome. After free calicheamicin is released, it translocates to the nucleus where it cleaves double-stranded DNA and induces cell death. The product was however, voluntarily withdrawn in 2010, when post approval study required by the FDA did not show evidence of clinical benefit in AML patients nor did it demonstrate improved survival (Bethan, 2010). Limitations with ADCs include their inadequate cellular uptake (< 1%) and residual off-target effects which continue to pose challenges.

5   Development in Production Methodologies

Production of Abs for preclinical and CTs has been evaluated in numerous expression systems, including bacteria, yeast, plant, insect and mammalian cells. For most therapeutic Ab products the doses required for these products are much higher than for other biologic products, resulting in the need for large-scale production and efficient, cost-effective manufacturing processes. When mAb products were first developed and approved, expression levels of MAbs were typically on the order of 100–500 milligrams per liter. In the past decade, improvements have been made in critical areas, such as cell line generation and large-scale cell culture production, to maximize specific Ab productivity from a given cell line and improve overall productivity in bioreactors. These advances include the use of new expression vectors and transfection technology to introduce the genes into cells and improve cell line generation; and high-throughput, robust screening technologies to select the highest producing clones rapidly and more effectively. As a result, the production of cell lines expressing multigram quantities of antibody per liter of culture medium is now routine. These advances, coupled with improvements in cell culture media and greatly optimized bioreactor processes, have made the large-scale production of mAbs economically viable (Susan *et al.*, 2007). The biological activity of mAbs is closely linked to their structural, conformational and chemical stability. Physical or chemical degradation may occur at various stages of development, which could interfere with the intended biological activity, as the site of degradation may involve a domain critical for biological function (Sumit *et al.*, 2013).

6   Targeting Tumors and their Microenviornment

The killing of tumor cells using mAbs can result from direct action of the Ab (e.g., through receptor blockade), immune-mediated cell killing mechanisms, payload delivery, and specific effects of an Ab on the tumor vasculature and stroma. In addition, Abs that target the tumor microenvironment and inhibit processes such as angiogenesis have shown therapeutic promise. They may also inhibit cytokines or other factors that are necessary for cell survival. Many mechanisms have been proposed to explain their clinical antitumor activity.

6.1   Antibody-dependent Cellular Cytotoxicity (ADCC)

ADCC is a well-recognized immune effector mechanism which occurs when an IgG that is bound to the cell surface is recognized by Fc receptors on natural killer (NK) cells and monocytes, resulting in cell-mediated lysis of the target cell. The ADCC is a tripartite process and requires three components viz.

   a)   The expression of the target antigen on cancer cells,

   b)   The presence of the antigen-specific Abs of the appropriate isotype, and

c)   Fc receptor-bearing effector cells.

This cytolytic effector mechanism of Abs relies on the engagement of FcγRs (FcγRIIIa in humans) and recruitment of immune effector cells in an Fc dependent manner, leading to the destruction of target cells by exocytosis of the cytolytic granule complex perforin/granzyme from NK cells (Carter, 2001).

6.2   Complement-dependent Cytotoxicity (CDC)

Most clinically approved mAbs that mediate ADCC also activate the complement system. CDC is a cytolytic cascade known as the 'classical pathway' of the complement system, and is mediated by a series of complement proteins (C1–C9) that are abundantly present in the serum. CDC occurs after complement binds to the Fc portion of the Ab that is bound to the target cell, and results in cell lysis and recruitment of effector cells to tumor cells.

6.3   Targeting Immune Cells

In addition to directly targeting tumor cells, numerous Ab-based therapeutic strategies have been developed to target cells of the immune system with the goal of enhancing antitumor immune responses.

6.4   Combination Approaches

The antitumor efficacy of many therapeutic Abs can be enhanced by their use in combination with other immunomodulatory approaches such as chemotherapy, radiotherapy, targeted therapy agents, vaccines or other immunomodulators. The relative importance of each of these mechanisms varies with the type of tumor and the treatment administered.

7   Limitations and Toxicities

Apart from their prohibitive costs, therapeutic mAbs have some limitations *viz* inability to target intracellular molecules, less efficient tissue penetration, and poor bioavailability when given orally. Modern Ab design has strived to create small Abs that can penetrate to cancerous sites but maintain their affinity and avidity. A variety of factors can reduce Ab efficacy (Reilly *et al.*, 1995). These include:

- Limited penetration of the Ab into a large solid tumor or into vital regions such as brain;

- Reduced extravasation of Abs into target sites owing to decreased vascular permeability;

- Cross-reactivity and nonspecific binding of Ab to normal tissues, reducing the targeting effect;

- Heterogeneous tumor uptake resulting in untreated zones;

- Increased metabolism of injected Abs, reducing therapeutic effects; and

- Rapid formation of HAMA and human antihuman Abs, inactivating the therapeutic Ab.

One of the major challenges in using mAbs for the delivery of cytotoxic agents to tumors has been to achieve high tumor-to-non-tumor ratios, because non-targeted conjugates can lead to dose limiting toxicities. Cross-reactivity with healthy tissues can cause substantial side effects for unconjugated Abs, which can be enhanced when the Abs are conjugated with toxins or radioisotopes. The toxicities noted with mAbs in cancer treatment include gastrointestinal perforation; wound healing complications; hemorrhage; cardiotoxicity, arterial and venous thromboembolism; proteinuria; hypertension; acneiform rash; diarrhea; hypomagnesemia; hypocalcemia; nausea and vomiting; lymphocytopenia; Hepatitis B virus (HBV) reactivation; severe mucocutaneous reactions etc (David, 2008). Immune-mediated complications include dyspnea from pulmonary toxic effects, occasional central and peripheral nervous system complications, and decreased liver and renal function. Radioimmunotherapy with isotopic conjugated Abs also can cause bone marrow suppression

8   Biosimiar mAbs–resisting Tyranny

Conventional generic drugs are defined by the U.S. Food and Drug Administration (FDA) as " identical, or bioequivalent to a brand name drug in dosage form, safety, strength, route of administration, quality, performance characteristics and intended use". The term generic, as applied to conventional non-protein small molecule drugs, is not used to describe biosimilar versions of biopharmaceuticals including mAbs due to their complexity. Developing a biosimilar mAb has its inherent set of concerns/challenges. Defining the comparability of two mAbs (test and reference product) will require consideration of a wide range of aspects, including analytical and physicochemical characterization by several orthogonal methods, comparative biological assays and comparative immunogenicity assessment. Due to variability in the manufacturing process, drug complexity, and the inability to completely characterize the resulting biosimilar product to the same degree as done for conventional generic drugs, one must rely on comparability exercises at all steps in the biosimilar development process.

Designs for the production platform and processes for biosimilar Abs must be carefully considered for their ability to produce a highly consistent, comparable product. Adding to this challenge, the production methods, characterization, and formulation are often kept as trade secrets or are protected by 'patent thickets'. One needs to screen and navigate through the myriad of multiple patents which cover not only the product itself, but also the formulation and the associated manufacturing processes (McCabe, 2009; Holliday, 2009), the technologies used to generate the mAbs, and the vectors as well as cell lines used to produce them (Chartrain and Chu, 2008). Estimated patent expiration dates for blockbuster mAbs and related products in the near offering are 2014 for infliximab (in EU); 2015 for rituximab, trastuzumab and palivizumab; 2016 for adalimumab; and 2017 for bevacizumab.

Originators are trying to keep the biosimilar players at bay by carrying out studies/CTs to support newer indications to the approved list and making efforts to extend their patent protection period. Avastin®, an anti–vascular endothelial growth factor (VEGF) mAb, originally approved to treat metastatic colorectal cancer in 2004, became a blockbuster just one year after its approval. In October 2006, Avastin® was approved for an additional indication, non-small cell lung cancer (NSCLC). Genentech later submitted a supplementary application for breast cancer and got the approval. Another example being Rituxan®, which has been approved for both oncology and autoimmune indications. Targeting the CD20 antigen, Rituxan® was originally approved in the late 1990s for NHL. In addition to pursuing several more oncology indications, the marketers of Rituxan®, were successful in garnering approval for moderately to severely active rheumatoid arthritis (RA) as part of a combination treatment.

Given the escalating development costs of novel mAbs, the high degree of risk from attrition in developing a molecule against a novel target and the imminent expiration of patents for some currently marketed mAb products, the decision of developing mAbs that recognize known, validated targets is becoming more lucrative. Despite these challenges, biosimilar mAbs are going after the blockbuster mAbs. In fact a couple of biosimilar mAbs have already been approved in few of the emerging markets for firms such as M/s Dr. Reddy's Labs of India (Reditux® as a biosimilar version of rituximab) and M/s ISU Abxisof South Korea (Clotinab®, as a biosimilar form of abciximab). European Medicines Agency (EMA) approved in June 2013 the first two biosimilar versions of infliximab namely Celltrion Healthcare's Remsima™ and Hospira's Inflectra™. Both have been approved for the same indications as Remicade, including RA, Crohn's disease, ulcerative colitis, ankylosing spondylitis, psoriatic arthritis and psoriasis.

9   Partnerships and Licensing Deals

The technologies enabling the generation of human mAbs are also now accessible through partnerships or licensing from the companies that have developed these approaches (Aaron *et al.* 2010). Large pharmaceutical companies are in the process of acquiring a number of companies that focus on mAb R&D. For example, Abmaxis, Morphotek and Agensys were acquired by pharmaceutical firms Merck, Eisai and Astellas, respectively. In addition, Cambridge Antibody Technology and MedImmune were both acquired by AstraZeneca. There have also been a multitude of collaborations and partnering deals between pharmaceutical and biotechnology firms focused on mAb R&D, such as Sanofi-Aventis' collaboration with Regeneron and GlaxoSmithKline's deal with OncoMed (Janice, 2008). In 2009, Hospira entered into agreement with South Korean based Celltrion for biosmilar mAbs. Under the distribution agreement, the parties would collaborate on manufacturing and supply of the products. After regulatory approval, Hospira and Celltrion would co-exclusively market the drugs, with the products independently commercialized under each party's brand name. More recent partnerships include Pfizer, Sanofi, GSK, Amgen, Bayer, Takeda and Biogen Idec, all of whom have participated in multiple deals. Pfizer has had three deals in 2011 alone, partnering with MedImmune (for tremelimumab), Theraclone Sciences (for I-STAR technology to discover broadly protective mAbs in the areas of infectious disease and cancer) and Seattle Genetics (for ADC technology). Eli Lilly has entered into two deals in 2011, partnering with Immunogen (for maytansinoid targeted Ab Payload (TAP) technology with mAbs to develop ADC anticancer therapeutics) and Mentrik Biotech (for AME-133v humanized Fc-engineered anti-CD20mAb). BoehringerIngelheim also signed two deals in 2011, partnering with Aveo (for manufacturing Ficlatuzumab) and Morphosys (for manufacturing MOR208, a potent monoclonal anti-CD19 Ab). ImmunoGen is also having multiple collaborations with companies like Genentech, Sanofi-Aventis, Amgen, Biogen Idec, Biotest and Bayer Schering (Bethan, 2010). Switzerland based Roche has signed a manufacturing contract with Emcure Pharmaceuticals, India in March 2012 for its blockbuster biologics drugs Herceptin® and MabThera®, wherein Emcure will manufacture these drugs for the Indian market and depending on the success of this drug it will be taken to other developing countries. In January 2014, Ranbaxy Laboratories signed a licensing pact with EPIRUS Switzerland GmbH for "BOW015", a biosimilar version of Infliximab for marketing in India and other Emerging Markets. With so many companies active in this domain, the field is all set to take-off.

10   Regulatory Framework

EMA has been at the forefront of regulatory agency activities concerning mAbs and development of bio-similars/similar biological products. As regards general regulatory requirements, European Pharmacopoeia (EP) documentation is available for mAbs, like the monograph for mAbs (EP Monograph 2031) or the monograph for products of recombinant DNA technology (EP Monograph 0784). Further guidance from CHMP for production and quality control of mAbs and on immunogenicity assessment for *in vivo* clinical use (EMA/CHMP/BMWP/86289/2010) is also available. EMA has laid down guidelines on non-clinical and clinical development for similar biological medicinal products containing mAbs (EMEA/CHMP/403543/2010). The principles mentioned in the above guideline can be applied to related products/substances like, for example, fusion proteins. It is highly recommend that companies intending to develop biosimilar mAbs seek regulatory scientific advice early in the development process. Some other countries have also come up with regulations/guidelines for governing biologics/biosimilars, drawing heavily from the EMA and World health organization (WHO) guidelines, however none including the US FDA has guidelines/regulations exclusively on mAbs. The implementation of "quality by design" (QbD) and other new regulatory concepts would help in reducing the cost and development timelines. The key principles of regulating biologics/biosimilars have been the same across different agencies. They all emphasize a stepwise, risk based approach (Bobby, 2012a).

11   The Next Frontier

Advances in mAb engineering are driving a transformation in this field, resulting in new drugs with decreased immunogenicity and improved potency, specificity, stability and lower production costs. The newer classes of mAbs being developed are directed against immunogenic tumor specific antigens (TSA's) which are present on the surface of tumor cells and absent in normal tissues. These are expected to have greater potential for effective tumor control in metastic cancer (Arlen *et al.*, 2010). The use of Abs, immunoconjugates and mAb-targeted nanoparticle drug delivery systems, such as immunoliposomes, that offer effective tumor targeting and provide diverse effector functions has emerged as a promising new treatment option for refractory malignancies. Ab-enzyme fusions have also been developed for prodrug activation, primarily for cancer therapy. Smaller recombinant fragments, for example, classic monovalent Ab fragments (Fab, scFv and engineered variants; diabodies, triabodies, minibodies and single-domain Abs) are now being engineered as credible alternatives to mAbs. These fragments retain the targeting specificity of whole mAbs but can be produced more economically and possess other unique and superior properties for a range of diagnostic and therapeutic applications (Holliger and Hudson, 2005). For example nanobodies are distinguished from other conventional Abs by their unique properties of size (15 KDa), solubility, intrinsic stability, easy tailoring into pluripotent constructs, recognition of uncommon or hidden epitopes, binding into cavities or active sites of enzyme targets, ease and speed of drug discovery and ease of manufacture. Their technological and biophysical advantages enable them to outperform conventional Abs in several areas. Nanobodies may add value to cancer diagnostic tests used at present for example, early detection and staging of prostate cancer (Khalissa *et al.*, 2009). Several nanobody therapies are also being developed for treatment of oncology or inflammatory diseases based on blocking molecular interactions. Nanobodies binding to epidermal growth factor receptor (EGFR) can block EGF binding to its receptor, which can be used to treat solid tumors (Roovers *et al.*, 2007).

There is clearly need to continue to improve and accelerate the translation of preclinical research into improved therapeutic strategies for cancer patients. The use of biomarkers in early CTs can increase the possibility of patient benefit, accelerate the drug development process, maximize the ability to generate important biological information about human cancer, and decrease the risk of late and costly drug attrition. Critical to future progress will be an increased understanding of tumor biology, the identification of disease 'driver' molecular targets, the discovery of rationally designed anticancer drugs and their clinical development either as single agents or in rational combinations (de Bonno and Alan, 2010). New insights from animal models and CTs suggest a rationale for ADCC-based combination therapy, approaches that promote antigen presentation, co-stimulation and T cell activation or expansion. The next generation of unconjugated Ab therapies will undoubtedly yield effective new treatments for cancer over the coming years. These advances will arise from the identification and validation of new targets, the manipulation of tumor–host microenvironment interactions, and the optimization of Ab structure to promote the amplification of antitumor immune responses (Louis *et al.*, 2010). An imperative for successful drug development remains the need to identify targets that cancer cells are absolutely reliant on 'mission critical' so that when these functions are blocked there is a lethal or cytostatic effect. However, we need to recognize that our understanding of how a cancer cell is wired compared to normal cells is still far from complete!

Acknowledgments

I gratefully acknowledge the encouragement and support of Reliance Life Sciences Pvt. Ltd in carrying out this work (www.rellife.com).

References

Aaron, N.L., Eugen, D., Janice, M.R.(2010). *Development trends for human monoclonal antibody therapeutics. Nature Rev Drug Discov, Oct 9, 767–774.*

Alejandro, D.R. & Anthony, W.T. (2007). *Technology insight: Cytotoxic drug immunoconjugates for cancer therapy. Nat ClinPracOncol, 4, 245-255.*

Andrew, C.C. & Paul, J.C. (2010). *Therapeutic antibodies for autoimmunity and inflammation. Nature Rev Immunol, 10, May 301-316.*

Andrew, M.S., Jedd, D.W., Lloyd, J.O. (2012). *Antibody therapy of cancer. Nature Reviews, Apr 12, 278-287.*

Arlen, M., Arlen, P., Tsang, A., Wang, X., Gupta, R. (2010). *The therapeutic value of monclonal antibodies directed against immunogenic tumor glycoproteins. J Cancer, 1, 209-222.*

Bethan, H. (2010). Antibody-drug conjugates for cancer: Poised to deliver? Nature Rev. Drug Discov, Sep 9, 665–667.

Bobby, G. (2012a). Current regulations governing biosimilars. Pharma Times, May 44(05), 46-52.

Bobby, G. (2012b). Regulatory framework and challenges in developing biosimilar monoclonal antibodies and related biological products. International J. Pharmaceutical Sci and Nanotechnol, Oct-Dec. 5(3), 1765-1774

Carter, P. (2001). Improving the efficacy of antibody-based cancer therapies. Nat Rev Cancer, 1, 118–129.

Chartrain, M., & Chu, L. (2008). Development and production of commercial therapeutic monoclonal antibodies in mammalian cell expression systems: an overview of the current upstream technologies. Curr Pharm Biotechnol, 9, 447-467.

Datamonitor (2012). Biosimilar mAbs in Europe. Press release.

David EG (2008). Targeted Therapies: A New Generation of Cancer Treatments. Am Fam Physician, 77(3), 311-319.

de Bono, J.S.,&Alan, A.(2010). Translating cancer research into targeted therapeutics. Nature, 467, 30 Sep S43-S49.

EMA/CHMP/BMWP/403543/2010. Guideline on similar biological medicinal products containing monoclonal antibodies. 30th May 2012.

EMA/CHMP/BMWP/86289/2010. Guideline on immunogenicity assessment of monoclonal antibodies intended for in vivo clinical use. 24th May 2012.

Epenetos, A.A., Snook, D., Durbin, H., et al. (1986). Limitations of radiolabeled monoclonal antibodies for localization of human neoplasms. Cancer Res 46, 3183-3191.

European Pharmacopoeia.Monoclonal Antibodies for Human Use, Monograph 2031 (EP, Strausbourg, 2008).

European Pharmacopoeia.Recombinant DNA Technology, Products of, Monograph 0784 (EP, Strausbourg, 2008).

Hanahan, D., & Weinberg, R.A. (2000). The hallmarks of cancer. Cell, 100, 57–70.

Holliday, L. (2009). Patenting antibodies in Europe. mAbs, 1, 385-386.

Holliger, P.H., Hudson, J.P. (2005). Engineering antibody fragments and the rise of single domains. Nat Biotechnol,. 23, 1126-1136.

Houghton, A.N., & Scheinberg, D.A. (2000). Monoclonal antibody therapies - A 'constant' threat to cancer. Nat Med, 6, 373–374.

Janice, M.R. (2008). Monoclonal antibodies as innovative therapeutics. Curr Pharm Biotechnol, 9, 423–430.

Janice, M.R. (2012a). Marketed therapeutic antibodies compendium. mAbs, May 4(3), 1-3.

Janice, M.R. (2012b). Which are the antibodies to watch in 2012? mAbs, Jan/Feb 4(1), 1-3.

Jones, P.T., Dear, P.H., Foote, J., Neuberger, M.S., Winter, G. (1986). Replacing the complementarity-determining regions in a human antibody with those from a mouse. Nature, 321, 522–525.

Khalissa, D., Hengliang, S., Liang, L., Xingzhi, W., Xiaojuan, Z. (2009). Nanobodies - the new concept in antibody engineering. African J of Biotechnol, June, 8(12), 2645-2652.

Kohler, G. & Milstein, C. (1975). Continuous cultures of fused cells secreting antibody of predefined specificity. Nature, 256, 495-497.

Lonberg, N. (2008). Fully human antibodies from transgenic mouse and phage display platforms. Curr Opin Immunol, 20, 450–459.

Louis, M.W., Rishi, S., Shangzi, W. (2010). Monoclonal antibodies: versatile platforms for cancer immunotherapy. Nature Rev Immunol, 10, 317–327.

Luo, J., Solimini, N.L., Elledge, S.J. (2009). Principles of cancer therapy: Oncogene and non-oncogene addiction. Cell, 136, 823–837.

McCabe, K.W. (2009). Guardians at the gate: Patent protection for therapeutic monoclonal antibodies (Part 1). mAbs, 1, 382-384.

Mellstedt, H., Frodin, J.E., Massucci, G. (1989). Clinical status of monoclonal antibodies in the treatment of colorectal carcinoma. Oncology, 3, 25-31.

Michael, L.L., David, G.M., Irwin, D.B.(2002). Antibody-directed therapies for hematological malignancies. Trends in Molecular Med, Feb 8(2), 69-76.

Morrison, S.L., Johnson, M.J., Herzenberg, L.A., Oi, V.T. (1984). Chimeric human antibody molecules: mouse antigen-binding domains with human constant region domains. Proc Natl Acad Sci, 81, 6851–6855.

Nadler, L.M., Stashenko, P., Hardy, R., Kaplan, W.D., Button, L.N., Kufe, D.W., Antman, K.H., Schlossman, S.F.(1980). Serotherapy of a patient with a monoclonal antibody directed against a human lymphoma-associated antigen. Cancer Res, 40, 3147-3154.

Reilly, R.M., Sandhu, J., Alvarez-Diez, T.M. et al. (1995). Problems of delivery of monoclonal antibodies: Pharmaceutical and pharmacokinetic solutions. Clin Pharmacokinet, 28, 126-142.

Roovers, R.C., Laeremans, T., Huang, L., De Taeye, S., Verkleij, A.J., Revets, H., De Haard, H.J., Van Bergen en, H.P.M.P. (2007). Efficient inhibition of EGFR signaling and of tumor growth by antagonistic anti-EGFR nanobodies. Cancer Immunol Immunother, 56, 303-317.

Sumit, G., Wei, W., Tsutomu, A., Satoshi, O. (2013). Developments and Challenges for mAb-based therapeutics. Antibodies, 2, 452-500.

Susan, D.J., Francisco, J.C., Howard, L. (2007). Advances in the development of therapeutic monoclonal antibodies. BioPharm International, Oct. 96-114.

Theresa, M.A. (2002). Ligand-targeted therapeutics in anticancer therapy. Nature Reviews, Oct 2, 750-763.

Tsuguo, K., Rinpei, N., Mitsuo, S., Shiro, A., Kenya, S., Nobuo, H. (2009). Engineered therapeutic antibodies with improved effector functions. Cancer Sci, 100(9), 1566-1572.

Retargeting of Viruses to Generate Oncolytic Agents: Transductional Targeting Strategies and Challenges

Monique H. Verheije
Pathology Division, Department of Pathobiology
Faculty of Veterinary Medicine
Utrecht University, Utrecht, The Netherlands

Peter J.M. Rottier
Virology Division, Department of Infectious Diseases & Immunology
Faculty of Veterinary Medicine
Utrecht University Utrecht, The Netherlands

1   Cancer and Oncolytic Viruses

Cancer is one of the major health problems of our times. Though the prognosis for people diagnosed with, at least some forms of, cancer has increased considerably, it is more typical a disease of which treatment is initially effective, but which is often followed later by an irreversible and eventually fatal relapse. Already for decades cancer treatment is based on three types of approaches: surgery, radio- and chemotherapy. While the scientific and technological advancements have improved the efficacy of each of these classical approaches tremendously, and while also some new therapies have evolved including immunotherapy, the treatments apparently fail to eradicate all residual tumor cells or metastases completely. Therefore, additional means are urgently required to support or replace the conventional therapies. Hence a variety of new approaches is being explored one of which is based on the use of viruses.

The potential of viruses to reduce tumor burden was already noted more than a century ago (for a historical review on viruses as agents for tumor destruction, see (Kelly & Russell, 2007)). Cancer patients who accidently contracted an infectious disease showed brief periods of clinical remission, but it was not until the 1950s that researchers began to actively investigate the potential of viruses to cure cancer. By injecting virus preparations into patients they observed that, while most infections did not affect tumor growth and were likely cleared by the immune system, sometimes tumors regressed, especially in immunosuppressed patients (Southam, 1960). Despite the tremendous efforts in the 1950s and 1960s to make viruses more tumor-specific, successes were limited. The next era of oncolytic virus research basically started only in the 1990s, at the time when technological developments such as reverse genetics of viruses were coming of age. This enabled researchers to engineer viral genomes and to enhance their antitumor specificity in a more rational way. Nowadays, many different viruses are under investigation for their potential to specifically infect and kill tumor cells. Currently, already quite some genetically engineered viruses have reached phase I or II clinical trials (for an overview of current and recently completed clinical trials and targeted diseases see (Russell, Peng, & Bell, 2012; Zeyaullah *et al.*, 2012). So far, however, only one virus - a modified adenovirus H101 developed for the treatment of nasopharyngeal carcinoma - has been formally approved.

2   Tumor-Specific Targeting Strategies

Oncolytic viruses are replication competent viruses that are defined by their ability to specifically kill tumor cells while leaving the normal tissues unharmed. Their most characteristic features thus are their target specificity and their cytolytic capacity. Only very few viruses have a natural preference for replication in tumor cells. Some acquired such tropism by serial passage in culture cells; examples include measles virus, mumps virus and Newcastle disease virus (reviewed in (Lech & Russell, 2010)), vesicular stomatitis virus (Barber, 2004) and reovirus (Thirukkumaran & Morris, 2009). Most other viruses, however, need to be genetically modified to achieve tumor-specific infection.

Infection of cells by viruses depends on their successful entry and replication in these cells (a simplified scheme of the virus life cycle is shown in Figure 1). As a first step, virus binding to the cell relies on the specific interaction between the viral attachment protein(s) and the cellular receptor(s). Subsequently, the viral and cellular membranes fuse, upon which the viral genome is released into the cell. Depending on the nature of the virus, genome replication takes place in the nucleus or in the cytoplasm, to be followed by transcription and synthesis of the viral proteins. Successful viruses will ultimately encapsidate the viral genome and assemble their viral proteins in order to produce progeny virus, which can then spread and infect new target cells. During all steps of the viral life cycle, critical virus-host interactions are in play to determine the ultimate outcome of the infection. Though little is known yet about their nature and relevance, our understanding of virus-host interactions, particularly of oncolytic virus-host interactions, is rapidly increasing due to technological advances such as proteomics (Coiras *et al.*, 2008), as was recently reviewed in (Butt & Miggin, 2012). Ultimately, by exploiting cancer hallmarks (Hanahan & Weinberg, 2011) for one or more steps in the virus life cycle, researchers hope to provide oncolytic viruses with the so much needed tumor-specificity and cytolytic capacity.

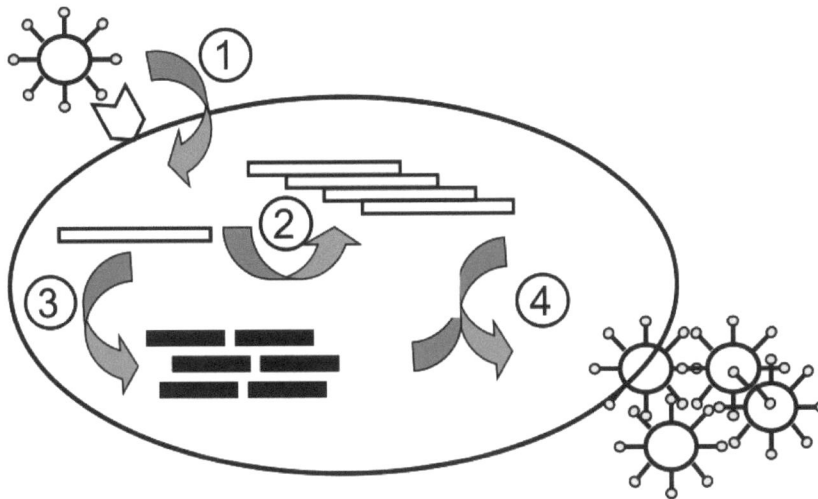

Figure 1: Schematic overview of the virus life cycle. A simplified overview of the virus life cycle, that is depicted in 4 steps: (-1-) virus binding to the host cell and entry; (-2-) replication of the viral genome; (-3-) transcription and translation in order to produce viral proteins; (-4-) assembly and release of progeny virus.

To achieve or enhance tumor-specific infection, several strategies can be employed to adapt the natural tropism of viruses. Up to date, four strategies can be distinguished. Below we first summarize each of these targeting strategies and, in the next section, we will provide a detailed overview of the most recent developments in transductional targeting currently employed to increase the tumor specificity of oncolytic viruses (as a review published in part in (Verheije & Rottier, 2012).

2.1   Transductional Targeting

For transductional targeting of viruses researchers make use of the differences in expression of cell surface antigens between normal and tumor cells. By enabling the specific binding of viruses to such tumor-specific or tumor-overexpressed antigens the virus can be specifically redirected towards the tumor cell (Figure 2A). This can be achieved by either changing a viral surface protein or by using so-called adapter proteins, which bridge the gap between the virus and the host cell. In addition it may be advantageous to selectively eliminate the undesirable tropism of the virus by ablating their binding to specific receptors

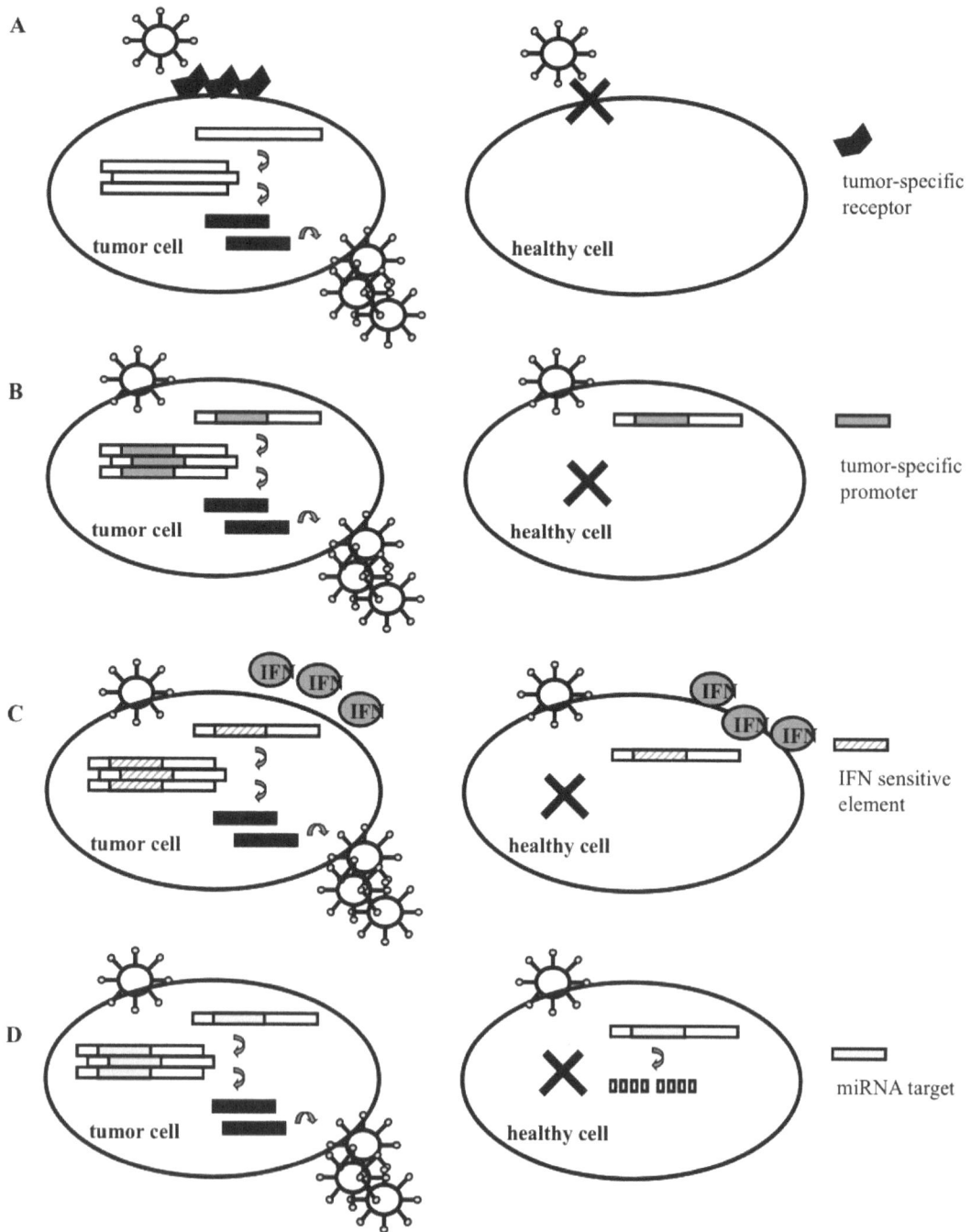

Figure 2: Schematic overview of the currently employed targeting strategies to achieve tumor specificity for oncolytic viruses. (A) Transductional targeting, based on the specific binding of the virus to specific or overexpressed cell membrane receptors on tumor cells; (B) Transcriptional targeting, based on cell specific transcription of an essential viral gene under control of a tissue- or tumor specific cellular promoter; (C) Physiological targeting, using the differences in innate immunity pathways between normal and tumor cells; (D) micro-RNA based targeting, focusing on tissue-specific degradation of the viral genome in healthy cells.

present on healthy tissue cells. As transductional targeting will be the focus of this book chapter, section 3 will provide a detailed overview of the currently applied targeting methods and will summarize all the viruses that are under investigation for oncolytic virus therapy.

2.2   Transcriptional/Translational Targeting

A second way to achieve tumor specificity is by transcriptional or translational targeting. For transcriptional targeting, which is only feasible for DNA viruses, the benefits of tissue- or tumor specific promoters are exploited. By placing an essential viral gene downstream of such cellular regulatory element in the viral genome, viral replication can be controlled (Figure 2B). Thus, progeny virus production will only be accomplished in cells expressing the selected promoter. Examples of promoters to control viral replication are the prostate-specific antigen (PSA) promoter, the first tissue-specific promoter used for oncolytic virus targeting (Rodriguez et al., 1997), and the human telomerase reversed transcriptase (hTERT) promoter (reviewed in (Ouellette, Wright, & Shay, 2011)). A detailed description of promoters, transcriptional targeting strategies and examples of oncolytic viruses targeted using this method is given in the recent overview by (Dorer & Nettelbeck, 2009). For RNA viruses, oncolytic virus specificity can be targeted by regulation of viral protein translation. Cellular IRES trans-acting factors can influence viral propagation in a cell type-specific manner; by placing either an IRES-dependent virus under the control of a tissue-specific element or by placing an essential viral gene under its control, viral protein translation and subsequent virus production can be regulated.

2.3   Physiological Targeting

A third strategy to increase tumor specificity exploits cancer cell defects and mainly targets the often deficient antiviral responses of tumor cells (Heiber & Barber, 2012). The approach is called physiological targeting, but is also referred to as viral gene inactivation or pro-apoptotic targeting. The most prominent example of physiological targeting exploits the interferon (IFN) signal transduction pathway (Figure 2C). Infected healthy cells often produce IFN leading to an antiviral state of neighboring cells, while tumor cells often have defects in IFN signaling pathways resulting in the lack of a proper innate immune response against the virus. Many viruses, on the other hand, have evolved strategies to counteract the inhibitory effects of innate immunity molecules likes IFN on their replication. By genetic engineering of the viral genome such that immunomodulatory proteins are abolished, one can generate a virus that is vulnerable to antiviral responses in normal cells, but accomplishes replication and virus dissemination in tumor cells. Another option to exploit the defective antiviral defense of tumor cells is pro-apoptotic targeting. Upon infection normal cells usually undergo apoptosis, thereby limiting virus propagation. Again, most viruses have strategies to combat this effect, but by engineering the viral genome in such a way that counteracting proteins are abolished, replication will be ensured in tumor cells, but aborted in normal cells. A recent overview of oncolytic viruses exploiting tumor specific defects in innate immune signaling pathways is given in (Naik & Russell, 2009).

2.4   Micro-RNA Targeting

Finally, the most recent oncolytic virus targeting strategy focuses on the differential expression of microRNAs (miRNAs) in normal and tumor cells. MiRNAs manipulate the expression of genes by interacting with complementary target sequences in cellular messenger RNAs, reducing their translation or initiating their destruction. By incorporating miRNA target sequences corresponding to sequences of tissue-specific cellular messenger RNAs into the viral genome, tumor-specific regulation of viral replication can be achieved (Figure 2D). This strategy is used to selectively eliminate the undesirable viral tropism by preventing its replication in normal tissues. Of particular interest in this respect is the possibility to ablate the viral tropism for liver cells, as systemic delivery of viruses *in vivo* often results in sequestration of the virus in this organ. An overview of the current field using miRNA targeting of oncolytic viruses is given in (Bell & Kirn, 2008; Russell *et al.*, 2012; Sakurai, Katayama, & Mizuguchi, 2011).

3   Transductional Targeting Strategies

This section will specifically focus on the three strategies for transductional retargeting of viruses that seem most promising for the development of new oncolytic viruses. The first part (3.1) will review the strategy through which viruses could be successfully provided new tropism by introducing targeting information into one of the viral surface proteins. As this strategy has been investigated most actively we will limit the overview of the examples to those viruses in which the new targeting specificity could be genomically encoded. In the second part (3.2) approaches are described by which scaffold-based modifications of viral surface proteins were applied to direct virions to new target cells, including the use of biotin or antibody-binding moieties. The third part (3.3) will review the use of bispecific adapter proteins as mediators of binding virions to tumor cells. Most often such adapters were simply combined with the respective viruses thereby enabling single-round infection. In some cases these targeting devices were incorporated genetically into the virus so as to generate self-targeted agents able to independently spread through a tumor.

3.1   Modification of Viral Surface Proteins

The most popular approach to generate oncolytic viruses has been by adapting their surface-exposed components. Viral surface proteins can be modified to express ligands that bind to receptors preferentially or exclusively expressed on tumor cells. Viruses can be genetically adapted to express those modifications to redirect them towards tumor cells (Figure 3A and 3B). The main advantage of this strategy is that the targeting specificity is inherent to the viral genome and will thus be maintained upon replication. Progeny virus is then able to infect neighboring cells harboring the target receptor, thereby establishing a multi-round infection that will be maintained until no further tumor target cells remain. For this strategy the ability to genetically modify the viral genome is crucial. Furthermore, detailed structural information about the viral surface protein to be modified is indispensible to predict at which location targeting motifs might be tolerated and will be exposed. Such motifs should not only allow binding of the modified virion to the cells, but should also not be detrimental to the entry mechanism of the particular virus, not interfering for instance with the fusion of viral and cellular membrane. In addition, the targeting ligand introduced into the viral protein will have to meet size limitations. Small peptides thus seem the first and most obvious choice. The development of targeting strategies of viruses is, however, severely limited by a shortage of naturally existing molecules available for use as targeting ligands. Therefore, other sources of binding ligands have been investigated and incorporated into viral proteins for this purpose. These include (parts of) antibodies, like scFvs (single chain variable fragments, composed of a fusion of the variable regions of the heavy (V_H) and light chains (V_L) of an immunoglobulin) or Fabs (antigen binding fragments, composed of one constant and one variable domain from each heavy and light chain of the antibody). The feasibility of modifying viral coat proteins has been demonstrated for a number of viruses as is summarized below.

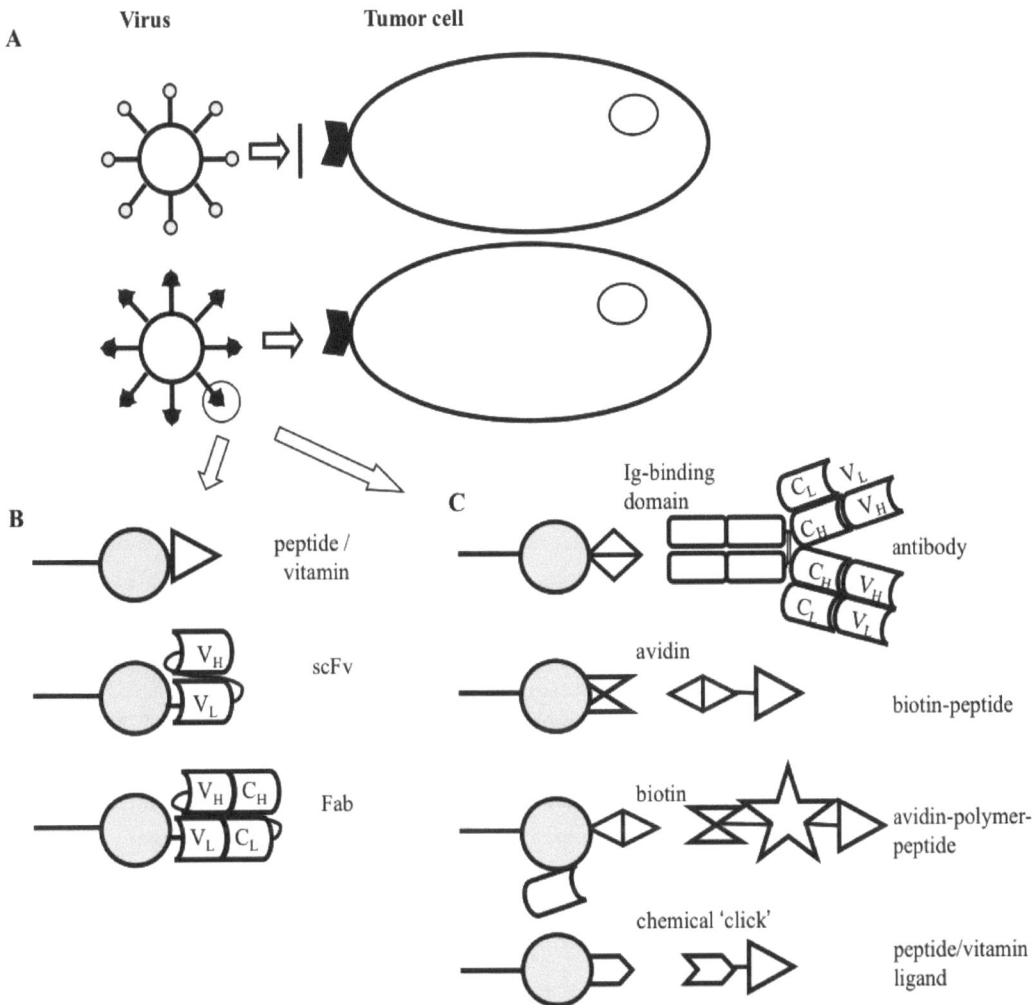

Figure 3: Transductional targeting through modification of viral surface proteins. (A) Principle of redirecting viruses by insertion of tumor-specific ligands into the viral coat: without modification of viral surface protein (upper part) no infection; (B) Schematic representation of a viral surface protein (represented by the grey-filled circle) on which tumor-binding peptides or antibodies are exposed. Ligands can be introduced at the N- or C-terminus of the protein or internally, provided that the correct folding of the viral protein and its accessibility for binding to the cell surface receptor are maintained; (C) Schematic representation of a viral surface protein on which a scaffold is exposed. The targeting ligand, examples of which are shown schematically, is then provided as a separate entity, binding on the one hand to the virion and on the other hand to the cell surface receptor of choice.

3.1.1   Adenoviruses

Adenoviruses are among the most extensively studied viruses for oncolytic viral therapy. In a wild-type infection, adenovirus binding to the cells is mediated by its major attachment factor, the fiber protein. Via its carboxy terminal knob domain this protein binds to the primary cellular receptor coxsackie/adenovirus receptor (CAR). Following viral attachment, internalization is mediated through interaction of RGD motifs in the penton base with cellular α_v integrins. In order to achieve CAR-independent infection by adenoviruses, the viral tropism can be modified via genetic engineering of adenovirus capsid proteins.

The list of reviews describing the development of genetically redirected adenoviruses through incorporation of ligands into viral surface proteins is numerous. In summary, heterologous peptide ligands have been successfully engineered into many adenoviral proteins, including the HI loop of the fiber, the C terminus of the fiber, the L1 loop in the hexon, the RGD loop in the penton base and in the minor capsid protein IX. Most commonly, targeting moieties are inserted in the HI loop of the fiber knob. For this protein, the importance of the insertion site of the ligand was demonstrated when introducing a model peptide CDCRGDCFC into the knob (Hesse, Kosmides, Kontermann, & Nettelbeck, 2007). Insertion of the ligand into three of five analyzed loops of the knob still allowed trimerization of the knob protein, and the resulting adenoviruses showed superior infectivity to that of viruses with the same peptide fused to the fiber C terminus. That the precise ligand positioning is pivotal was further demonstrated by the lack of enhancement of infectivity when the ligand-flanking linkers were extended and when tandem copies of the ligand peptide were inserted (Rein *et al.*, 2004). Targeted infection of tumor cells by adenoviruses can be further augmented by introduction of a cathepsin-cleavage site between the viral protein anchor and the ligand to increase the release from the receptor in the endosome (de Vrij *et al.*, 2011). Interestingly, also antibody-based targeting could be achieved for adenoviruses by generating fiber chimeras (Belousova, Mikheeva, Gelovani, & Krasnykh, 2008) or fusions of scFvs with the capsid protein IX *(Poulin et al.,* 2010). For the most recent reviews on transductionally targeted adenoviruses the reader is referred to (Coughlan *et al.*, 2010; Doronin & Shayakhmetov, 2012; Glasgow, Everts, & Curiel, 2006; Hall, Blair Zajdel, & Blair, 2010; Mathis, Stoff-Khalili, & Curiel, 2005; Waehler, Russell, & Curiel, 2007). For adenoviruses, the possibility to combine transductional with transcriptional targeting to increase adenoviral specificity makes this group of viruses particularly interesting for future therapy; however, their strong immunogenic nature might seriously hamper their efficacy *in vivo*.

3.1.2   Paramyxoviruses: Measles Virus

The measles virus is another virus well studied for oncolytic therapy, as the attenuated measles virus strain Edmonston has the ability to selectively destroy neoplastic tissue (reviewed in (Nakamura & Russell, 2004)). Measles virus has two envelope glycoproteins, the hemagglutinin (H) attachment protein and the fusion (F) protein. Virus attachment, entry and subsequent cell-cell fusion are mediated via the two measles receptors, CD46 and the signaling lymphocyte activation molecule (SLAM).

To improve the specificity of the infection, tumor-specific ligands have been introduced as C-terminal extensions of the H protein. A range of ligands including both peptides and scFvs were tolerated and, in addition, allowed the redirection of the virus to cells expressing the appropriate virus receptor. Again, the nature of the ligands was pivotal. Thus, though the length of the linkers separating the V_H and V_L domains was not of importance for scFvs to be incorporated into virions, it certainly affected the membrane fusion ability of the virus (Hammond *et al.*, 2001). For reviews on redirected measles virus, see (Blechacz & Russell, 2008; Galanis, 2010; Nakamura & Russell, 2004; Russell & Peng, 2009). As the

Edmonston strain has been used for vaccination for over 50 years now, its safety profile is impressive and might provide a good basis for future application in oncolytic therapy.

3.1.3   Herpesviruses: Herpes Simplex Virus (HSV)

Another field of active study involves the use of herpes simplex virus for tumor therapy (reviewed in (Campadelli-Fiume *et al.*, 2011; Shah & Breakefield, 2006)). Herpesvirus infects cells by attachment to heparan sulfate proteoglycans, mediated by the viral glycoproteins gC and gB, followed by interaction of the glycoprotein gD with one of two alternative protein receptors. One, designated herpesvirus entry- mediator, is a member of the family of tumor necrosis factors receptors. The second involves nectin1 and nectin2, both intercellular adhesion molecules belonging to the immunoglobulin (Ig) superfamily.

Retargeting of HSV could be achieved by insertion of ligands and scFvs into the gC and/ or the gD protein, with subsequent increased infectivity of target cells expressing the appropriate virus receptor. The current strategies to redirect HSV towards tumor cells have recently been reviewed (Campadelli-Fiume *et al.*, 2011; Manservigi, Argnani, & Marconi, 2010). For another herpesvirus, the gammaherpes virus saimiri, the native binding region of the viral glycoprotein ORF51 to heparan sulphate was replaced by that of a peptide sequence interacting with somatostatin receptors, known to be overexpressed on hepatocellular carcinoma cells. The subsequent recombinant virus appeared to infect the carcinoma cells as well as the wild type virus, while showing reduced infectivity for other cell lines. The reason for these observations is unclear (Turrell & Whitehouse, 2011). In conclusion, herpesviruses remain promising as candidates for oncolytic therapy as they can be redirected to tumor cells and are considered reasonably safe due to the induction of a self-limited disease in humans. On the other hand, their wide natural tropism and the presence of viral antibodies in the human population might hamper their effectiveness *in vivo*.

3.1.4   Parvoviruses: Adeno-Associated Virus (AAV) and Rat Parvovirus (H-1PV)

A less frequently studied candidate for development as oncolytic agent is AAV (reviewed in (K. Park *et al.*, 2008)). AAV has a broad host cell range due to the widespread distribution of its primary cellular receptor heparan sulfate proteoglycan. The viral capsid protein is responsible for the interaction with this host cell receptor.

Transductional targeting independent of the native tropism could be demonstrated by genetically incorporating the 14-amino-acid targeting peptide L14 (Girod *et al.*, 1999) into six different putative loops of the AAV2 capsid protein. The results showed that all mutant capsids were efficiently incorporated, that three mutants expressed L14 on the capsid surface, but that only one of these efficiently infected wild-type AAV2-resistant cell lines that expressed the integrin receptor recognized by L14. The importance of the incorporation site, the peptide sequence and the peptide length was further elucidated in other studies, showing that the assembly, the generation of infectious particles and the ability to transduce target cells depend both on the position in the capsid, the ligand introduced and the length of the targeting peptide (Grifman *et al.*, 2001; Naumer *et al.*, 2012; Shi, Arnold, & Bartlett, 2001). Successful targeting was demonstrated towards RGD (Shi & Bartlett, 2003) and towards the human luteinizing hormone receptor (Shi *et al.*, 2001). Recently it has been observed that target cell binding of AAV vectors displaying ligands in their viral capsid is just one factor determining the transduction of target cells; entry and post entry steps, including endocytosis and intracellular processing also appear to significantly affect the ultimate outcome of the transduction (Raupp *et al.*, 2012).

Recently, also a non-human parvovirus, H-1PV, was genetically engineered to explore its anti-tumor capacities. Amino acids of the capsid protein involved in native cell membrane binding and entry were removed while a cyclic RGD-4C peptide was inserted to allow specific infection of target cells. Indeed, viral infectivity could be rescued as observed by the infection of cells overexpressing αvβ5 integrins and efficient killing of these cells by the recombinant virus was achieved (Allaume *et al.*, 2012).

3.1.5   Retroviruses: Murine Leukemia Virus (MuLV)

Replication-competent retroviruses have gained interest as oncolytic agents, in particular because of their high transduction efficiency (reviewed in (Dalba, Klatzmann, Logg, & Kasahara, 2005; Tai & Kasahara, 2008)). Of MuLV different classes can be distinguished, of which the host range is based on the interaction between the envelope glycoprotein and a particular cell surface receptor. While the ecotropic MuLVs are particularly capable of infecting mouse and rat cells, amphotropic MuLV infects a range of mammalian, including human cells via the widely expressed Pit-2 receptor.

Initial studies to redirect ecotropic MuLV towards human tumor cells pointed towards the importance of the interaction between the envelope glycoprotein and its original virus receptor. Despite the correct folding of chimeric envelope glycoproteins displaying scFvs, their incorporation into viral particles, and the binding of pseudotyped virus particles carrying chimeric ecotropic Env to human cells, the resulting viruses were not infectious for the targeted cells (reviewed in (Russell & Cosset, 1999)). When expanding these studies using amphotropic MuLV, targeted infection could be achieved only when incorporating the high molecular weight melanoma associated antigen (HMWMAA), while targeting towards the EGF (Erlwein, Wels, & Schnierle, 2002), IGF (Chadwick, Morling, Cosset, & Russell, 1999) and folate (Pizzato *et al.*, 2001) receptors was unsuccessful, despite the observed binding to cells expressing those receptors. It was proposed that trafficking of the virus particles to lysosomes and subsequent degradation caused the lack of infectivity, but attempts to overcome this problem by inserting a translocation domain of exotoxin A of Pseudomonas aeruginosa into the envelope protein - in order to enhance the translocation of the virion from endosomes to the cytoplasm - were unsuccessful (Erlwein *et al.*, 2002). Recently it was demonstrated using pseudovirions of MuLV that the ligand insertion site is crucial for allowing the conformational changes needed to complete membrane fusion and targeted transduction (F. Li, Ryu, Krueger, Heldt, & Albritton, 2012). While this might open up new possibilities for successful targeting of retrovirus vectors towards tumor cells, clearly, the choice of receptor will be of ultimate importance.

3.1.6   Poxviruses: Vaccinia Virus

Vaccinia virus has been studied for its anti-tumor properties already for a long time. Despite its entry into a wide range of cells, for several vaccinia virus strains a natural preference for replication in cancer tissue has been reported. While the identity of the natural receptor is still under debate, it likely involves a widely expressed surface component, like heparan sulfate or chondroitin sulfate proteoglycans. Tumor targeting can be improved by deleting vaccinia virus genes that are necessary for replication in normal cells but not in cancer cells (recently reviewed in (Guse, Cerullo, & Hemminki, 2011)).

To increase the specificity of their tropism, tumor-specific scFvs have been displayed on the surface of vaccinia virus particles. Targeting moieties were introduced by fusing a scFv directed against the tumor-associated antigen ErbB2 to the N-terminus of the non-essential hemagglutinin HA protein in vaccinia virus strain IHD-J (Galmiche, Rindisbacher, Wels, Wittek, & Buchegger, 1997). Similarly, the non-essential p14 membrane-associated protein of vaccinia strain MVA could be replaced by a p14 fusion molecule carrying an inserted scFv directed against the tumor associated antigen MUC-1 (Paul *et al.*, 2007). The resulting fusion proteins could be expressed, were exposed on the envelope of the recombinant virus, and were able to bind the target cells. No preferential infection of the target cells was, however, observed, likely because the recombinant viruses still contained wild-type host cell attachment proteins, providing the infection with a broad cell range. Therefore, the future challenge for the transductional targeting of vaccinia virus towards tumor cells will lie in the elimination of its natural tropism.

3.1.7   Coronaviruses: Mouse Hepatitis Virus (MHV)

The favorable characteristics of - particularly the non-human - coronaviruses as potential oncolytic agents have been recognized only recently. In these viruses the spike (S) protein is responsible for receptor binding and subsequent cell entry through virus-cell membrane fusion. The amino-terminal S1 domain is required for virus binding to the cells and, while undergoing ordered structural changes, the S2 domain mediates fusion with the cell membrane. Infection of cells by coronaviruses depends on the expression of specific cellular receptors, which makes these viruses highly species-specific. For example, entry by MHV is mediated by the murine carcino-embryonic antigen (CEACAM1a) receptor.

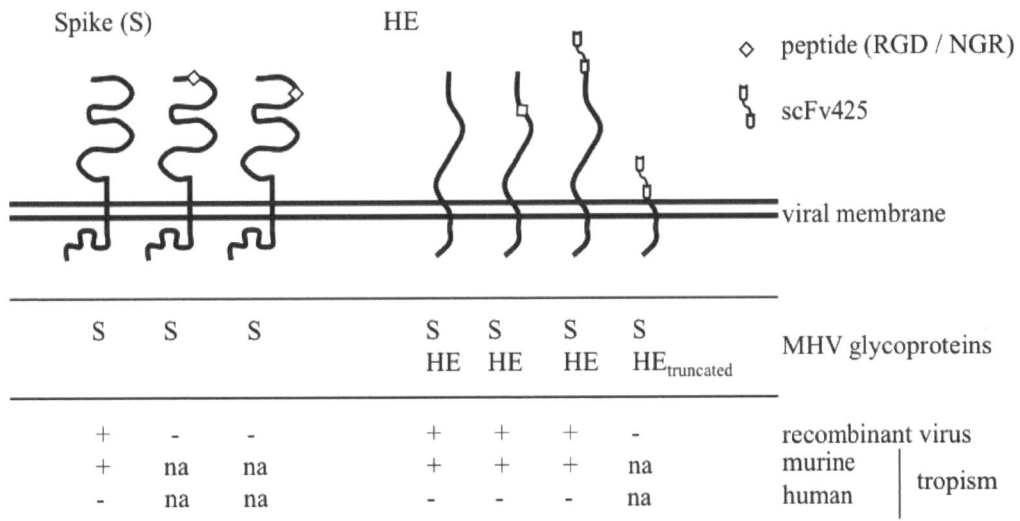

Figure 4: Modification of viral surface proteins for redirecting coronavirus to tumor cells. Schematic representation of MHV surface glycoproteins spike (S) and hemagglutinin-esterase (HE) and of modifications applied to redirect the virus to novel target cell antigens. Modifications tested include: insertion of small peptide ligands, including RGD and NGR, and extension with the anti-EGFR scFv425. Recombinant MHV viruses encoding such mutated S proteins or modified HE proteins (in the presence of wild type spike proteins) were generated by targeted recombination (Kuo *et al.*, 2000). Indicated is whether the intended recombinant viruses could actually be isolated (confirmed by RT-PCR and sequencing). Also indicated is the tropism of each successfully generated recombinant virus for murine and for human cells (Verheije and Rottier, unpublished data).

Attempts to redirect coronaviruses, in particular MHV, by mutation of the viral surface proteins were unsuccessful. Incorporation of ligands, such as RGD and NGR, into various non-conserved domains in the S1 domain of the spike protein appeared to be not tolerated, as selection of retargeted recombinant viruses based on the new binding properties of the modified spike was not successful (Figure 4; Verheije and Rottier, unpublished data). Obviously, without much knowledge of the tertiary structure of the coronavirus spike protein and of its conformational changes during cell entry, chances are high that the introduction of even small ligands affects its proper functioning. Some MHV strains carry an accessory hemagglutinin-esterase (HE) surface glycoprotein. Attempts to also use this glycoprotein for retargeting were equally unsuccessful. Though some HE gene modifications, such as insertions of small peptide ligands and terminal extensions with the anti-EGFR scFv425, could be incorporated into the viral genome, the resulting recombinant viruses were unable to redirect MHV to human tumor cells (Figure 4; Verheije and Rottier, unpublished data).

3.2   Introduction of Scaffolds into Viral Surface Proteins

Rather than incorporating specific tumor targeting information into a viral surface protein, an alternative approach involves the incorporation of a scaffold moiety into such a protein to which subsequently various types of targeting modules can be linked (schematically depicted in Figure 3A). The main strategic difference relative to the previous method is that the moiety incorporated is not a tumor ligand itself, but represents an attachment site for exogenously provided targeting moieties that, besides to the scaffold, also bind to the receptor of interest (compare Figure 3B and Figure 3C). An essential operational limitation is that this targeting strategy provides viruses that can only establish single-round infection, hence remaining dependent on the external supply of the targeting module. Yet, it has the advantage of flexibility as the targeting device, binding always to the same, previously modified viral protein, can be changed relatively easy. Some of these strategies are based on antibody targeting, giving the opportunity to redirect the oncolytic virus to virtually every tumor surface epitope. A particular application based on this principle relies on the biotin-(strept)avidin coupling method (reviewed in (Lesch, Kaikkonen, Pikkarainen, & Yla-Herttuala, 2010)).

3.2.1   Adenoviruses

For adenoviruses, single-round targeted virus particles could be generated by using the biotin-streptavidin coupling system. After incorporating a biotin-acceptor peptide into the fiber, metabolically biotinylated adenovirus was coupled to an EGF-streptavidin complex and found to successfully infect EGFR expressing target cells (Pereboeva, Komarova, Roth, Ponnazhagan, & Curiel, 2007). Similarly, a biotin-polyethylene glycol (PEG)-EGF conjugate coupled to an avidin-modified adenovirus could redirect the virus to a non-native receptor (J. W. Park, Mok, & Park, 2008). In another study, small protein ligands capable of selective binding to human IgG and IgA were incorporated as model ligands for tropism-modified adenoviruses. Viable viruses that had genetically incorporated scaffolds into their fiber gene could be rescued and were, after incubation with antibodies, able to enter cells displaying the Fc receptor on their surface (Henning et al., 2002). Recently, it was demonstrated that specific chemoselective modification of the adenoviral particle could also function as a scaffold for targeting devices. By metabolic incorporation of non-canonical monosaccharides and amino acids in adenoviral particles conjugation with a folate targeting motive in combination with a taxoid was achieved. Initial results demonstrated increased toxicity *in vitro* (Banerjee, Zuniga, Ojima, & Carrico, 2011).

3.2.2   Parvoviruses: Adeno-associated virus (AAV)

The Ig-binding fragment of protein A was tested as a possible scaffold to redirect AAV. The fragment was successfully introduced into the capsid protein providing a versatile platform for antibody-mediated AAV targeting (Gigout *et al.*, 2005). In a more recent study a biotin-acceptor peptide was incorporated into AAV particles. Subsequent biotin-labeling of the viruses with the biotin ligase BirA and attachment of an RGD peptide to target integrins resulted in a significant increase in the transduction of endothelial cells, demonstrating again the feasibility of this approach (Stachler, Chen, Ting, & Bartlett, 2008).

3.2.3   Togaviruses: Sindbis Virus (SV)

Sindbis virus has inherent oncolytic properties and has been studied quite extensively as an oncolytic virus (reviewed in (Quetglas *et al.*, 2010)). One of the surface proteins on mammalian cells to mediate the Sindbis virus infection is the laminin receptor, which is overexpressed on various human tumors. The envelope protein E2 of Sindbis virus is responsible for receptor-binding.

To increase the specificity of the infection, researchers combined the introduction of ligands into the viral envelope with the use of targeting molecules. To this end, virus particles were generated which contained the IgG-binding domain of protein A inserted into their envelope protein E2. When combined with antibodies that bound to specific surface antigens on non-susceptible cells the chimeric virus was able to infect these otherwise refractory cells (Ohno, Sawai, Iijima, Levin, & Meruelo, 1997). A comparable combination approach was taken by introducing Ig-binding domains as N-terminal extensions of the E2 glycoprotein. After adding species-matched antibodies, Fc receptor-positive cell lines could be successfully infected (Klimstra, Williams, Ryman, & Heidner, 2005).

3.2.4   Retroviruses: Murine Leukemia Virus (MLV)

Also for MLV studies were performed to introduce the IgG-binding domain of protein A to enable modular use of antibodies of various specificities for vector targeting. By inserting this binding domain into the hinge region of the viral envelope protein virions were generated that were capable of capturing anti-ErbB2 antibodies. Subsequent efficient binding of the virus-antibody complex to ErbB2-positive target cells and enhancement of transduction of these cells was observed (Tai *et al.*, 2003).

3.2.5   Poxviruses: Vaccinia Virus

Biotin-avidin-biotin linkers have been used successfully to redirect vaccinia virus to target cells. In particular, a biotinylated vaccinia viral vector was cross-linked using avidin to biotinylated antibodies. In this way, the virus could infect murine cells artificially expressing a murine class I MHC molecule or a co-stimulatory molecule for T-cells. Interestingly, addition of the targeting coat also diminished the infectivity of the modified vaccinia virus for control cells (Purow & Staveley-O'Carroll, 2005).

4   Transductional Targeting of Viruses using Bispecific Adapters

An elegant strategy currently employed to target viruses towards tumor cells makes use of bispecific adapters. Such proteins consist of two domains ('arms'), one binding to the virion, the other to a cell surface epitope of interest, thereby enabling indirect interaction of virus and tumor cell. The composition of the adapter proteins can vary greatly, depending on the design of the arms. The virus binding domains that have been used include soluble receptor fragments (so-called pseudoreceptors), polymers like PEG, (parts of) antibodies, including scFvs or Fabs. Moieties that have been applied for cell-binding are natural peptide or vitamin ligands for receptors, and again scFvs or Fabs directed against a cell epitope of interest. The specificity for two different antigens is achieved either by joining the arms together chemically or by combining the two moieties in one fusion protein, often with a flexible linker, the targeting arm typically being at the C-terminus. The principle of redirecting viruses towards non-native cells using bispecific proteins is shown in Figure 5A, with typical examples of the two domains being depicted in Figure 5B. In Table 1 an overview is provided of combinations of arms in bispecific adapter proteins actually generated to target viruses to tumor cells.

The use of adapters to redirect viruses towards tumor cells has several advantages over the introduction of targeting or scaffold moieties into viral attachment proteins. First, no detailed structural information is required about the viral surface proteins, as manipulation of these proteins is not required. Second, as the size of the targeting part of the adapter protein seems less crucial than when introducing this moiety into a viral protein, the choice of targets can easily be expanded by using (parts of) antibodies. In this way, the selection of targeting receptors becomes virtually unlimited, as antibodies can be generated relatively easy, once the receptor of interest has been identified. Third, as adapter proteins are straightforward to construct, expanding the repertoire of target receptors becomes fairly simple. Finally, the binding of adapter proteins to the virion has, at least in some cases, been reported to ablate the virus' natural tropism, which is especially useful when the oncolytic virus of choice has a preference for normal cells in the host.

There are also disadvantages of using bispecific proteins in targeting oncolytic viruses. As bispecific proteins are artificial polypeptides composed of parts that do not occur linked together naturally, their proper biogenesis with independent folding of both moieties and efficient secretion may be impaired. Moreover, unless expressed by the oncolytic virus itself, production and purification of the adaptors may be a challenge.

To redirect oncolytic viruses towards tumor cells, bispecific proteins can be applied in two ways. First, after recombinant production or chemical synthesis the proteins can be precomplexed with virions before applying them *in vitro* or *in vivo*. A major drawback of this approach is, however, that it allows single-round infection only; progeny virus will not be able to infect neighboring cells as the amount of adapter protein will be limiting. Consequently, the use of such adapter-precomplexed viruses *in vivo* is likely to be restricted to local, rather than systemic application. It will probably also require repeated administration of high doses of the adapter proteins. Little is known about the potential risks of such approach.

As an alternative, the genetic information for the adapter protein can be incorporated into the viral genome. When properly expressed, this ensures the local production of the targeting device together with the progeny virus in the infected cell. This approach will enable multi-round infection and lateral spread of the oncolytic virus. The time span and, hence, the efficacy of this kind of therapy will be limited by the emergence of immunity against the bispecific protein and/or the virus. The feasibility of this strategy depends on the availability of a genetic modification system to introduce the adapter-encoding gene into the viral genome as an additional expression cassette. While such modification systems are currently available for most viruses, the capacity of the genome to accept such insertions can be limited; hence, the size of the targeting moiety might be restricted. Finally, the genetic stability of such recombinant viruses might be an issue, in particular when the adapter protein is used to ablate the natural tropism of the virus.

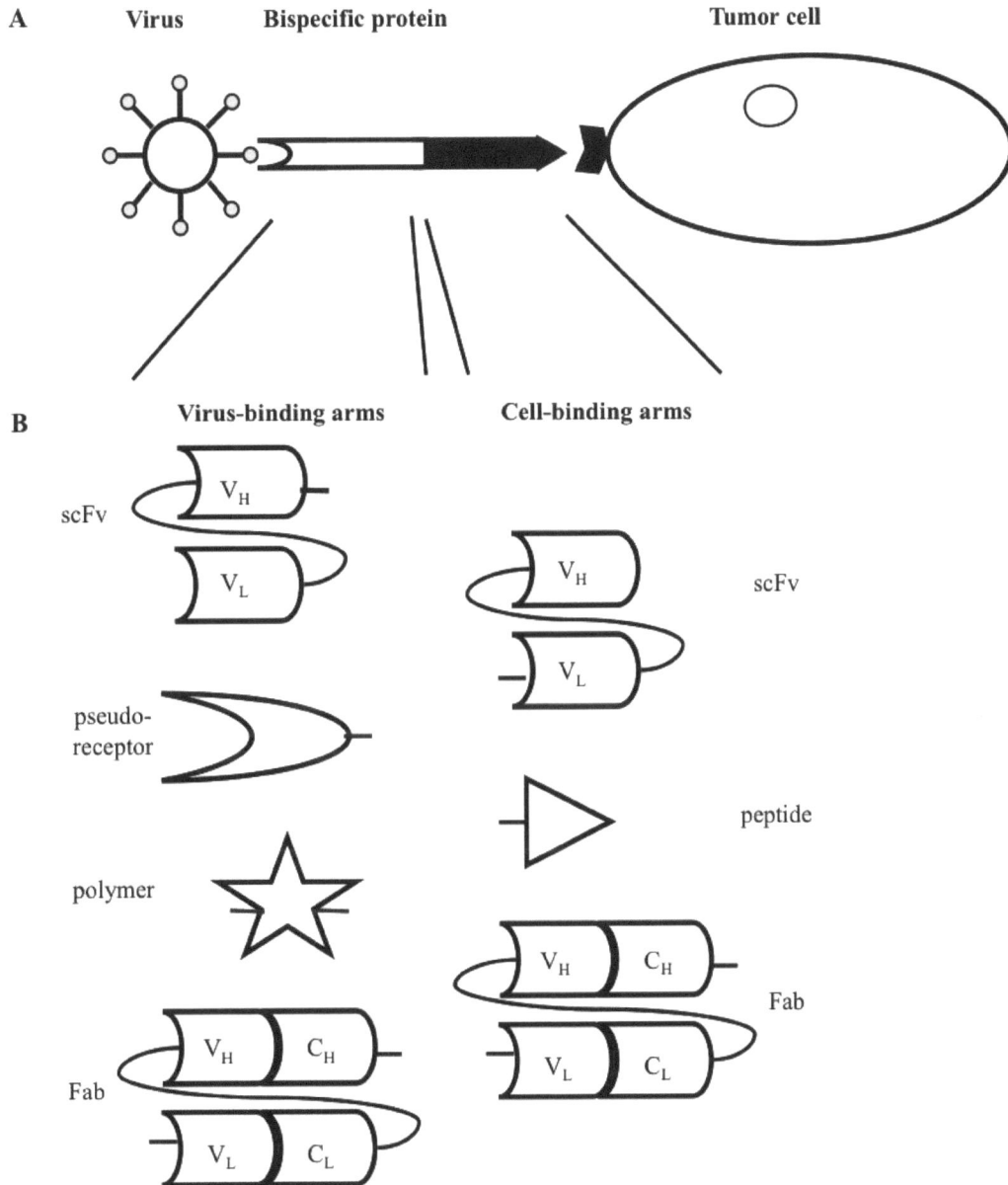

Figure 5: Bispecific adapter targeting principle and composition. (A) Principle of targeting viruses towards tumor cells using bispecific adapters; (B) Typical examples of virus-binding moieties (left) and cell-binding moieties (right) of bispecific adapters. In theory, all combinations of virus-binding and cell-binding arms are possible. An overview of the composition of the bispecific adapters used to target particular viruses to tumor cells is provided in Table 1.

The feasibility of using adapter proteins for oncolytic viral therapy has been explored for a number of viruses. Below we first present an overview of the studies in which targeting to tumor cells was performed by co-administration of viruses and adaptor proteins (4a). Thereafter we discuss the studies describing genetic targeting of oncolytic viruses generated by the incorporation of genes coding for bispecific proteins into the viral genome (4b).

Arm of the adapter protein binding to virion	Cell	Targeting demonstrated for
antibody (scFv or Fab)	antibody (scFv or Fab)	adenovirus adeno-associated virus coronavirus
antibody (scFv or Fab)	ligand peptide	adenovirus paramyxovirus
soluble receptor/ pseudoreceptor	antibody (scFv or Fab)	adenovirus herpesvirus coronavirus
soluble receptor/ pseudoreceptor	ligand peptide	adenovirus coronavirus
polymer	antibody (scFv or Fab)	adenovirus
polymer	ligand peptide	adenovirus

Table 1: Overview of the composition of bispecific adapters used to re-route viruses for oncolytic purposes

4.1   Single-Round Transductional Targeting using Bispecific Adapters

4.1.1   Adenoviruses

To redirect adenoviruses to tumor cells, virus-neutralizing anti-knob fiber antibodies have been used extensively. The first demonstration of their potential application for retargeting of these viruses to a non-adenovirus cellular receptor was in 1996, when such antibodies were chemically conjugated to folate and shown to mediate infection of folate-receptor expressing cells (Douglas *et al.*, 1996). Many non-native receptors have since been targeted by conjugating an anti-knob antibody fragment to either ligand peptides or antibody domains directed against a cellular receptor. This resulted in successful targeting towards the EGF receptor (EGFR) (Miller *et al.*, 1998; Watkins, Mesyanzhinov, Kurochkina, & Hawkins, 1997), FGF receptor (Goldman *et al.*, 1997; Gu *et al.*, 1999; Rogers *et al.*, 1997), integrins (Haisma *et al.*, 2010; Wickham *et al.*, 1996), EGP-2 (also known as EpCAM) (Haisma *et al.*, 1999; Heideman *et al.*, 2001), the melanoma-associated antigen HMWMAA receptor (Nettelbeck *et al.*, 2004), carbonic anhydrase IX protein G250 (Jongmans *et al.*, 2003), CD40 (Tillman *et al.*, 1999; Tillman, Hayes, DeGruijl, Douglas, & Curiel, 2000), various organ- and tumor homing peptide receptors (Trepel, Grifman, Weitzman, & Pasqualini, 2000), mesothelin MSLN (Breidenbach *et al.*, 2005), prostate-specific membrane antigen PSMA (Kraaij, van Rijswijk, Oomen, Haisma, & Bangma, 2005), (Haisma *et al.*, 2010), VEGFR2 (Haisma *et al.*, 2010), Ly-6D (van Zeeburg *et al.*, 2010) and Tie2 receptors (Haisma *et al.*, 2010).

Similar approaches have been explored using antibodies directed against other adenoviral proteins. Thus, Fabs directed against the penton base of the fiber in combination with targeting ligands, such as

EGF, IGF, and TNFα could mediate infection of target cells expressing the appropriate receptors (E. Li, Brown, Von Seggern, Brown, & Nemerow, 2000). Also Fabs directed against the hexon protein chemically linked to Fabs specifically binding to an antigen highly overexpressed on human hepatocellular carcinoma were successfully applied to redirect adenoviruses to a non-native receptor (Yoon *et al.*, 2000).

Another strategy successfully employed for the same purpose made use of pseudoreceptors. In this approach, bispecific proteins were generated by fusion of a soluble form of CAR (sCAR) to EGF (Dmitriev, Kashentseva, Rogers, Krasnykh, & Curiel, 2000; Wesseling *et al.*, 2001), to the Fc region of human IgG1 (Ebbinghaus *et al.*, 2001), and to scFvs against ErbB2 (Kashentseva, Seki, Curiel, & Dmitriev, 2002) and CEA (H. J. Li *et al.*, 2007).

In yet another approach polymers were exploited as targeting ligands in a single round fashion. Here, adenovirus particles were coated to inhibit their natural tropism after which ligands, including peptides and scFvs, were attached. Several types of polymers have been used (Bachtarzi *et al.*, 2011; Fisher *et al.*, 2007; Green *et al.*, 2008; Han *et al.*, 2010; Moselhy *et al.*, 2007; Stevenson *et al.*, 2007), including polyethylene and metacrylamide derivatives, to successfully target adenoviruses to FGF2 (Lanciotti *et al.*, 2003), RGD (Eto *et al.*, 2005), TNFα (Gao *et al.*, 2007) and the ErbB2 receptor (Jung *et al.*, 2007). It has been proposed that adenoviral coating with polymers might have enhanced potential for systemic delivery, as it prolongs the viral plasma half-live and reduces the hepatotoxicity *in vivo* (Gao *et al.*, 2007).

Another type of bispecific molecule based on the binding ability of the Gla domain of coagulation factor X to the hexon was subsequently exploited for targeting. Upon fusion of Gla to scFv proteins, increased infection of tumor cells by adenovirus could be observed. However, the anticipated reduction in liver transduction was not observed (Chen, May, & Barry, 2010).

As an alternative for antibodies recently ankyrin repeat proteins (DARPins) were investigated for their applicability to redirect adenovirus to alternative receptors. Target-specific DARPins against the Ad5 fiber and the human ErbB2 complexed with adenovirions were found to guide the virus to ErbB2 receptor-expressing cells, resulting in single round target-specific infection (Dreier *et al.*, 2011). DARPins can be generated against any target and might provide a versatile strategy for targeting towards a broad range of tumors. However, it is yet unknown whether such sequences are tolerated in the context of the viral genome.

Finally and interestingly, it has recently been observed that adenoviral vectors transductionally retargeted using bispecific adaptor molecules displayed an increase in transcription, rather than in transduction. In this case, reducing the non-target delivery by adding soluble fiber knob raised the number of transduced cells in the tumor and apparently improved the overall effectiveness of the approach (Hogg, Thorpe, & Gerard, 2011).

4.1.2   Adeno-Associated Viruses (AAV)

AAV has a broad host cell range due to the widespread distribution of its primary cellular receptor heparan sulfate proteoglycan. To achieve a more specific infection, a bispecific Fab was tested of which one arm recognized the cell-surface integrins αIIbβ3 while the other bound to the AAV capsid (Bartlett, Kleinschmidt, Boucher, & Samulski, 1999). Targeting this way did not inhibit downstream steps required for productive infection. Moreover, a decrease of infection of normally permissive cells was observed, indicating that the bispecific protein was able to ablate the normal tropism.

4.1.3   Herpesviruses: Herpes simplex virus (HSV)

HSV binding to the cell is mediated by several widely expressed cell surface receptors, including heparan sulfate, nectin1 and herpesvirus entry mediator (HVEM). HSV was successfully redirected to the EGFR by means of a soluble adapter protein comprising the N-terminal domain of nectin1 fused to a scFv directed against EGFR (Nakano *et al.*, 2005). Adapter-mediated entry was, however, promoted by the presence of heparan sulfate proteoglycans on cells, which are also required for wild type HSV infection. An alternative approach was taken by using an adapter consisting of the HSV gD-binding domain of HVEM linked to a scFv directed to the carcinoembryonic antigen (CEA), while detargeting the virus for recognition of nectin1 (Baek *et al.*, 2011). The targeted infection was demonstrated *in vitro* and *in vivo* by reduction of growth of gastric adenocarcinoma tumors in nude mice after repeated injection of virus.

4.1.4   Paramyxoviruses: Newcastle Disease virus (NDV)

In the avian paramyxovirus NDV the hemagglutinin-neuraminidase (HN) protein is responsible for sialic acid receptor attachment, while the F protein mediates the fusion of viral envelope and cellular membrane. NDV has oncolytic properties by nature, however, it has a broad cell tropism due to the widespread occurrence of sialic acids on many cells. To narrow its specificity the use of bispecific adapter proteins has been investigated. Preincubation of NDV with a recombinant bispecific protein composed of an scFv against HN that blocks the native receptor binding site and the interleukin-2 peptide clearly enhanced the specificity of the virus (Bian, Fournier, Moormann, Peeters, & Schirrmacher, 2005) and reduced its side-effects when applied systemically *in vivo* (Bian, Wilden, Fournier, Peeters, & Schirrmacher, 2006).

4.1.5   Coronaviruses: Mouse Hepatitis Coronavirus (MHV) and Feline Infectious Peritonitis Virus (FIPV)

The first demonstration of retargeting of coronaviruses was achieved by exchanging the viral spike ectodomains. Thus, felinized MHV (fMHV) (Haijema, Volders, & Rottier, 2003) and murinized FIPV (mFIPV) (Kuo, Godeke, Raamsman, Masters, & Rottier, 2000) were generated in which the murine viruses carried the feline S ectodomain and *vice versa*. These otherwise highly species-specific recombinant viruses were able to cross species barriers: fMHV had acquired feline cell tropism but completely lost its murine cell tropism while the opposite was true for mFIPV. To extend the species tropism of non-human coronaviruses towards human tumor cells, bispecific adapter proteins were generated. Proteins composed of a bispecific scFv directed against both the feline spike protein and the EGFR could mediate FIPV and fMHV infection of EGFR-expressing human cancer cells, with subsequent syncytia formation typical of a productive coronavirus infection (Wurdinger, Verheije, Raaben *et al.*, 2005).

Subsequent studies to redirect murine coronavirus MHV to human tumor cells were based on an adapter protein that consisted of a pseudoreceptor, composed of the N-terminal domain of murine CEA-CAM1a (soluble receptor; soR), fused to an scFv directed against the EGFR (Wurdinger, Verheije, Broen *et al.*, 2005) or to the EGF ligand (Verheije *et al.*, 2009). Again, such adapter proteins could mediate EGFR-specific entry of MHV into human cancer cells. However, in contrast to many of the previous examples, no ablation of the natural tropism of the virus was observed.

4.2   Multiple-round Transductional Targeting using Bispecific Adapters

To overcome the major drawback inherent to single-round targeting, a number of investigations focused on the expression of the bispecific adapters from the viral genome in order to allow the recombinant viruses to produce their own targeting device and sustain the infection. The feasibility of this approach has so far only been demonstrated for some adenoviruses and coronaviruses.

4.2.1   Adenoviruses

To redirect adenoviruses to non-native surface receptors, conditionally replicating adenoviruses (CRAds) seem to be the viruses of choice, due to their selective replication in tumor cells. The first experiments demonstrating the ability to redirect CRAds towards tumor cells were performed using dual-virus mixtures consisting of a CRAd and an adenovirus secreting a bispecific adapter protein consisting of a fusion between the soluble CAR receptor and the EGF ligand (Hemminki *et al.*, 2001). Dual virus infections resulted in increased oncolytic activity *in vitro* and improved therapeutic efficacy *in vivo*.

Subsequently, CRAds were engineered to express the bispecific adapter proteins by themselves. Van Beusechem *et al.* (van Beusechem *et al.*, 2003) developed such a CRAd encoding a bispecific protein composed of the anti-EGFR scFv 425 and anti-fiber knob scFv s11. The resulting virus AdΔ24-425S11 produced the bispecific protein 425-s11 during replication in cancer cells, yielding progeny virus with enhanced infectivity and oncolytic properties on EGFR-positive, CAR-deficient tumor cells. However, in addition to infection mediated by EGFR, the virus retained its capacity to infect cells through binding to the native receptors CAR and integrins. To abolish the native tropism, mutations were introduced that eliminated CAR- and integrin-binding (Carette *et al.*, 2007), resulting in a recombinant virus with a strictly EGFR-dependent targeting profile and reduced replication in EGFR-negative cells. Both viruses displayed similar oncolytic potency in cell lines and tissue specimens (Carette *et al.*, 2007). Also when applied in a mouse model by intrajugular or intramuscular injection, the native tropism of adenoviruses appeared to be reduced after removal of both the CAR and integrin binding sites (Einfeld *et al.*, 2001). Strikingly, however, when expressing the soluble CAR-EGF targeting moiety from a CRAd rather than from a dual virus system, its oncolytic potential was severely impaired (Hemminki *et al.*, 2003), suggesting that the expression of biologically active proteins can be counterproductive to virus replication.

To overcome the biosynthetic differences between the bispecific proteins -translated and secreted via the ER-Golgi route- and the adenovirus -with translation in the cytoplasm but assembly in the nucleus-, an elegant strategy was developed by tagging of the adenovirus fiber and the scFv each with a synthetic leucine zipper-like dimerization domain (Glasgow, Mikheeva, Krasnykh, & Curiel, 2009). Tagging of the proteins with the zipper peptide sequences preserved both the trimerization capability of the adenovirus fiber and the recognition of the EGFR by the zipper-scFv protein but, most importantly, it gave rise to receptor-specific infection of the target cells.

Several studies have shown the feasibility of using bispecific proteins for redirecting adenoviruses towards target cells *ex vivo* or *in vivo* in laboratory animal models, including (Barker *et al.*, 2003; Everts *et al.*, 2005; H. J. Li *et al.*, 2007; H. J. Li, Everts, Yamamoto, Curiel, & Herschman, 2009; Reynolds *et al.*, 2000; Reynolds *et al.*, 2001; van Beusechem *et al.*, 2002; van Beusechem *et al.*, 2003). Although quite effective, these studies were all based on a two-component strategy, requiring the mixing of virions with bispecific proteins before administration. To our knowledge, no *in vivo* studies have yet been performed using recombinant adenoviruses expressing a bispecific adapter from their viral genome to establish whether they have superior targeting and cell killing abilities.

4.2.2   Coronaviruses

To generate self-targeted coronaviruses, initially the coding sequence for a bispecific adapter protein composed of the soluble mCEACAM1a receptor linked to a His-tag was incorporated into the MHV viral genome by targeted recombination, creating the virus designated MHVsoR-His (Verheije *et al.*, 2006). The presence of this additional expression cassette was tolerated and the resulting recombinant viruses indeed expressed the adapter protein. Inoculation of target cells expressing the artificial His-receptor on their surface showed the recombinant viruses to be able to establish a multi-round, receptor-dependent infection. Furthermore, extensive cell-cell fusion and rapid cell killing of infected target cells was observed, demonstrating the possibility of generating genetically redirected coronaviruses (Verheije *et al.*, 2006).

The expression cassette was subsequently extended by inserting the sequence encoding the EGF peptide between that of the soluble receptor and the His-tag (Verheije *et al.*, 2009). Again, the generated recombinant MHVsoR-EGF-His thereby acquired the ability to cause multi-round infection of otherwise non-susceptible, EGFR-expressing cell cultures *in vitro*, with subsequent efficient cytolytic activity (Verheije *et al.*, 2009). More importantly, the redirected virus demonstrated oncolytic capacity also *in vivo* in an orthotopic U87dEGFR xenograft mouse model. Survival rates of the mice were significantly longer when the tumor-bearing animals were treated with MHVsoR-EGF-His than after treatment with control virus MHVsoR-His or with PBS (Figure 6A). In none of the MHVsoR-EGF-His treated mice recurrent tumor load could be detected, demonstrating the strong oncolytic capacity of such viruses *in vivo* (Verheije *et al.*, 2009) (Figure 6B). Despite the impressive oncolytic effect *in vivo* of the redirected MHV, replication of MHV in non-tumor tissue of the natural host was observed (Figure 6C), presumably because the natural tropism of MHV was not ablated.

Further experiments demonstrated that the composition of the bispecific protein is of critical importance for the success of generating recombinant oncolytic coronaviruses. In particular, viable recombinant coronaviruses expressing a bispecific scFv from an additional expression cassette in the viral genome could not be rescued (Fig. 7; Verheije and Rottier, unpublished data). Subsequent introduction of a bispecific gene encoding the soR fused to a scFv against the EGFR did generate viable viruses; however, such viruses were genetically highly unstable, loosing the foreign gene usually already within one passage (Figure 7; Verheije and Rottier, unpublished data). As successful incorporation of other, even larger, foreign genes at the same position in the MHV genome has been reported (including for example the gene encoding luciferase (de Haan, van Genne, Stoop, Volders, & Rottier, 2003)), the instability of the scFvs is likely due to their particular sequence composition rather than to their size.

In conclusion, oncolytic coronaviruses expressing a soluble receptor that is C-terminally extended with a peptide ligand have great potential for oncolytic therapy. By expanding the targeting repertoire through exchange of peptide ligands, coronaviruses can probably be redirected towards various tumor epitopes, provided that the binding and fusion ability of the viral proteins are maintained. As murine coronaviruses display great species-specificity in their infection, ablation of the natural tropism will probably not be required, making MHV a safe candidate oncolytic agent for use in other mammals, including humans.

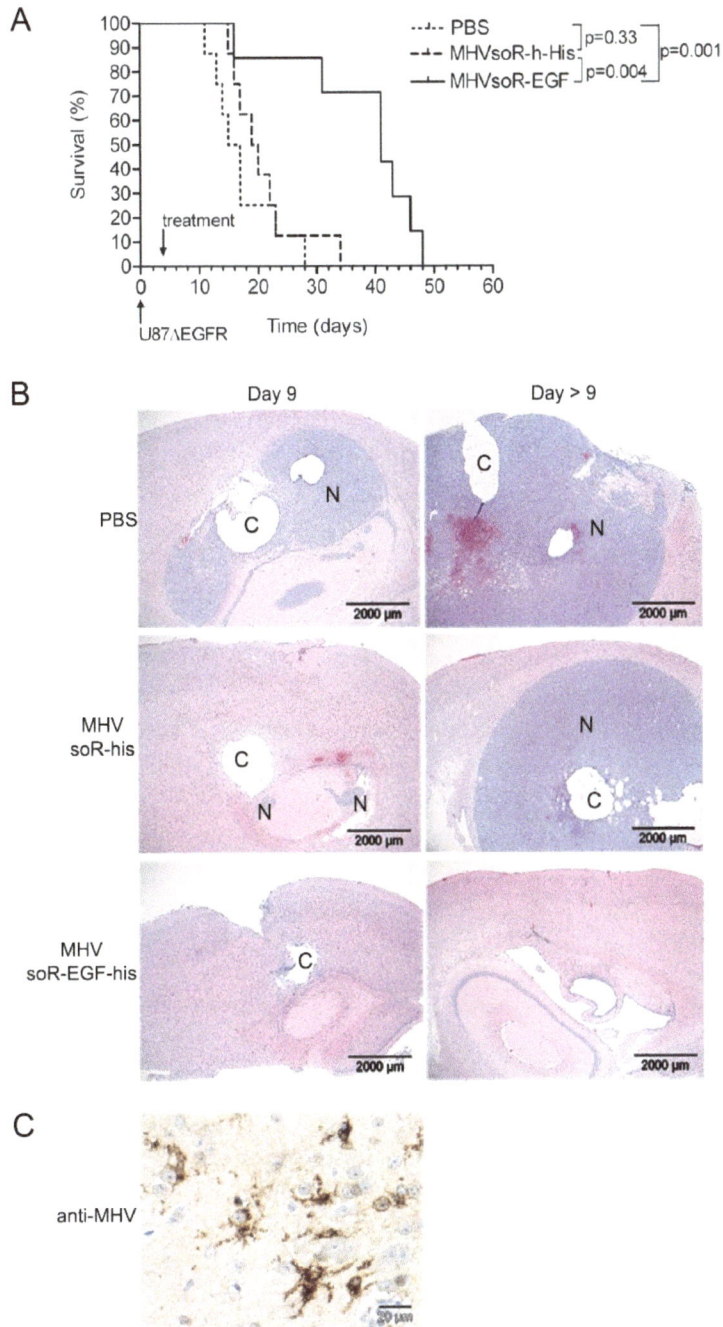

Figure 6: *In vivo* oncolytic activity of murine coronavirus MHV. Mice with established intracranial U87ΔEGFR tumors were treated with MHV genetically redirected to the EGFR (MHVsoR-EGF-his), the His-receptor (MHVsoR-his) or with PBS. (A) Survival curves; (B) Histopathological analysis of brains at day 9 post treatment and at the day of euthanasia (day>9). Large neoplasms and cystic structures are indicated by "N" and "C," respectively; (C) Immunostaining of brains after treatment with MHVsoR-EGF-his using polyclonal anti-MHV antibodies (Copyright © American Society for Microbiology, Journal of Virology, Vol. 83, No. 15, P. 7507-16, 2009, DOI 10.1128/JVI.00495-09).

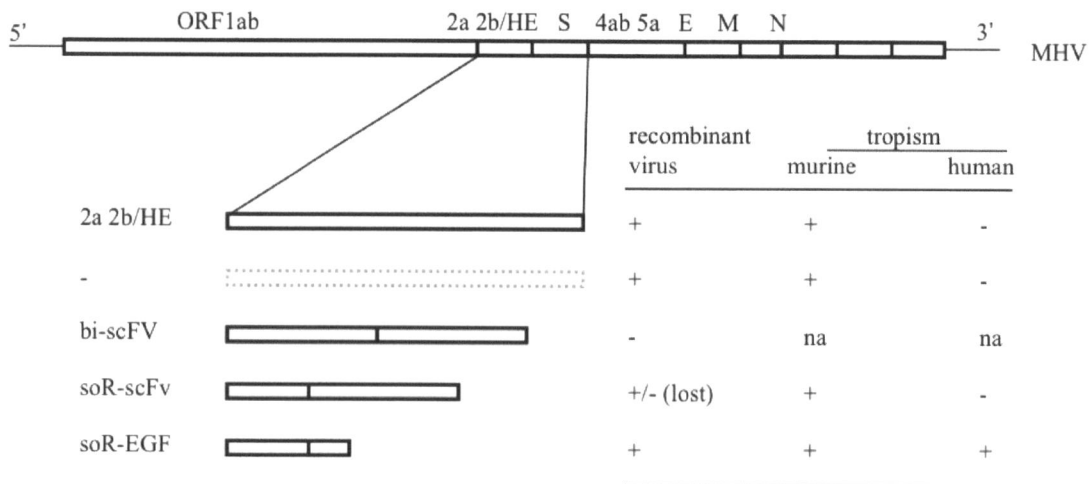

recombinant virus	tropism	
	murine	human
2a 2b/HE +	+	-
- +	+	-
bi-scFV -	na	na
soR-scFv +/- (lost)	+	-
soR-EGF +	+	+

Figure 7: Introduction of bispecific adapter cassettes into the coronaviral genome. Schematic representation of the MHV genome and of the bispecific expression cassettes introduced herein. The plus-strand RNA genome contains, from 5' to 3', the polymerase precursor gene (ORF1ab), the accessory genes 2a and 2b/HE, the S gene, the non-essential genes 4ab and 5a, and the genes encoding the virion proteins E, M and N. In the recombinant viruses the gene cluster 2a + 2b/HE was replaced by an expression cassette downstream of the transcription regulatory sequence for protein 2a. Recombinant MHV viruses were generated by targeted recombination (Kuo *et al.*, 2000). Indicated is whether the particular recombinant virus could be isolated, as confirmed by RT-PCR on virus RNA. In addition, the ability of such viruses to infect murine and human cells is depicted (Verheije and Rottier, unpublished data). Abbreviations of adapters: as specified in the text; "na": not applicable.

5   Conclusions and Perspectives on Transductional Virus Targeting

What this overview emphatically reveals is that the field of transductional retargeting of viruses for therapeutic use is in its early infancy. In fact, for the majority of the viruses studied, scientists are still struggling with the most fundamental aspects of changing their cell tropism. Robust platforms for retargeting have actually not been established yet for any of the viruses. On the positive side, the feasibility of retargeting was, at least *in vitro,* demonstrated for an increasing number of viruses in the past years. Clearly the most attractive goal will be to generate oncolytic viruses that carry the retargeting information in their genome. Only then will the viruses be able to sustain their replication in the tumor tissue, irrespective of the retargeting principle used, i.e. whether through modification of the viral attachment protein or through expression of an adapter protein.

Although clinical application of transductionally targeted oncolytic viruses is still disconcertingly remote, the oncolytic virus field has made tremendous progress in the last decade. Currently, the appealing characteristics of numerous viruses are exploited in order to develop improved tumor therapeutics. Clinical trials performed with oncolytic viruses have provided a wealth of information from which the transductional targeting field can benefit in order to maximize their therapeutic index. The lessons learned from clinical trials are summarized below, followed by an overview of the various aspects that will need to be addressed to solve the two most important challenges for the field: increasing the oncolytic virus' tumor specificity and enhancing its oncolytic potency.

6   Lessons Learned from Clinical Trials using Oncolytic Viruses

Clinical trials have been performed with quite a variety of different oncolytic viruses by which diverse tumor types were targeted (recently reviewed in (Russell *et al.*, 2012)). Yet, currently only one oncolytic virus has been clinically approved for the treatment of head and neck cancer in China. Despite this still limited success the many clinical trials have provided a wealth of useful information to help the field further (summarized in (Liu, Galanis, & Kirn, 2007; Parato, Senger, Forsyth, & Bell, 2005; Russell *et al.*, 2012)).

From dose escalation studies it became clear that the maximum tolerable dose was often not yet reached, likely due to current limitations in the manufacturing systems. So to certain extend, concerns about toxicity have been alleviated although it is too early to judge the side effects when oncolytic virotherapy will be applied at higher, more effective, doses. Another safety aspect concerns the spread of the oncolytic virus to other people. So far, transmission to contacts and caretakers has not yet been observed, though virus shedding has been detected in urine or respiratory secretions (Liu *et al.*, 2007). Nevertheless, safety remains an extremely important aspect of new therapeutics, hence further steps to ensure the safety and specificity when using higher virus titers will be required.

Another lesson learned from the many clinical trials is that the therapeutical outcome might benefit from amplification of cytolytic capacities of the oncolytic virus. Typically, cytolytic destruction of tumor cells by oncolytic viruses does not overlap with the mechanisms induced by traditional therapies. Therefore, currently oncolytic virus trials are often combined with chemotherapeutic or radiation therapy to enhance the oncolytic effect. While relatively high frequencies of response have been observed, the contribution of the oncolytic virus to the outcome is, however, difficult to assess in such studies.

Finally, it becomes clear that human clinical trials often fall short and that more reliable predictive preclinical models are needed to test oncolytic viruses before they enter a phase I or II study. The current models, including cultured cells and human xenograft models in immune compromised animals, cannot take into account the effects of the immune system on the oncolytic virus and on the tumor. Other animal models might be limited in their predictive capacity for safety aspects as they are not susceptible to the particular virus. The ultimate challenge for the field is therefore the development of orthotopic cancer models in immunocompetent animals, in which the animal should be susceptible to the oncolytic virus and the disease and virus replication should mirror human pathogenesis. This will be, however, extremely difficult, and other options, like including the application of mathematical and computational models (Hiss & Fielding, 2012), should be considered to better predict the outcome when translating therapeutics from animal to human patients.

7   Challenges for the Oncolytic Virus Field

7.1   Increasing Safety and Specificity of Transductionally Targeted Viruses

7.1.1   Target Receptors

One major challenge fundamental to the idea of oncolytic virotherapy is the availability of suitable target receptors on tumor cells. Ideally such receptors are unique or highly overexpressed in order to provide sufficient specificity for the infection. Recent developments in the proteomics field have already recognized various proteins that are overexpressed in tumor cells as compared to normal tissues and many more will hopefully be identified. It remains, however, questionable whether truly unique tumor surface proteins exist. This stresses the need to increase the specificity of oncolytic viruses in other ways. One such strategy might involve dual-receptor targeting, in which the virus is redirected to more than one receptor. This approach has been shown to be feasible for adenovirus, in which dual-ligand-targeted fibers improved transduction specificity in cell culture (Rein *et al.*, 2004).

7.1.2   Combining Targeting Strategies

Another strategy to increase the specificity of oncolytic viruses is the exploitation of different cancer hallmarks. In this respect, combining transductional targeting with translational or physiological targeting could increase the therapeutic index of the engineered oncolytic virus. The feasibility of combining both transductional and translational targeting has already been demonstrated for DNA viruses, including an adenovirus studied in clinical trials (Kimball *et al.*, 2010), while for RNA viruses investigations rather focus on the transductional targeting of attenuated viruses. Another strategy that holds promise to increase tumor specificity is the reduction of undesired replication in healthy cells by means of miRNA targeting. Although to our knowledge no studies have yet addressed the feasibility of combining transductional with miRNA targeting, from a theoretical point of view it should both be feasible and result in increased selectivity of replication once target cells are infected.

A notable example in which tumor selectivity is achieved by exploitation of different pathways is JX-594, the lead product within the oncolytic poxviruses field (Parato *et al.*, 2012). Here, the viral thymidine kinase (TK) gene is disrupted for attenuation, and the virus is armed with a transgene encoding the granulocyte-macrophage colony-stimulating factor (GM-CSF) under the control of a synthetic promoter. In phase I and II clinical trials intratumoral and systemic application of JX-594 were found to be well-tolerated, indicating that multifactorial targeting may indeed add to the safety of oncolytic viruses.

7.1.3   Ablation of Natural Tropism

The natural tropism of the therapeutic virus is another important aspect that needs to be taken into account with regard to safety. Ablation of the native tropism might be required for those viruses naturally infecting humans, to prevent infection of normal tissues, but also when the virus has a preference for binding, for instance, to blood substances or when it exhibits hepatic tropism, both being a major cause of loss of infectious virus *in vivo*.

Modification of the natural tropism of a virus might be achieved by replacement of a viral attachment protein by that of another virus or serotype, provided that the resulting recombinant virus remains viable. This approach has been successfully applied for both adenoviruses (Ranki & Hemminki, 2010) and measles virus (Miest *et al.*, 2011), the latter by exchange of the viral glycoproteins with those of the related canine distemper virus.

Until now, detargeting the natural tropism of oncolytic viruses has mainly been studied for adenoviruses. A recent comparative study has shed more light on the feasibility of methods to reduce the virus' broad tropism and high liver infectivity. Competition with the soluble fiber knob for adenovirus receptor binding had only little effect on tumor and liver specific infection. On the contrary, ablation of the CAR and HSG-binding sites in the fiber knob and fiber shaft, respectively, not only reduced liver tropism, but also the infection of tumor cells. The same result was observed upon co-administration of coagulation factor X, known to be involved in the transduction of liver cells, with adenoviruses (Hogg *et al.*, 2011).

Thus, for adenoviruses, but perhaps also for other viruses, elimination of native interactions with receptors is unlikely to improve the tumor specificity of the infection. Overall, these results indicate that strategies to ablate the undesirable tropism of viruses should be combined with additional retargeting strategies to improve the overall therapeutic index of these approaches (summarized in (Coughlan *et al.*, 2010)). An alternative strategy to detarget adenoviruses is polymer coating of particles before systemic application. For wild type adenovirus this has resulted in decreased hepatic toxicity, increased plasma half live, and improved therapeutic index over uncoated viruses (Green *et al.*, 2012). Yet, technically this strategy can only be performed upon virus administration and not during lateral spread of the virus.

7.2   Increasing Potency and Efficacy of Transductionally Targeted Viruses

7.2.1   Replication Competency

In order to achieve effective eradication of all tumor cells, a desirable characteristic of oncolytic viruses is their ability to cause sustained, multi-round infection. In this respect, replication competent viruses, including viruses genetically redirected through incorporation of tumor-binding ligands and those having incorporated a bispecific adapter into their viral genome, seem the best choice. The stability of such recombinant viruses might, however, be a matter of concern, in particular when the targeting protein is required to ablate the natural human tropism. In general, DNA viruses are considered to be more stable than RNA viruses in which, in addition, the mutation rate is relatively high.

7.2.2   Immune Suppression

The history of the oncolytic virus field suggests that immune suppressed patients generally respond better to oncolytic virus therapy than patients with an intact immune system. Irrespective of the origin of the virus, immunity induced upon (repeated) viral treatment against viral antigens but also against introduced foreign proteins including bispecific adapter proteins expressed from the viral genome, might limit the effectiveness of the therapy. Therefore, combining virotherapy with immunosuppressive drugs is appealing to prolong the virus' antitumor activity. However, there is probably a delicate balance between the favorable effect of suppressing the adaptive antiviral immune response and the undesirable cytotoxicity of the oncolytic virus for normal tissues in immune compromised patients.

To overcome the limitations of pre-existing immunity in the use of oncolytic viruses for therapy, comparable but antigenically unrelated viruses from different hosts might be used. The use of non-human viruses for oncolytic therapy gains interest, as such viruses are usually non-pathogenic for humans and, in addition, no pre-existing antibodies circulate that might limit their efficacy. Their use may, however, also be the cause of new safety concerns as these viruses might adapt to their new host, cause unexpected disease and spread to non-patient humans and the environment. For a review on these issues see (Koppers-Lalic & Hoeben, 2011).

7.2.3   Promoting Cytotoxicity of Oncolytic Viruses

In clinical trials oncolytic virus treatment is often combined with conventional immuno-, chemo-, or radiation therapy. Although the outcome seemed to be improved in the treatment of several cancers, it is, however, difficult to assess the contribution of the oncolytic virus to the observed increased therapeutic index. Currently, it is believed that the increased oncolytic capacity is due to synergistic interactions, as oncolytic viruses act by antitumor mechanisms distinct from the conventional therapies,

To further exploit the differences, oncolytic viruses can be therapeutically armed to increase their potency of killing the infected tumor cell (reviewed in (Cattaneo, Miest, Shashkova, & Barry, 2008)). This might be achieved by the introduction into the viral genome of transgenes encoding therapeutic proteins which are hence produced selectively within tumor cells upon their infection. Transgenes for this purpose are numerous, and might include virulence genes from other viruses or strains to increase cytolysis, additional viral fusion genes to recruit neighboring uninfected tumor cells, pro-apoptotic genes causing cell death at late stages of the viral infection, pro-drug convertases capable of converting a harmless prodrug into a cytotoxic compound at the site of infection (recently reviewed in (Wennier, Liu, & McFadden, 2011), small molecules that suppress the innate immune responses to the virus, immune stimulatory molecules or tumor-associated antigens to increase the antitumor response (recently reviewed in (Altomonte & Ebert, 2012), transporters allowing local radiotherapy (recently reviewed in (Touchefeu, Franken, & Harrington, 2012), molecules inhibiting the tumor neoangiogenesis, and proteases or collagenases that digest the tumor extracellular matrix to allow increased penetration of the virus into the tumor mass.

7.2.4   Barriers for Delivery and Spread in the Body

Intravenous application is a major goal of oncolytic virus therapy in the treatment of metastatic cancer. However, in order to achieve sufficient virus to actually reach the tumor and cause tumor destruction, a certain dose threshold needs to be exceeded. In a recent clinical trial with vaccinia virus, therapeutic virus could only be recovered from tumor biopsies from patients inoculated with the highest virus dose (Breitbach, Thorne, Bell, & Kirn, 2011). While currently for many viruses the manufacturing systems likely limit the maximum application dose, systemic oncolytic therapy will particularly benefit from strategies to improve viral delivery to the tumor. To achieve this, sequestration in the liver and spleen needs to be minimized, and efforts should be undertaken to avoid opsonization of virus by phagocytic cells and neutralization by serum antibodies or other immune factors. Other strategies to improve transduction of tumor cells include the targeting of viruses to endothelial cells surrounding the vascular system of the tumor and selectively enhancing the vessel permeability of the tumor vasculature. All these strategies (reviewed in (Russell *et al.*, 2012)) might increase the local viral dose and in this way enhance its oncolytic effects.

Clearly, overcoming barriers for delivery and spread of oncolytic viruses coincides with reducing humoral and cellular immunity against oncolytic viruses. Next to shielding viruses from antibodies by using polymers to mask natural attachment proteins (Green *et al.*, 2004; Green *et al.*, 2012), the delivery of oncolytic virus to tumor cells might be increased by the use of carrier cells, including stem cells and tumor cells, which have the ability to home to the tumor (Nakashima, Kaur, & Chiocca, 2010).

Finally, detargeting the native tropism of viruses can also substantially increase the effective virus dose. As mentioned, this can be achieved by genetic ablation of native receptor-binding determinants, inhibition of specific interactions between viral proteins and serum factors, or by polymer coating of virions upon inoculation. Furthermore, depletion of particular cell types in the blood might increase the amount of virus in the vascular system as has been demonstrated for adenovirus (Koski *et al.*, 2009). However, this might cause serious side effects of the oncolytic virus, resulting in decreased safety of the virus for patients.

8   Summarizing Remarks

In conclusion, transductionally targeted viruses may provide a much needed tumor-specific therapy, but researchers will have to face, besides the technological challenges, a delicate balance between safety and effectiveness during development of such new viruses for clinical use. Yet, despite all problems and concerns, the importance of the ultimate goal of winning the fight against cancer warrants the sacrifice of all the energy and creativity needed for its realization.

References

Allaume, X., El-Andaloussi, N., Leuchs, B., Bonifati, S., Kulkarni, A., Marttila, T., et al. (2012). Retargeting of rat parvovirus H-1PV to cancer cells through genetic engineering of the viral capsid. Journal of Virology, 86(7), 3452-3465. doi:10.1128/JVI.06208-11

Altomonte, J., & Ebert, O. (2012). Replicating viral vectors for cancer therapy: Strategies to synergize with host immune responses. Microbial Biotechnology, 5(2), 251-259. doi:10.1111/j.1751-7915.2011.00296.x; 10.1111/j.1751-7915.2011.00296.x

Bachtarzi, H., Stevenson, M., Subr, V., Ulbrich, K., Seymour, L. W., & Fisher, K. D. (2011). Targeting adenovirus gene delivery to activated tumour-associated vasculature via endothelial selectins. Journal of Controlled Release : Official Journal of the Controlled Release Society, 150(2), 196-203. doi:10.1016/j.jconrel.2010.10.011

Baek, H., Uchida, H., Jun, K., Kim, J. H., Kuroki, M., Cohen, J. B., et al. (2011). Bispecific adapter-mediated retargeting of a receptor-restricted HSV-1 vector to CEA-bearing tumor cells. Molecular Therapy : The Journal of the American Society of Gene Therapy, 19(3), 507-514. doi:10.1038/mt.2010.207

Banerjee, P. S., Zuniga, E. S., Ojima, I., & Carrico, I. S. (2011). Targeted and armed oncolytic adenovirus via chemoselective modification. Bioorganic & Medicinal Chemistry Letters, doi:10.1016/j.bmcl.2011.05.039

Barber, G. N. (2004). Vesicular stomatitis virus as an oncolytic vector. Viral Immunology, 17(4), 516-527. doi:10.1089/vim.2004.17.516

Barker, S. D., Dmitriev, I. P., Nettelbeck, D. M., Liu, B., Rivera, A. A., Alvarez, R. D., et al. (2003). Combined transcriptional and transductional targeting improves the specificity and efficacy of adenoviral gene delivery to ovarian carcinoma. Gene Therapy, 10(14), 1198-1204. doi:10.1038/sj.gt.3301974

Bartlett, J. S., Kleinschmidt, J., Boucher, R. C., & Samulski, R. J. (1999). Targeted adeno-associated virus vector transduction of nonpermissive cells mediated by a bispecific F(ab'gamma)2 antibody. Nature Biotechnology, 17(2), 181-186. doi:10.1038/6185

Bell, J. C., & Kirn, D. (2008). MicroRNAs fine-tune oncolytic viruses. Nature Biotechnology, 26(12), 1346-1348. doi:10.1038/nbt1208-1346

Belousova, N., Mikheeva, G., Gelovani, J., & Krasnykh, V. (2008). Modification of adenovirus capsid with a designed protein ligand yields a gene vector targeted to a major molecular marker of cancer. Journal of Virology, 82(2), 630-637. doi:10.1128/JVI.01896-07

Bian, H., Fournier, P., Moormann, R., Peeters, B., & Schirrmacher, V. (2005). Selective gene transfer in vitro to tumor cells via recombinant newcastle disease virus. Cancer Gene Therapy, 12(3), 295-303. doi:10.1038/sj.cgt.7700774

Bian, H., Wilden, H., Fournier, P., Peeters, B., & Schirrmacher, V. (2006). In vivo efficacy of systemic tumor targeting of a viral RNA vector with oncolytic properties using a bispecific adapter protein. International Journal of Oncology, 29(6), 1359-1369.

Blechacz, B., & Russell, S. J. (2008). Measles virus as an oncolytic vector platform. Current Gene Therapy, 8(3), 162-175.

Breidenbach, M., Rein, D. T., Everts, M., Glasgow, J. N., Wang, M., Passineau, M. J., et al. (2005). Mesothelin-mediated targeting of adenoviral vectors for ovarian cancer gene therapy. Gene Therapy, 12(2), 187-193. doi:10.1038/sj.gt.3302404

Breitbach, C. J., Thorne, S. H., Bell, J. C., & Kirn, D. H. (2011). Targeted and armed oncolytic poxviruses for cancer: The lead example of JX-594. Current Pharmaceutical Biotechnology,

Butt, A. Q., & Miggin, S. M. (2012). Cancer and viruses: A double-edged sword. Proteomics, 12(13), 2127-2138. doi:10.1002/pmic.201100526; 10.1002/pmic.201100526

Campadelli-Fiume, G., De Giovanni, C., Gatta, V., Nanni, P., Lollini, P. L., & Menotti, L. (2011). Rethinking herpes simplex virus: The way to oncolytic agents. Reviews in Medical Virology, doi:10.1002/rmv.691; 10.1002/rmv.691

Carette, J. E., Graat, H. C., Schagen, F. H., Mastenbroek, D. C., Rots, M. G., Haisma, H. J., et al. (2007). A conditionally replicating adenovirus with strict selectivity in killing cells expressing epidermal growth factor receptor. Virology, 361(1), 56-67. doi:10.1016/j.virol.2006.11.011

Cattaneo, R., Miest, T., Shashkova, E. V., & Barry, M. A. (2008). Reprogrammed viruses as cancer therapeutics: Targeted, armed and shielded. Nature Reviews.Microbiology, 6(7), 529-540. doi:10.1038/nrmicro1927

Chadwick, M. P., Morling, F. J., Cosset, F. L., & Russell, S. J. (1999). Modification of retroviral tropism by display of IGF-I. Journal of Molecular Biology, 285(2), 485-494. doi:10.1006/jmbi.1998.2350

Chen, C. Y., May, S. M., & Barry, M. A. (2010). Targeting adenoviruses with factor x-single-chain antibody fusion proteins. Human Gene Therapy, 21(6), 739-749. doi:10.1089/hum.2009.190

Coiras, M., Camafeita, E., Lopez-Huertas, M. R., Calvo, E., Lopez, J. A., & Alcami, J. (2008). Application of proteomics technology for analyzing the interactions between host cells and intracellular infectious agents. Proteomics, 8(4), 852-873. doi:10.1002/pmic.200700664

Coughlan, L., Alba, R., Parker, A. L., Bradshaw, A. C., McNeish, I. A., Nicklin, S. A., et al. (2010). Tropism-modification strategies for targeted gene delivery using adenoviral vectors. Viruses, 2(10), 2290-2355. doi:10.3390/v2102290

Dalba, C., Klatzmann, D., Logg, C. R., & Kasahara, N. (2005). Beyond oncolytic virotherapy: Replication-competent retrovirus vectors for selective and stable transduction of tumors. Current Gene Therapy, 5(6), 655-667.

de Haan, C. A., van Genne, L., Stoop, J. N., Volders, H., & Rottier, P. J. (2003). Coronaviruses as vectors: Position dependence of foreign gene expression. J Virol, 77(21), 11312-23.

de Vrij, J., Dautzenberg, I. J., van den Hengel, S. K., Magnusson, M. K., Uil, T. G., Cramer, S. J., et al. (2011). A cathepsin-cleavage site between the adenovirus capsid protein IX and a tumor-targeting ligand improves targeted transduction. Gene Therapy, doi:10.1038/gt.2011.162; 10.1038/gt.2011.162

Dmitriev, I., Kashentseva, E., Rogers, B. E., Krasnykh, V., & Curiel, D. T. (2000). Ectodomain of coxsackievirus and adenovirus receptor genetically fused to epidermal growth factor mediates adenovirus targeting to epidermal growth factor receptor-positive cells. J Virol, 74(15), 6875-84.

Dorer, D. E., & Nettelbeck, D. M. (2009). Targeting cancer by transcriptional control in cancer gene therapy and viral oncolysis. Advanced Drug Delivery Reviews, 61(7-8), 554-571. doi:10.1016/j.addr.2009.03.013

Doronin, K., & Shayakhmetov, D. M. (2012). Construction of targeted and armed oncolytic adenoviruses. Methods in Molecular Biology (Clifton, N.J.), 797, 35-52. doi:10.1007/978-1-61779-340-0_3

Douglas, J. T., Rogers, B. E., Rosenfeld, M. E., Michael, S. I., Feng, M., & Curiel, D. T. (1996). Targeted gene delivery by tropism-modified adenoviral vectors. Nat Biotechnol, 14(11), 1574-8.

Dreier, B., Mikheeva, G., Belousova, N., Parizek, P., Boczek, E., Jelesarov, I., et al. (2011). Her2-specific multivalent adapters confer designed tropism to adenovirus for gene targeting. Journal of Molecular Biology, 405(2), 410-426. doi:10.1016/j.jmb.2010.10.040

Ebbinghaus, C., Al-Jaibaji, A., Operschall, E., Schoffel, A., Peter, I., Greber, U. F., et al. (2001). Functional and selective targeting of adenovirus to high-affinity fcgamma receptor I-positive cells by using a bispecific hybrid adapter. J Virol, 75(1), 480-9.

Einfeld, D. A., Schroeder, R., Roelvink, P. W., Lizonova, A., King, C. R., Kovesdi, I., et al. (2001). Reducing the native tropism of adenovirus vectors requires removal of both CAR and integrin interactions. Journal of Virology, 75(23), 11284-11291. doi:10.1128/JVI.75.23.11284-11291.2001

Erlwein, O., Wels, W., & Schnierle, B. S. (2002). Chimeric ecotropic MLV envelope proteins that carry EGF receptor-specific ligands and the pseudomonas exotoxin A translocation domain to target gene transfer to human cancer cells. Virology, 302(2), 333-341.

Eto, Y., Gao, J. Q., Sekiguchi, F., Kurachi, S., Katayama, K., Maeda, M., et al. (2005). PEGylated adenovirus vectors containing RGD peptides on the tip of PEG show high transduction efficiency and antibody evasion ability. The Journal of Gene Medicine, 7(5), 604-612. doi:10.1002/jgm.699

Everts, M., Kim-Park, S. A., Preuss, M. A., Passineau, M. J., Glasgow, J. N., Pereboev, A. V., et al. (2005). Selective induction of tumor-associated antigens in murine pulmonary vasculature using double-targeted adenoviral vectors. Gene Therapy, 12(13), 1042-1048. doi:10.1038/sj.gt.3302491

Fisher, K. D., Green, N. K., Hale, A., Subr, V., Ulbrich, K., & Seymour, L. W. (2007). Passive tumour targeting of polymer-coated adenovirus for cancer gene therapy. Journal of Drug Targeting, 15(7-8), 546-551. doi:10.1080/10611860701501014

Galanis, E. (2010). Therapeutic potential of oncolytic measles virus: Promises and challenges. Clinical Pharmacology and Therapeutics, 88(5), 620-625. doi:10.1038/clpt.2010.211

Galmiche, M. C., Rindisbacher, L., Wels, W., Wittek, R., & Buchegger, F. (1997). Expression of a functional single chain antibody on the surface of extracellular enveloped vaccinia virus as a step towards selective tumour cell targeting. J Gen Virol, 78 (Pt 11), 3019-27.

Gao, J. Q., Eto, Y., Yoshioka, Y., Sekiguchi, F., Kurachi, S., Morishige, T., et al. (2007). Effective tumor targeted gene transfer using PEGylated adenovirus vector via systemic administration. Journal of Controlled Release : Official Journal of the Controlled Release Society, 122(1), 102-110. doi:10.1016/j.jconrel.2007.06.010

Gigout, L., Rebollo, P., Clement, N., Warrington, K. H.,Jr, Muzyczka, N., Linden, R. M., et al. (2005). Altering AAV tropism with mosaic viral capsids. Molecular Therapy : The Journal of the American Society of Gene Therapy, 11(6), 856-865. doi:10.1016/j.ymthe.2005.03.005

Girod, A., Ried, M., Wobus, C., Lahm, H., Leike, K., Kleinschmidt, J., et al. (1999). Genetic capsid modifications allow efficient re-targeting of adeno-associated virus type 2. Nat Med, 5(9), 1052-6.

Glasgow, J. N., Everts, M., & Curiel, D. T. (2006). Transductional targeting of adenovirus vectors for gene therapy. Cancer Gene Therapy, 13(9), 830-844. doi:10.1038/sj.cgt.7700928

Glasgow, J. N., Mikheeva, G., Krasnykh, V., & Curiel, D. T. (2009). A strategy for adenovirus vector targeting with a secreted single chain antibody. PloS One, 4(12), e8355. doi:10.1371/journal.pone.0008355

Goldman, C. K., Rogers, B. E., Douglas, J. T., Sosnowski, B. A., Ying, W., Siegal, G. P., et al. (1997). Targeted gene delivery to kaposi's sarcoma cells via the fibroblast growth factor receptor. Cancer Res, 57(8), 1447-51.

Green, N. K., Hale, A., Cawood, R., Illingworth, S., Herbert, C., Hermiston, T., et al. (2012). Tropism ablation and stealthing of oncolytic adenovirus enhances systemic delivery to tumors and improves virotherapy of cancer. Nanomedicine (London, England), doi:10.2217/nnm.12.50

Green, N. K., Herbert, C. W., Hale, S. J., Hale, A. B., Mautner, V., Harkins, R., et al. (2004). Extended plasma circulation time and decreased toxicity of polymer-coated adenovirus. Gene Therapy, 11(16), 1256-1263. doi:10.1038/sj.gt.3302295

Green, N. K., Morrison, J., Hale, S., Briggs, S. S., Stevenson, M., Subr, V., et al. (2008). *Retargeting polymer-coated adenovirus to the FGF receptor allows productive infection and mediates efficacy in a peritoneal model of human ovarian cancer.* The Journal of Gene Medicine, 10(3), 280-289. doi:10.1002/jgm.1121

Grifman, M., Trepel, M., Speece, P., Gilbert, L. B., Arap, W., Pasqualini, R., et al. (2001). *Incorporation of tumor-targeting peptides into recombinant adeno-associated virus capsids.* Mol Ther, 3(6), 964-75.

Gu, D. L., Gonzalez, A. M., Printz, M. A., Doukas, J., Ying, W., D'Andrea, M., et al. (1999). *Fibroblast growth factor 2 retargeted adenovirus has redirected cellular tropism: Evidence for reduced toxicity and enhanced antitumor activity in mice.* Cancer Res, 59(11), 2608-14.

Guse, K., Cerullo, V., & Hemminki, A. (2011). *Oncolytic vaccinia virus for the treatment of cancer.* Expert Opinion on Biological Therapy, 11(5), 595-608. doi:10.1517/14712598.2011.558838

Haijema, B. J., Volders, H., & Rottier, P. J. (2003). *Switching species tropism: An effective way to manipulate the feline coronavirus genome.* J Virol, 77(8), 4528-38.

Haisma, H. J., Kamps, G. K., Bouma, A., Geel, T. M., Rots, M. G., Kariath, A., et al. (2010). *Selective targeting of adenovirus to alphavbeta3 integrins, VEGFR2 and Tie2 endothelial receptors by angio-adenobodies.* International Journal of Pharmaceutics, 391(1-2), 155-161. doi:10.1016/j.ijpharm.2010.02.032

Haisma, H. J., Pinedo, H. M., Rijswijk, A., der Meulen-Muileman, I., Sosnowski, B. A., Ying, W., et al. (1999). *Tumor-specific gene transfer via an adenoviral vector targeted to the pan-carcinoma antigen EpCAM.* Gene Ther, 6(8), 1469-74.

Hall, K., Blair Zajdel, M. E., & Blair, G. E. (2010). *Unity and diversity in the human adenoviruses: Exploiting alternative entry pathways for gene therapy.* The Biochemical Journal, 431(3), 321-336. doi:10.1042/BJ20100766

Hammond, A. L., Plemper, R. K., Zhang, J., Schneider, U., Russell, S. J., & Cattaneo, R. (2001). *Single-chain antibody displayed on a recombinant measles virus confers entry through the tumor-associated carcinoembryonic antigen.* J Virol, 75(5), 2087-96.

Han, J., Zhao, D., Zhong, Z., Zhang, Z., Gong, T., & Sun, X. (2010). *Combination of adenovirus and cross-linked low molecular weight PEI improves efficiency of gene transduction.* Nanotechnology, 21(10), 105106. doi:10.1088/0957-4484/21/10/105106

Hanahan, D., & Weinberg, R. A. (2011). *Hallmarks of cancer: The next generation.* Cell, 144(5), 646-674. doi:10.1016/j.cell.2011.02.013

Heiber, J. F., & Barber, G. N. (2012). *Evaluation of innate immune signaling pathways in transformed cells.* Methods in Molecular Biology (Clifton, N.J.), 797, 217-238. doi:10.1007/978-1-61779-340-0_15

Heideman, D. A., Snijders, P. J., Craanen, M. E., Bloemena, E., Meijer, C. J., Meuwissen, S. G., et al. (2001). *Selective gene delivery toward gastric and esophageal adenocarcinoma cells via EpCAM-targeted adenoviral vectors.* Cancer Gene Ther, 8(5), 342-51.

Hemminki, A., Dmitriev, I., Liu, B., Desmond, R. A., Alemany, R., & Curiel, D. T. (2001). *Targeting oncolytic adenoviral agents to the epidermal growth factor pathway with a secretory fusion molecule.* Cancer Res, 61(17), 6377-81.

Hemminki, A., Wang, M., Hakkarainen, T., Desmond, R. A., Wahlfors, J., & Curiel, D. T. (2003). *Production of an EGFR targeting molecule from a conditionally replicating adenovirus impairs its oncolytic potential.* Cancer Gene Ther, 10(8), 583-8.

Henning, P., Magnusson, M. K., Gunneriusson, E., Hong, S. S., Boulanger, P., Nygren, P. A., et al. (2002). *Genetic modification of adenovirus 5 tropism by a novel class of ligands based on a three-helix bundle scaffold derived from staphylococcal protein A.* Human Gene Therapy, 13(12), 1427-1439. doi:10.1089/10430340260185067

Hesse, A., Kosmides, D., Kontermann, R. E., & Nettelbeck, D. M. (2007). *Tropism modification of adenovirus vectors by peptide ligand insertion into various positions of the adenovirus serotype 41 short-fiber knob domain.* Journal of Virology, 81(6), 2688-2699. doi:10.1128/JVI.02722-06

Hiss, D. C., & Fielding, B. C. (2012). Optimization and preclinical design of genetically engineered viruses for human oncolytic therapy. Expert Opinion on Biological Therapy, doi:10.1517/14712598.2012.707183

Hogg, R. T., Thorpe, P., & Gerard, R. D. (2011). Retargeting adenoviral vectors to improve gene transfer into tumors. Cancer Gene Therapy, 18(4), 275-287. doi:10.1038/cgt.2010.78

Jongmans, W., van den Oudenalder, K., Tiemessen, D. M., Molkenboer, J., Willemsen, R., Mulders, P. F., et al. (2003). Targeting of adenovirus to human renal cell carcinoma cells. Urology, 62(3), 559-565.

Jung, Y., Park, H. J., Kim, P. H., Lee, J., Hyung, W., Yang, J., et al. (2007). Retargeting of adenoviral gene delivery via herceptin-PEG-adenovirus conjugates to breast cancer cells. Journal of Controlled Release : Official Journal of the Controlled Release Society, 123(2), 164-171. doi:10.1016/j.jconrel.2007.08.002

Kashentseva, E. A., Seki, T., Curiel, D. T., & Dmitriev, I. P. (2002). Adenovirus targeting to c-erbB-2 oncoprotein by single-chain antibody fused to trimeric form of adenovirus receptor ectodomain. Cancer Res, 62(2), 609-16.

Kelly, E., & Russell, S. J. (2007). History of oncolytic viruses: Genesis to genetic engineering. Molecular Therapy : The Journal of the American Society of Gene Therapy, 15(4), 651-659. doi:10.1038/sj.mt.6300108

Kimball, K. J., Preuss, M. A., Barnes, M. N., Wang, M., Siegal, G. P., Wan, W., et al. (2010). A phase I study of a tropism-modified conditionally replicative adenovirus for recurrent malignant gynecologic diseases. Clinical Cancer Research : An Official Journal of the American Association for Cancer Research, 16(21), 5277-5287. doi:10.1158/1078-0432.CCR-10-0791

Klimstra, W. B., Williams, J. C., Ryman, K. D., & Heidner, H. W. (2005). Targeting sindbis virus-based vectors to fc receptor-positive cell types. Virology, 338(1), 9-21. doi:10.1016/j.virol.2005.04.039

Koppers-Lalic, D., & Hoeben, R. C. (2011). Non-human viruses developed as therapeutic agent for use in humans. Reviews in Medical Virology, 21(4), 227-239. doi:10.1002/rmv.694; 10.1002/rmv.694

Koski, A., Rajecki, M., Guse, K., Kanerva, A., Ristimaki, A., Pesonen, S., et al. (2009). Systemic adenoviral gene delivery to orthotopic murine breast tumors with ablation of coagulation factors, thrombocytes and kupffer cells. The Journal of Gene Medicine, 11(11), 966-977. doi:10.1002/jgm.1373

Kraaij, R., van Rijswijk, A. L., Oomen, M. H., Haisma, H. J., & Bangma, C. H. (2005). Prostate specific membrane antigen (PSMA) is a tissue-specific target for adenoviral transduction of prostate cancer in vitro. The Prostate, 62(3), 253-259. doi:10.1002/pros.20150

Kuo, L., Godeke, G. J., Raamsman, M. J., Masters, P. S., & Rottier, P. J. (2000). Retargeting of coronavirus by substitution of the spike glycoprotein ectodomain: Crossing the host cell species barrier. J Virol, 74(3), 1393-406.

Lanciotti, J., Song, A., Doukas, J., Sosnowski, B., Pierce, G., Gregory, R., et al. (2003). Targeting adenoviral vectors using heterofunctional polyethylene glycol FGF2 conjugates. Molecular Therapy : The Journal of the American Society of Gene Therapy, 8(1), 99-107.

Lech, P. J., & Russell, S. J. (2010). Use of attenuated paramyxoviruses for cancer therapy. Expert Review of Vaccines, 9(11), 1275-1302. doi:10.1586/erv.10.124

Lesch, H. P., Kaikkonen, M. U., Pikkarainen, J. T., & Yla-Herttuala, S. (2010). Avidin-biotin technology in targeted therapy. Expert Opinion on Drug Delivery, 7(5), 551-564. doi:10.1517/17425241003677749

Li, E., Brown, S. L., Von Seggern, D. J., Brown, G. B., & Nemerow, G. R. (2000). Signaling antibodies complexed with adenovirus circumvent CAR and integrin interactions and improve gene delivery. Gene Ther, 7(18), 1593-9.

Li, F., Ryu, B. Y., Krueger, R. L., Heldt, S. A., & Albritton, L. M. (2012). Targeted entry via somatostatin receptors using a novel modified retrovirus glycoprotein that delivers genes at levels comparable to those of wild-type viral glycoproteins. Journal of Virology, 86(1), 373-381. doi:10.1128/JVI.05411-11

Li, H. J., Everts, M., Pereboeva, L., Komarova, S., Idan, A., Curiel, D. T., et al. (2007). Adenovirus tumor targeting and hepatic untargeting by a coxsackie/adenovirus receptor ectodomain anti-carcinoembryonic antigen bispecific adapter. Cancer Research, 67(11), 5354-5361. doi:10.1158/0008-5472.CAN-06-4679

Li, H. J., Everts, M., Yamamoto, M., Curiel, D. T., & Herschman, H. R. (2009). Combined transductional untargeting/retargeting and transcriptional restriction enhances adenovirus gene targeting and therapy for hepatic colorectal cancer tumors. Cancer Research, 69(2), 554-564. doi:10.1158/0008-5472.CAN-08-3209

Liu, T. C., Galanis, E., & Kirn, D. (2007). Clinical trial results with oncolytic virotherapy: A century of promise, a decade of progress. Nature Clinical Practice.Oncology, 4(2), 101-117. doi:10.1038/ncponc0736

Manservigi, R., Argnani, R., & Marconi, P. (2010). HSV recombinant vectors for gene therapy. The Open Virology Journal, 4, 123-156. doi:10.2174/1874357901004030123

Mathis, J. M., Stoff-Khalili, M. A., & Curiel, D. T. (2005). Oncolytic adenoviruses - selective retargeting to tumor cells. Oncogene, 24(52), 7775-7791. doi:10.1038/sj.onc.1209044

Miest, T. S., Yaiw, K. C., Frenzke, M., Lampe, J., Hudacek, A. W., Springfeld, C., et al. (2011). Envelope-chimeric entry-targeted measles virus escapes neutralization and achieves oncolysis. Molecular Therapy : The Journal of the American Society of Gene Therapy, 19(10), 1813-1820. doi:10.1038/mt.2011.92; 10.1038/mt.2011.92

Miller, C. R., Buchsbaum, D. J., Reynolds, P. N., Douglas, J. T., Gillespie, G. Y., Mayo, M. S., et al. (1998). Differential susceptibility of primary and established human glioma cells to adenovirus infection: Targeting via the epidermal growth factor receptor achieves fiber receptor-independent gene transfer. Cancer Res, 58(24), 5738-48.

Moselhy, J., Sarkar, S., Chia, M. C., Mocanu, J. D., Taulier, N., Liu, F. F., et al. (2007). Evaluation of copolymers of N-isopropylacrylamide and 2-dimethyl(aminoethyl)methacrylate in nonviral and adenoviral vectors for gene delivery to nasopharyngeal carcinoma. International Journal of Nanomedicine, 2(3), 461-478.

Naik, S., & Russell, S. J. (2009). Engineering oncolytic viruses to exploit tumor specific defects in innate immune signaling pathways. Expert Opinion on Biological Therapy, 9(9), 1163-1176. doi:10.1517/14712590903170653

Nakamura, T., & Russell, S. J. (2004). Oncolytic measles viruses for cancer therapy. Expert Opinion on Biological Therapy, 4(10), 1685-1692. doi:10.1517/14712598.4.10.1685

Nakano, K., Asano, R., Tsumoto, K., Kwon, H., Goins, W. F., Kumagai, I., et al. (2005). Herpes simplex virus targeting to the EGF receptor by a gD-specific soluble bridging molecule. Mol Ther, 11(4), 617-26.

Nakashima, H., Kaur, B., & Chiocca, E. A. (2010). Directing systemic oncolytic viral delivery to tumors via carrier cells. Cytokine & Growth Factor Reviews, 21(2-3), 119-126. doi:10.1016/j.cytogfr.2010.02.004

Naumer, M., Ying, Y., Michelfelder, S., Reuter, A., Trepel, M., Muller, O. J., et al. (2012). Development and validation of novel AAV2 random libraries displaying peptides of diverse lengths and at diverse capsid positions. Human Gene Therapy, 23(5), 492-507. doi:10.1089/hum.2011.139

Nettelbeck, D. M., Rivera, A. A., Kupsch, J., Dieckmann, D., Douglas, J. T., Kontermann, R. E., et al. (2004). Retargeting of adenoviral infection to melanoma: Combining genetic ablation of native tropism with a recombinant bispecific single-chain diabody (scDb) adapter that binds to fiber knob and HMWMAA. International Journal of Cancer.Journal International Du Cancer, 108(1), 136-145. doi:10.1002/ijc.11563

Ohno, K., Sawai, K., Iijima, Y., Levin, B., & Meruelo, D. (1997). Cell-specific targeting of sindbis virus vectors displaying IgG-binding domains of protein A. Nat Biotechnol, 15(8), 763-7.

Ouellette, M. M., Wright, W. E., & Shay, J. W. (2011). Targeting telomerase-expressing cancer cells. Journal of Cellular and Molecular Medicine, 15(7), 1433-1442. doi:10.1111/j.1582-4934.2011.01279.x; 10.1111/j.1582-4934.2011.01279.x

Parato, K. A., Breitbach, C. J., Le Boeuf, F., Wang, J., Storbeck, C., Ilkow, C., et al. (2012). The oncolytic poxvirus JX-594 selectively replicates in and destroys cancer cells driven by genetic pathways commonly activated in cancers. Molecular Therapy : The Journal of the American Society of Gene Therapy, 20(4), 749-758. doi:10.1038/mt.2011.276; 10.1038/mt.2011.276

Parato, K. A., Senger, D., Forsyth, P. A., & Bell, J. C. (2005). Recent progress in the battle between oncolytic viruses and tumours. Nature Reviews.Cancer, 5(12), 965-976. doi:10.1038/nrc1750

Park, J. W., Mok, H., & Park, T. G. (2008). Epidermal growth factor (EGF) receptor targeted delivery of PEGylated adenovirus. Biochemical and Biophysical Research Communications, 366(3), 769-774. doi:10.1016/j.bbrc.2007.12.045

Park, K., Kim, W. J., Cho, Y. H., Lee, Y. I., Lee, H., Jeong, S., et al. (2008). Cancer gene therapy using adeno-associated virus vectors. Frontiers in Bioscience : A Journal and Virtual Library, 13, 2653-2659.

Paul, S., Geist, M., Dott, K., Snary, D., Taylor-Papadimitriou, J., Acres, B., et al. (2007). Specific tumor cell targeting by a recombinant MVA expressing a functional single chain antibody on the surface of intracellular mature virus (IMV) particles. Viral Immunology, 20(4), 664-671. doi:10.1089/vim.2007.0058

Pereboeva, L., Komarova, S., Roth, J., Ponnazhagan, S., & Curiel, D. T. (2007). Targeting EGFR with metabolically biotinylated fiber-mosaic adenovirus. Gene Therapy, 14(8), 627-637. doi:10.1038/sj.gt.3302916

Pizzato, M., Blair, E. D., Fling, M., Kopf, J., Tomassetti, A., Weiss, R. A., et al. (2001). Evidence for nonspecific adsorption of targeted retrovirus vector particles to cells. Gene Ther, 8(14), 1088-96.

Poulin, K. L., Lanthier, R. M., Smith, A. C., Christou, C., Risco Quiroz, M., Powell, K. L., et al. (2010). Retargeting of adenovirus vectors through genetic fusion of a single-chain or single-domain antibody to capsid protein IX. Journal of Virology, 84(19), 10074-10086. doi:10.1128/JVI.02665-09

Purow, B., & Staveley-O'Carroll, K. (2005). Targeting of vaccinia virus using biotin-avidin viral coating and biotinylated antibodies. The Journal of Surgical Research, 123(1), 49-54. doi:10.1016/j.jss.2004.04.022

Quetglas, J. I., Ruiz-Guillen, M., Aranda, A., Casales, E., Bezunartea, J., & Smerdou, C. (2010). Alphavirus vectors for cancer therapy. Virus Research, 153(2), 179-196. doi:10.1016/j.virusres.2010.07.027

Ranki, T., & Hemminki, A. (2010). Serotype chimeric human adenoviruses for cancer gene therapy. Viruses, 2(10), 2196-2212. doi:10.3390/v2102196

Raupp, C., Naumer, M., Muller, O. J., Gurda, B. L., Agbandje-McKenna, M., & Kleinschmidt, J. A. (2012). The threefold protrusions of AAV8 are involved in cell surface targeting as well as post attachment processing. Journal of Virology, doi:10.1128/JVI.00209-12

Rein, D. T., Breidenbach, M., Wu, H., Han, T., Haviv, Y. S., Wang, M., et al. (2004). Gene transfer to cervical cancer with fiber-modified adenoviruses. International Journal of Cancer.Journal International Du Cancer, 111(5), 698-704. doi:10.1002/ijc.20295

Reynolds, P. N., Nicklin, S. A., Kaliberova, L., Boatman, B. G., Grizzle, W. E., Balyasnikova, I. V., et al. (2001). Combined transductional and transcriptional targeting improves the specificity of transgene expression in vivo. Nature Biotechnology, 19(9), 838-842. doi:10.1038/nbt0901-838

Reynolds, P. N., Zinn, K. R., Gavrilyuk, V. D., Balyasnikova, I. V., Rogers, B. E., Buchsbaum, D. J., et al. (2000). A targetable, injectable adenoviral vector for selective gene delivery to pulmonary endothelium in vivo. Molecular Therapy : The Journal of the American Society of Gene Therapy, 2(6), 562-578. doi:10.1006/mthe.2000.0205

Rodriguez, R., Schuur, E. R., Lim, H. Y., Henderson, G. A., Simons, J. W., & Henderson, D. R. (1997). Prostate attenuated replication competent adenovirus (ARCA) CN706: A selective cytotoxic for prostate-specific antigen-positive prostate cancer cells. Cancer Research, 57(13), 2559-2563.

Rogers, B. E., Douglas, J. T., Ahlem, C., Buchsbaum, D. J., Frincke, J., & Curiel, D. T. (1997). Use of a novel crosslinking method to modify adenovirus tropism. Gene Ther, 4(12), 1387-92.

Russell, S. J., & Cosset, F. L. (1999). Modifying the host range properties of retroviral vectors. The Journal of Gene Medicine, 1(5), 300-311. doi:2-T

Russell, S. J., & Peng, K. W. (2009). Measles virus for cancer therapy. Current Topics in Microbiology and Immunology, 330, 213-241.

Russell, S. J., Peng, K. W., & Bell, J. C. (2012). Oncolytic virotherapy. Nature Biotechnology, 30(7), 658-670. doi:10.1038/nbt.2287; 10.1038/nbt.2287

Sakurai, F., Katayama, K., & Mizuguchi, H. (2011). MicroRNA-regulated transgene expression systems for gene therapy and virotherapy. Frontiers in Bioscience : A Journal and Virtual Library, 17, 2389-2401.

Shah, K., & Breakefield, X. O. (2006). HSV amplicon vectors for cancer therapy. Current Gene Therapy, 6(3), 361-370.

Shi, W., Arnold, G. S., & Bartlett, J. S. (2001). Insertional mutagenesis of the adeno-associated virus type 2 (AAV2) capsid gene and generation of AAV2 vectors targeted to alternative cell-surface receptors. Hum Gene Ther, 12(14), 1697-711.

Shi, W., & Bartlett, J. S. (2003). RGD inclusion in VP3 provides adeno-associated virus type 2 (AAV2)-based vectors with a heparan sulfate-independent cell entry mechanism. Mol Ther, 7(4), 515-25.

Southam, C. M. (1960). Present status of oncolytic virus studies. Transactions of the New York Academy of Sciences, 22, 657-673.

Stachler, M. D., Chen, I., Ting, A. Y., & Bartlett, J. S. (2008). Site-specific modification of AAV vector particles with bio-physical probes and targeting ligands using biotin ligase. Molecular Therapy : The Journal of the American Society of Gene Therapy, 16(8), 1467-1473. doi:10.1038/mt.2008.129

Stevenson, M., Hale, A. B., Hale, S. J., Green, N. K., Black, G., Fisher, K. D., et al. (2007). Incorporation of a laminin-derived peptide (SIKVAV) on polymer-modified adenovirus permits tumor-specific targeting via alpha6-integrins. Cancer Gene Therapy, 14(4), 335-345. doi:10.1038/sj.cgt.7701022

Tai, C. K., & Kasahara, N. (2008). Replication-competent retrovirus vectors for cancer gene therapy. Frontiers in Bioscience : A Journal and Virtual Library, 13, 3083-3095.

Tai, C. K., Logg, C. R., Park, J. M., Anderson, W. F., Press, M. F., & Kasahara, N. (2003). Antibody-mediated targeting of replication-competent retroviral vectors. Human Gene Therapy, 14(8), 789-802. doi:10.1089/104303403765255174

Thirukkumaran, C., & Morris, D. G. (2009). Oncolytic viral therapy using reovirus. Methods in Molecular Biology (Clifton, N.J.), 542, 607-634.

Tillman, B. W., de Gruijl, T. D., Luykx-de Bakker, S. A., Scheper, R. J., Pinedo, H. M., Curiel, T. J., et al. (1999). Maturation of dendritic cells accompanies high-efficiency gene transfer by a CD40-targeted adenoviral vector. J Immunol, 162(11), 6378-83.

Tillman, B. W., Hayes, T. L., DeGruijl, T. D., Douglas, J. T., & Curiel, D. T. (2000). Adenoviral vectors targeted to CD40 enhance the efficacy of dendritic cell-based vaccination against human papillomavirus 16-induced tumor cells in a murine model. Cancer Res, 60(19), 5456-63.

Touchefeu, Y., Franken, P., & Harrington, K. J. (2012). Radiovirotherapy: Principles and prospects in oncology. Current Pharmaceutical Design, 18(22), 3313-3320.

Trepel, M., Grifman, M., Weitzman, M. D., & Pasqualini, R. (2000). Molecular adaptors for vascular-targeted adenoviral gene delivery. Hum Gene Ther, 11(14), 1971-81.

Turrell, S. J., & Whitehouse, A. (2011). Mutation of herpesvirus saimiri ORF51 glycoprotein specifically targets infectivity to hepatocellular carcinoma cell lines. Journal of Biomedicine & Biotechnology, 2011, 785158. doi:10.1155/2011/785158

van Beusechem, V. W., Grill, J., Mastenbroek, D. C., Wickham, T. J., Roelvink, P. W., Haisma, H. J., et al. (2002). Efficient and selective gene transfer into primary human brain tumors by using single-chain antibody-targeted adenoviral vectors with native tropism abolished. J Virol, 76(6), 2753-62.

van Beusechem, V. W., Mastenbroek, D. C., van den Doel, P. B., Lamfers, M. L., Grill, J., Wurdinger, T., et al. (2003). Conditionally replicative adenovirus expressing a targeting adapter molecule exhibits enhanced oncolytic potency on CAR-deficient tumors. Gene Therapy, 10(23), 1982-1991. doi:10.1038/sj.gt.3302103

van Zeeburg, H. J., van Beusechem, V. W., Huizenga, A., Haisma, H. J., Korokhov, N., Gibbs, S., et al. (2010). Adenovirus retargeting to surface expressed antigens on oral mucosa. The Journal of Gene Medicine, 12(4), 365-376. doi:10.1002/jgm.1447

Verheije, M. H., Lamfers, M. L., Wurdinger, T., Grinwis, G. C., Gerritsen, W. R., van Beusechem, V. W., et al. (2009). Coronavirus genetically redirected to the epidermal growth factor receptor exhibits effective antitumor activity against a malignant glioblastoma. J Virol, 83(15), 7507-16.

Verheije, M. H., & Rottier, P. J. (2012). Retargeting of viruses to generate oncolytic agents. Advances in Virology, 2012, 798526. doi:10.1155/2012/798526

Verheije, M. H., Wurdinger, T., van Beusechem, V. W., de Haan, C. A., Gerritsen, W. R., & Rottier, P. J. (2006). Redirecting coronavirus to a nonnative receptor through a virus-encoded targeting adapter. J Virol, 80(3), 1250-60.

Waehler, R., Russell, S. J., & Curiel, D. T. (2007). Engineering targeted viral vectors for gene therapy. Nat Rev Genet, 8(8), 573-87.

Watkins, S. J., Mesyanzhinov, V. V., Kurochkina, L. P., & Hawkins, R. E. (1997). The 'adenobody' approach to viral targeting: Specific and enhanced adenoviral gene delivery. Gene Ther, 4(10), 1004-12.

Wennier, S. T., Liu, J., & McFadden, G. (2011). Bugs and drugs: Oncolytic virotherapy in combination with chemotherapy. Current Pharmaceutical Biotechnology,

Wesseling, J. G., Bosma, P. J., Krasnykh, V., Kashentseva, E. A., Blackwell, J. L., Reynolds, P. N., et al. (2001). Improved gene transfer efficiency to primary and established human pancreatic carcinoma target cells via epidermal growth factor receptor and integrin-targeted adenoviral vectors. Gene Ther, 8(13), 969-76.

Wickham, T. J., Segal, D. M., Roelvink, P. W., Carrion, M. E., Lizonova, A., Lee, G. M., et al. (1996). Targeted adenovirus gene transfer to endothelial and smooth muscle cells by using bispecific antibodies. J Virol, 70(10), 6831-8.

Wurdinger, T., Verheije, M. H., Broen, K., Bosch, B. J., Haijema, B. J., de Haan, C. A., et al. (2005). Soluble receptor-mediated targeting of mouse hepatitis coronavirus to the human epidermal growth factor receptor. J Virol, 79(24), 15314-22.

Wurdinger, T., Verheije, M. H., Raaben, M., Bosch, B. J., de Haan, C. A., van Beusechem, V. W., et al. (2005). Targeting non-human coronaviruses to human cancer cells using a bispecific single-chain antibody. Gene Ther, 12(18), 1394-404.

Yoon, S. K., Mohr, L., O'Riordan, C. R., Lachapelle, A., Armentano, D., & Wands, J. R. (2000). Targeting a recombinant adenovirus vector to HCC cells using a bifunctional fab-antibody conjugate. Biochemical and Biophysical Research Communications, 272(2), 497-504. doi:10.1006/bbrc.2000.2788

Zeyaullah, M., Patro, M., Ahmad, I., Ibraheem, K., Sultan, P., Nehal, M., et al. (2012). Oncolytic viruses in the treatment of cancer: A review of current strategies. Pathology Oncology Research : POR, doi:10.1007/s12253-012-9548-2

Development of Therapies for Ewing Sarcoma: Strategies for Treating a Chemosensitive Pediatric Sarcoma

Thomas C. Badgett
Pediatric Hematology-Oncology
University of Kentucky, USA

Lars Wagner
Pediatric Hematology-Oncology
University of Kentucky, USA

1   Introduction

Ewing sarcoma was first described in the early twentieth century by James Ewing, who identified a small round cell malignancy that typically arose in the bones of adolescents and young adults(Ewing 1972). Over the years, many variations of this tumor have been appreciated, including differences in location of the primary tumor (bone vs. soft tissue) as well as the degree of histologic differentiation. However, despite these differences, the clinical course and response to therapy has been remarkably similar between these subtypes. One explanation for this similarity has been the consistent identification of translocations involving the *EWS* gene on chromosome 22 and members of the *ETS* oncogene family, suggesting the underlying biology of these malignancies is the same. These similar clinical and molecular findings have resulted in the previously described entities of classic Ewing sarcoma of bone, Askin tumors of the chest wall, and extraskeletal primitive neuroectodermal tumors all being now considered as part of the broader Ewing's family of tumors (EFT) (Delattre, Zucman *et al.* 1994).

EFT has a reported incidence of 2.93 per million in the US population under 20 years, making it the second most common bone cancer in children and young adults behind osteosarcoma (Esiashvili, Goodman *et al.* 2008). There is a slight male predominance, and most patients are diagnosed in their teenage years or early twenties. Patients generally present with a mass or tumor-related pain. The pelvis and femur are the two most common locations for primary tumors, although virtually any area of the body can be affected. Metastases are evident at the time of diagnosis in approximately one-fourth of patients, with the lungs being the most common site followed by other bones and/or bone marrow.

Tissue biopsy is required to establish the diagnosis. Pathologic findings suggestive of EFT include sheets of small round blue cells which have membranous staining for CD99, a cell surface marker which is invariably expressed but not specific to this tumor type. Immunohistochemistry is used to distinguish these tumors from other small round blue cell malignancies of childhood, such as rhabdomyosarcoma. In most cases, the diagnosis is confirmed by identification of an *EWS*-containing translocation, such as the *EWS-FLI-1* translocation that is seen in approximately 85% of Ewing sarcoma family of tumors (de Alava and Gerald 2000). There are multiple other partners for EWS that are seen at a much lower frequency. *EWS* is a RNA-binding protein that, when fused to the transcription factor *FLI-1*, results in upregulation or downregulation of target gene transcription, leading to malignant transformation (Erkizan, Uversky *et al.* 2010).

One critical feature of Ewing sarcoma is the high likelihood for patients to develop distant metastases even if they undergo complete surgical resection or radiotherapy of what appears to be a localized tumor. For example, only 10% of patients can be cured with surgery or irradiation alone, even in the absence of identifiable metastatic disease on imaging or conventional bone marrow analysis at the time of diagnosis (Johnson and Humphreys 1969). The cause of recurrence in this situation is felt to be occult tumor cells that are present in the blood or bone marrow at levels below the limits of routine detection. These residual tumor cells escape local therapies and eventually go on to form fatal lung metastases. Chemotherapy is now used to help eradicate this so-called micrometastatic disease, and since the use of systemic chemotherapy began in the 1970s, 5-year survival rates have steadily improved to the point that up to three-fourths of newly-diagnosed patients with localized tumors can be expected to be long-term survivors with current therapies (Balamuth and Womer 2010).

Because EFT is more responsive to chemotherapy than other adult-type bone or soft tissue sarcomas, the current treatment paradigm is that all patients receive a combination of systemic chemotherapy as well as local treatment with surgery and/or radiation. While this approach has been helpful for many

ESFT patients, treatment still fails in some cases, and cure rates remain low for those with recurrent or initially metastatic tumors. In the following sections, we outline the treatment philosophies and regimens that have been used in the past and are currently being employed. In addition, we discuss how the identification of new therapeutic targets can be exploited through the use of novel tumor-specific agents.

2   Evolution of Treatment Strategies for EFT

As mentioned, cure was quite uncommon for patients treated prior to the use of adjuvant chemotherapy (Johnson and Humphreys 1969). Beginning in the late 1960s, early reports of responses to single-agent chemotherapy in patients with metastatic EFT began to emerge. There were a limited number of chemotherapy agents available at that time, and their use was mainly empiric. Interestingly, many of those initial agents are still used today, including vinca alkaloids (vincristine), anthracyclines (doxorubicin), and alkylators (cyclophosphamide). Nevertheless, drug resistance to single agents developed rapidly, and survival rates were not consistently improved until the advent of multi-agent regimens (Rosen, Wollner et al. 1974; Jaffe, Paed et al. 1976). For example, in one small series, adjuvant combination chemotherapy using vincristine, dactinomycin, and cyclophosphamide (VAC) in addition to radiation for local control resulted in 7 of 9 patients with local disease surviving for more than four years after therapy, a dramatic increase from 27% survival in patients treated with single-agent chemotherapy and radiation (Jaffe, Paed et al. 1976). This study, and others like it, highlights the role of both local control and systemic multiagent chemotherapy to eradicate micrometastatic disease and overcome drug resistance.

The advances in survival noted in small retrospective studies using historical controls led to more robust prospective studies using combination chemotherapy in the adjuvant setting. Because of the rarity of EFT, randomized studies to convincingly establish the efficacy of therapy required collaboration between multiple institutions. One of the first such trials was the Intergroup Ewing's Sarcoma Study (IESS), which randomized patients with localized EFT following radiation to receive one of the following regimens: 1) VAC, 2) VAC plus doxorubicin (VACA), or 3) VACA plus bilateral pulmonary radiation (VACA + BPR). Patients treated with VACA had a 5-year relapse-free survival (RFS) rate of 60% and 5-year overall survival (OS) rate of 65%, which was significantly better than the other two arms(Nesbit, Gehan et al. 1990). These results highlighted the importance of including doxorubicin in the treatment regimen, and also showed that prophylactic lung irradiation did not help prevent fatal lung metastases in patients with localized disease. Based on the results of this study, VACA then became the standard chemotherapy regimen for non-metastatic EFT. The second intergroup study, IESS-2, demonstrated improved relapse-free and overall survival with higher intermittent doses of doxorubicin (5-year RFS 73%, OS 77%) versus lower continuous dosing (5-year RFS 56%, OS 63%), establishing that anthracycline dose intensity was important for optimizing treatment (Burgert, Nesbit et al. 1990).

The next logical step was to consider adding further agents as they became available, such as ifosfamide and etoposide (IE), to the VACA backbone. In the INT-0091 study conducted by the combined Children's Cancer Group and Pediatric Oncology Group cooperative groups, VACA + IE demonstrated an 5-year event-free survival (EFS) of 69% and an OS 72% compared with the standard VACA (54% and 61%, respectively)(Grier, Krailo et al. 2003). Interestingly, patients with metastatic disease treated on this study showed no benefit to the addition of IE to the standard VACA backbone.

Attempts to further improve efficacy of standard cytotoxic regimens focused on escalating the intensity of therapy either by increasing the doses of the alkylating agents (cyclophosphamide and ifosfamide), or by decreasing the interval between cycles. While increasing alkylator doses at set intervals of 3 weeks did not improve outcomes (Granowetter, Womer *et al.* 2009), the recently completed Children's Oncology Group (COG) study AEWS0031 did show that compressing the intervals of standard-dose chemotherapy from 3 to 2 weeks improved the 3-year EFS to 76% compared to 65% with 3 week cycles (Womer, West *et al.* 2008). These encouraging results from AEWS0031 have helped to establish this regimen using interval compression as the current standard of care for localized EFT in North America.

3   Current Therapeutic Strategies

3.1   Localized Disease

The presence of identifiable metastatic disease at initial diagnosis is one of the strongest prognostic factors in EFT. For example, roughly 3 in 4 patients with localized tumors can be long-term survivors, compared to approximately 1 in 4 patients with identifiable metastases(Balamuth and Womer 2010) Therefore, current clinical trials generally stratify patients based on this important risk factor. The usual strategy for incorporation of new agents is to first demonstrate activity in the relapsed setting, and then add these drugs onto a standard therapeutic backbone so as not to compromise the efficacy for newly-diagnosed patients with potentially curable tumors. Current strategies in North America for localized EFT build on the backbone of vincristine/doxorubicin/cyclophosphamide alternating with ifosfamide/etoposide, using interval compression as discussed above. The Children's Oncology Group is now performing a randomized Phase III trial comparing this standard treatment with the same regimen + cassettes of cyclophosphamide/topotecan, based on two studies showing responses in approximately one-third of patients with recurrent EFT who were treated with this drug pair (Saylors, Stine *et al.* 2001; Hunold, Weddeling *et al.* 2006). Topotecan is a camptothecin agent which poisons the topoisomerase I enzyme that relieves torsional strain in DNA, and has shown activity against other "small round blue cell tumors" of childhood such as neuroblastoma (London, Frantz *et al.* 2010). The activity of camptothecins is enhanced when using DNA-damaging agents like cyclophosphamide, which is an important observation given that topotecan alone had insufficient activity to be developed as a single agent (Blaney, Needle *et al.* 1998). Children and young adults treated on this international COG Phase III study undergo 6 cycles of induction chemotherapy, followed by local control of the primary tumor with either surgery and/or radiotherapy. Patients then go on to complete11 remaining cycles of chemotherapy.

In Europe, the treatment strategy also factors in other known risk factors, such as the size of the primary tumor and the histologic response of the primary tumor to induction chemotherapy. A four-drug combination of vincristine/ifosfamide/doxorubicin/etoposide (VIDE regimen) is administered in three-week cycles, followed by local control of the primary tumor site. Patients with smaller tumors and favorable histologic response to induction chemotherapy go on to receive maintenance therapy with either VAC, or with vincristine/actinomycin/ifosfamide (VAI). No randomized trials have directly compared these two similar but somewhat different cooperative group chemotherapy strategies.

3.2   Metastatic Disease

Unfortunately, progress has lagged behind in the treatment of patients with metastatic disease, with long-term cure rates being frustratingly stable over the decades. Interventions that improve survival in patients with localized disease, such as the addition of ifosfamide and etoposide, do not have proven benefit in metastatic patients (Grier, Krailo *et al.* 2003), presumably because of inherent biological differences in metastatic tumors that make them less responsive to conventional therapy. Interestingly, the site of metastases has impact on the prognosis, as patients with metastases limited to the lungs have improved outcomes compared to those with bone or bone marrow metastases, who rarely survive(Pinkerton, Bataillard *et al.* 2001). This difference in prognosis is likely not just related to tumor burden, but also reflects underlying biological differences between these patients.

Because alkylating agents have a steep dose-response curve, there has been investigation of very high-dose, myeloablative chemotherapy followed by rescue with peripheral blood stem cells as a way to further intensify treatment. This so-called "megatherapy" with alkylating drugs like busulfan and melphalan has theoretical appeal, but has not consistently showed improvement in the highest-risk patients such as those with bone or bone marrow metastases (Ladenstein, Lasset *et al.* 1995; Meyers, Krailo *et al.* 2001). The ongoing European EuroEWING-99 study is the first to address the issue of autologous transplantation in a prospective randomized fashion, comparing megatherapy after local control with continued standard-dose chemotherapy in patients with unfavorable histologic response to induction or lung metastases.

In the US, new trials are being developed that will likely incorporate targeted agents described in detail below, as well as a different alkylator/camptothecin combination. In the same way the drug pair of cyclophosphamide/topotecan showed activity in relapsed patients and is now being incorporated into front-line trials, the combination of the alkylating agent temozolomide and the camptothecin irinotecan has also shown responses in patients with recurrent disease, including those resistant to topotecan (Wagner, McAllister *et al.* 2007; Casey, Wexler *et al.* 2009; Wagner 2011).

It is for this high-risk population of patients with metastatic disease that new therapies are most needed. Over the past two decades, at least a dozen other conventional chemotherapy agents apart have been studied in Phase II trials, including cytarabine, vinorelbine, pemetrexed, ixabepilone, oxaliplatin, vinblastine, and the combination of gemcitabine and docetaxel. While occasional responses have been seen, in general the results are disappointing and suggest that further benefit is unlikely to come from either conventional cytotoxic agents or additional manipulation of dose intensity or dose density. Thus, interest has now turned to so-called "targeted therapies," which in contrast to conventional cytotoxics that indiscriminately kill rapidly dividing cells, are purported to selectively interfere with key pathways that are uniquely activated in tumor cells. The promise of targeted therapies is that they can more effectively eradicate tumor cells, while reducing life-affecting or life-threatening toxicities associated with conventional therapies such as severe infection, cardiomyopathy, or secondary cancers. In the following section, we present some examples of targeted therapies and their potential application for EFT.

4   Potential Molecular Targets for Therapy

4.1   Direct Inhibition of the EWS-FLI1 Fusion Protein

Perhaps the most appealing target in Ewing's sarcoma is the oncogenic fusion protein EWS-FLI1 which results from the t(11:22) translocation seen in 85% of EFTs. Oncogenic fusion proteins are attractive targets due to their presence in tumor cells and absence in normal tissues. In fact, the age of targeted therapy was ushered in with the development of imatinib and related compounds, which target the t(9;22) translocation that characterizes chronic myelogenous leukemia (Yeung and Hughes 2012).

EWS-FLI1 is a dysregulated transcriptional protein which can transform mesenchymal stem cells so they produce colonies with morphological, immunhistochemical and gene expression profiles similar to Ewing sarcoma tumors (Erkizan, Uversky *et al.* 2010). Historically, transcription factors have been considered "undruggable," but new strategies using anti-sense DNA and siRNA targeting *EWS-FLI1* have shown promise in cell lines and xenografts (Takigami, Ohno *et al.* 2011). However, while the delivery of anti-sense DNA and siRNAs is an excellent way to demonstrate proof of principle, clinical application of this strategy has been limited by feasibility. Recently, high through-put screening of chemical libraries have identified small molecule inhibitors of the EWS-FLI1 protein, including the antitumor antibiotic mithramycin and the DNA-modulating agent trabectidin (Erkizan, Kong *et al.* 2009; Grohar, Griffin *et al.* 2011; Grohar, Woldemichael *et al.* 2011). Of note, mithramycin is an older agent used in the 1960s to treat testicular cancer and malignancy-associated hypercalcemia, and it is now being currently investigated in clinical trials for EFT based on these preclinical findings. On the other hand, a Phase II trial of trabectidin has recently been completed by the Children's Oncology Group, and showed very little activity despite the encouraging preclinical results (Baruchel, Pappo *et al.* 2012). A similar experience has been seen with cytarabine, a nucleoside analogue used to treat leukemia. A signature-based small molecule screening process suggested that this agent may have activity against EFT, and preclinical studies showed that cytarabine downregulated EWS-FLI1 protein expression *in vitro*, producing gene expression patterns similar to when EFT cells are treated with RNA interference to knock down EWS-FLI1 (Stegmaier, Wong *et al.* 2007). Further, those investigators showed that use of cytarabine to treat mouse xenografts harboring human EFT resulted in significant growth inhibition. However, despite this strong preclinical rationale, a recent Phase II trial also showed disappointing results for this agent (DuBois, Krailo *et al.* 2009). These examples demonstrate that compelling rationale and activity seen in the laboratory does not always translate into clinical effectiveness.

4.2   PARP Inhibition

Leveraging the power of high-throughput cell line screening against genomic analysis has identified heretofore unappreciated targets. This functional genomics approach recently identified Poly (ADP-ribose) polymerase (PARP) as a target for inhibition in Ewing's cell lines that harbor the *EWS-FLI1* translocation. In one screen, 630 cells lines from adult and pediatric cancers were tested against 130 compounds, including traditional cytotoxic chemotherapeutics and molecularly targeted agents which were both approved drugs and experimental agents. In total, over 48,000 drug/cell line combinations were tested. Genomic characterization of the 630 cells lines was performed, including exon sequencing of 64 known cancer-causing genes, copy number analysis by Affymetrix SNP6.0 microarrays, and expression profiling using Affymetrix HT-U133A microarrays. Of note, cell lines containing the *EWS-FLI1* translocation were sensitive to PARP inhibition with experimental agents such as olaparib and AG-014699 (Garnett, Edelman *et al.* 2012). PARP inhibitors interfere with the ability of cells to repair single-stranded breaks in their DNA, which lead to double-stranded breaks during DNA replication. Cells with deficient homologous recombination repair pathways, like those with *BRCA* mutations, are particularly sensitive to PARP inhibition, because they accumulate irreparable double-stranded breaks that lead to cell death. PARP inhibitor activity had been identified in *BRCA1* and *BRCA2* deficient cancers, but not previously in Ewing sarcoma cells, which were thought to have intact homologous recombination repair pathways. In a separate study, PARP inhibition with the investigational agent olaparib was shown to disrupt survival and invasion capacity of multiple Ewing sarcoma cell lines harboring the *EWS-FLI1* translocation. Additionally,

EFT xenografts showed significant growth delay with olaparib monotherapy, and synergy with sustained complete responses for 30 days with combined temozolomide treatment (Brenner, Feng *et al.* 2012). In this study, olaparib appears to function by both potentiating DNA damage and by inhibiting transcription of the *EWS-FLI1* fusion gene by interfering with a PARP1: EWS-FLI1 positive feedback loop. These results show the promise of a functional genomics approach where high-throughput drug screening is coupled with genomic analysis to identify novel targets in specific tumor types, although these results have not yet been confirmed in the clinic.

4.3   Insulin-like Growth Factor Type 1 Receptor Antibodies

The insulin-like growth factor type 1 Receptor (IGF-1R) has long been considered a promising target for the treatment of EFT. IGF-1R is a transmembrane tyrosine kinase receptor that when bound to either of its two ligands, IGF-1 or IGF-2, activates pathways involved in proliferation (Ras/Raf/MAPK) and survival (PI3K/AKT/mTOR) (Olmos, Tan *et al.* 2010). EFT cell lines and primary tumors strongly express IGF-1R as well as both ligands, suggesting there may be an autocrine stimulation driving tumor growth (Scotlandi, Benini *et al.* 1996). Preclinical studies targeting IGF-1R with either monoclonal antibodies or small molecule inhibitors have shown activity in cell lines and xenograft models (Scotlandi, Manara *et al.* 2005). Early small molecule inhibitors to IGF-1R also had substantial inhibition of the insulin receptor, which can impair glucose control. Therefore, monoclonal antibodies reached clinical development first, and impressive tumor reduction and prolonged stable disease was seen in these early trials (Tolcher, Sarantopoulos *et al.* 2009; Olmos, Postel-Vinay *et al.* 2010; Malempati, Weigel *et al.* 2012). These responses, as well as the presence of IGF-1R expression in a wide variety of solid tumors other than sarcoma, led to the clinical development of at least 8 different IGF-1R antibodies. Unfortunately, larger Phase II trials did not confirm high response rates in relapsed EFT patients in the three studies reported to date. For example, response rates have ranged from 6-14%, with median progression-free survival of 1.9-7.9 months (Juergens, Daw *et al.* 2011; Pappo, Patel *et al.* 2011; Tap, Demetri *et al.* 2012). These results have dampened enthusiasm for the use of IGF-1R antibodies as a single-agent, but it remains possible that they might be useful in the right clinical context, such as in combination with other agents, or in the setting of very low tumor burden.

5   Role of Biomarkers to Predict Response

The clinical experience with IGF-1R has been a good demonstration of how rational targets can be identified through basic science research, evaluated preclinically in xenograft models through translational research, and then tested in patients through clinical research. The development of this class of agents also highlights the difficulties in determining the optimal application of a drug. For example, although some striking and durable clinical responses have been achieved with IGF-1R antibodies, the overall activity in larger studies has been relatively low, and does not justify further investigation as a single agent to treat patient with bulky tumors. However, it is possible that such a drug could be synergistic with other chemotherapy agents, or could be beneficial as maintenance therapy in high-risk patients who appear to be in remission and have completed all of planned conventional chemotherapy. More importantly, if there was a way to prospectively identify the 10 – 15% of patients with recurrent Ewing sarcoma who benefit from this treatment, then clinical trials could be "enriched" for these patients and it would be predicted that response rates would be much higher. Such a strategy has been seen with other targeted therapies used in adult cancers (Sequist, Bell *et al.* 2007), although this usually involves identification of a mutation in the therapeutic target, which has not been described with IGF-1R in Ewing sarcoma. Thus, there is a focused effort to identify other potential predictive biomarkers that could suggest a response to this therapy.

Expression of IGF-1R on tumor cells intuitively seems a necessary requirement for benefit from IGF-1R antibodies, but it is clear that this factor alone cannot be used to stratify patients. In fact, most Ewing sarcoma primary tumors express this target (Scotlandi, Benini *et al.* 1996), but responses are seen in only a minority. Assuming the receptor is effectively neutralized by the antibody, how then can growth of tumor cells be maintained? One possibility is redundant growth signaling through other cell surface receptors. Recent preclinical work has suggested that signaling of IGF-2 through the structurally similar insulin receptor (IR) is not abrogated using conventional anti-IGF-1R antibodies, and may serve as a mechanism of resistance to this therapy. For example, Garofalo *et al.* report that tumors with a low IGF-1R:IR ratio are unlikely to benefit from IGF-1R antibody therapy (Garofalo, Manara *et al.* 2011). When examining 109 archival Ewing sarcoma tumor samples by immunohistochemistry, 60% were determined to have high IGF-1R expression, while 81% had high expression of insulin receptor A, and an inverse correlation was present such that tumors with great expression of IR had less IGF-1R expression. These findings would be consistent with the relatively low rate of objective responses to single-agent IGF-1R antibodies. The clinical impact of insulin receptor expression in still unknown, but will be assessed prospectively in a study of an IGF-1R antibody combined with an inhibitor of mammalian target of rapamycin (mTOR) currently being conducted through the Children's Oncology Group. That study will also use immunohistochemistry to assess for other potential signaling pathways that could contribute to resistance from IGF-1R antibodies, such as ERK (Subbiah, Naing *et al.* 2011) and RON (Potratz, Saunders *et al.* 2010). It is likely that identification of predictive biomarkers will be necessary for these agents to continue to be used in the clinic.

The trial mentioned above reflects the growing enthusiasm to combine targeted agents to maximize efficacy and circumvent tumor cell resistance. This can be done by targeting multiple cell surface receptors, using a so-called "horizontal inhibition" approach. For example, the small molecule OSI-906 is designed to inhibit both the IGF-1R as well as the insulin receptor, which theoretically may eliminate one mechanism of tumor cell resistance (Mulvihill, Cooke *et al.* 2009). Alternatively, one can inhibit two separate targets within the same pathway, using "vertical inhibition." This strategy has been effective in preclinical testing which shows that upstream blockade of IGF-1R is synergistic with downstream inhibition of mTOR in preclinical models of Ewing sarcoma (Kurmasheva, Dudkin *et al.* 2009). Benefits have been seen with either simultaneous administration, or as demonstrated by Cao *et al.*, the later addition of rapamycin to treat mice bearing rhabdomyosarcoma xenografts which were failing therapy with IGF-1R antibody (Cao, Yu *et al.* 2008). Similar findings were also seen in Ewing sarcoma patients, who benefitted from the addition of an mTOR inhibitor following progression with single-agent IGF-1R antibody therapy (Subbiah, Naing *et al.* 2011). This synergy is presumably from either IGF-1R blockade working upstream of Akt, or mTOR inhibition working downstream of Akt, suggesting that these two agents function together to abrogate escape pathways that result from single-agent therapy. Promising activity in early adult clinical trials has now been reported with this combination (Naing, LoRusso *et al.* 2012; Schwartz, Tap *et al.* 2012), and will be further assessed by the ongoing COG study. Of note, one of the recently completed adult trials of an IGF-1R antibody and an mTOR inhibitor stratified patients based on the presence or absence of IGF-1R expression in tumor tissue. Rates of disease stabilization were similar between groups (Schwartz, Tap *et al.* 2012), again demonstrating the complexity of this process and that expression of the purported "target" is not the only factor which determines clinical benefit.

6   Conclusions

When compared to many adult-type sarcomas, EFT is different in both its tendency for metastatic disease to develop despite adequate local control, and its relative responsiveness to chemotherapy. These features have underscored the need for systemic therapy, and thoughtful clinical testing of well-formed hypotheses has resulted in up to three-fourths of patients with localized tumors remaining free of disease five years after diagnosis. However, patients with identifiable metastases at diagnosis, or those with recurrent tumors after initial therapy, generally have resistant tumors for which new therapies are necessary, as further modifications of conventional agents are unlikely to result in substantial improvement. Instead, the current focus is on identifying new molecular targets which can be therapeutically exploited, with the potential for improved efficacy and less toxicity. The examples offered here show not only the promise but also the complexity and frustrations of targeted therapy, and underscore our need for better understanding of the mechanisms of action and resistance of these drugs so that we can more effectively develop these agents and apply them to the specific population most likely to benefit.

References

Balamuth, N. J. and R. B. Womer (2010). "Ewing's sarcoma." The Lancet Oncology 11(2): 184-192.

Baruchel, S., A. Pappo, et al. (2012). "A phase 2 trial of trabectedin in children with recurrent rhabdomyosarcoma, Ewing sarcoma and non-rhabdomyosarcoma soft tissue sarcomas: a report from the Children's Oncology Group." European Journal of Cancer 48(4): 579-585.

Blaney, S. M., M. N. Needle, et al. (1998). "Phase II trial of topotecan administered as 72-hour continuous infusion in children with refractory solid tumors: a collaborative Pediatric Branch, National Cancer Institute, and Children's Cancer Group Study." Clinical Cancer Research 4(2): 357-360.

Brenner, J. C., F. Y. Feng, et al. (2012). "PARP-1 inhibition as a targeted strategy to treat Ewing's sarcoma." Cancer Research 72(7): 1608-1613.

Burgert, E. O., Jr., M. E. Nesbit, et al. (1990). "Multimodal therapy for the management of nonpelvic, localized Ewing's sarcoma of bone: intergroup study IESS-II." Journal of Clinical Oncology 8(9): 1514-1524.

Cao, L., Y. Yu, et al. (2008). "Addiction to elevated insulin-like growth factor I receptor and initial modulation of the AKT pathway define the responsiveness of rhabdomyosarcoma to the targeting antibody." Cancer Research 68(19): 8039-8048.

Casey, D. A., L. H. Wexler, et al. (2009). "Irinotecan and temozolomide for Ewing sarcoma: the Memorial Sloan-Kettering experience." Pediatric Blood & Cancer 53(6): 1029-1034.

de Alava, E. and W. L. Gerald (2000). "Molecular biology of the Ewing's sarcoma/primitive neuroectodermal tumor family." Journal of Clinical Oncology 18(1): 204-213.

Delattre, O., J. Zucman, et al. (1994). "The Ewing family of tumors--a subgroup of small-round-cell tumors defined by specific chimeric transcripts." The New England Journal of Medicine 331(5): 294-299.

DuBois, S. G., M. D. Krailo, et al. (2009). "Phase II study of intermediate-dose cytarabine in patients with relapsed or refractory Ewing sarcoma: a report from the Children's Oncology Group." Pediatric Blood & Cancer 52(3): 324-327.

Erkizan, H. V., Y. Kong, et al. (2009). "A small molecule blocking oncogenic protein EWS-FLI1 interaction with RNA helicase A inhibits growth of Ewing's sarcoma." Nature Medicine 15(7): 750-756.

Erkizan, H. V., V. N. Uversky, et al. (2010). "Oncogenic partnerships: EWS-FLI1 protein interactions initiate key pathways of Ewing's sarcoma." Clinical Cancer Research **16**(16): 4077-4083.

Esiashvili, N., M. Goodman, et al. (2008). "Changes in incidence and survival of Ewing sarcoma patients over the past 3 decades: Surveillance Epidemiology and End Results data." Journal of Pediatric Hematology/Oncology **30**(6): 425-430.

Ewing, J. (1972). "Classics in oncology. Diffuse endothelioma of bone. James Ewing. Proceedings of the New York Pathological Society, 1921." CA**22**(2): 95-98.

Garnett, M. J., E. J. Edelman, et al. (2012). "Systematic identification of genomic markers of drug sensitivity in cancer cells." Nature**483**(7391): 570-575.

Garofalo, C., M. C. Manara, et al. (2011). "Efficacy of and resistance to anti-IGF-1R therapies in Ewing's sarcoma is dependent on insulin receptor signaling." Oncogene **30**(24): 2730-2740.

Granowetter, L., R. Womer, et al. (2009). "Dose-intensified compared with standard chemotherapy for nonmetastatic Ewing sarcoma family of tumors: a Children's Oncology Group Study." Journal of Clinical Oncology **27**(15): 2536-2541.

Grier, H. E., M. D. Krailo, et al. (2003). "Addition of ifosfamide and etoposide to standard chemotherapy for Ewing's sarcoma and primitive neuroectodermal tumor of bone." The New England Journal of Medicine **348**(8): 694-701.

Grohar, P. J., L. B. Griffin, et al. (2011). "Ecteinascidin 743 interferes with the activity of EWS-FLI1 in Ewing sarcoma cells." Neoplasia **13**(2): 145-153.

Grohar, P. J., G. M. Woldemichael, et al. (2011). "Identification of an inhibitor of the EWS-FLI1 oncogenic transcription factor by high-throughput screening." Journal of the National Cancer Institute **103**(12): 962-978.

Hunold, A., N. Weddeling, et al. (2006). "Topotecan and cyclophosphamide in patients with refractory or relapsed Ewing tumors." Pediatric Blood & Cancer **47**(6): 795-800.

Jaffe, N., D. Paed, et al. (1976). "Improved outlook for Ewing's sarcoma with combination chemotherapy (vincristine, actinomycin D and cyclophosphamide) and radiation therapy." Cancer **38**(5): 1925-1930.

Johnson, R. and S. R. Humphreys (1969). "Past failures and future possibilities in Ewing's sarcoma. Experimental and preliminary clinical results." Cancer **23**(1): 161-166.

Juergens, H., N. C. Daw, et al. (2011). "Preliminary efficacy of the anti-insulin-like growth factor type 1 receptor antibody figitumumab in patients with refractory Ewing sarcoma." Journal of Clinical Oncology **29**(34): 4534-4540.

Kurmasheva, R. T., L. Dudkin, et al. (2009). "The insulin-like growth factor-1 receptor-targeting antibody, CP-751,871, suppresses tumor-derived VEGF and synergizes with rapamycin in models of childhood sarcoma." Cancer Research**69**(19): 7662-7671.

Ladenstein, R., C. Lasset, et al. (1995). "Impact of megatherapy in children with high-risk Ewing's tumours in complete remission: a report from the EBMT Solid Tumour Registry." Bone Marrow Transplantation **15**(5): 697-705.

London, W. B., C. N. Frantz, et al. (2010). "Phase II randomized comparison of topotecan plus cyclophosphamide versus topotecan alone in children with recurrent or refractory neuroblastoma: a Children's Oncology Group study." Journal of Clinical Oncology **28**(24): 3808-3815.

Malempati, S., B. Weigel, et al. (2012). "Phase I/II trial and pharmacokinetic study of cixutumumab in pediatric patients with refractory solid tumors and Ewing sarcoma: a report from the Children's Oncology Group." Journal of Clinical Oncology **30**(3): 256-262.

Meyers, P. A., M. D. Krailo, et al. (2001). "High-dose melphalan, etoposide, total-body irradiation, and autologous stem-cell reconstitution as consolidation therapy for high-risk Ewing's sarcoma does not improve prognosis." Journal of Clinical Oncology **19**(11): 2812-2820.

Mulvihill, M. J., A. Cooke, et al. (2009). "Discovery of OSI-906: a selective and orally efficacious dual inhibitor of the IGF-1 receptor and insulin receptor." Future Medicinal Chemistry **1**(6): 1153-1171.

Naing, A., P. LoRusso, et al. (2012). "Insulin growth factor-receptor (IGF-1R) antibody cixutumumab combined with the mTOR inhibitor temsirolimus in patients with refractory Ewing's sarcoma family tumors." Clinical Cancer Research 18(9): 2625-2631.

Nesbit, M. E., Jr., E. A. Gehan, et al. (1990). "Multimodal therapy for the management of primary, nonmetastatic Ewing's sarcoma of bone: a long-term follow-up of the First Intergroup study." Journal of Clinical Oncology 8(10): 1664-1674.

Olmos, D., S. Postel-Vinay, et al. (2010). "Safety, pharmacokinetics, and preliminary activity of the anti-IGF-1R antibody figitumumab (CP-751,871) in patients with sarcoma and Ewing's sarcoma: a phase 1 expansion cohort study." The Lancet Oncology 11(2): 129-135.

Olmos, D., D. S. Tan, et al. (2010). "Biological rationale and current clinical experience with anti-insulin-like growth factor 1 receptor monoclonal antibodies in treating sarcoma: twenty years from the bench to the bedside." Cancer Journal 16(3): 183-194.

Pappo, A. S., S. R. Patel, et al. (2011). "R1507, a monoclonal antibody to the insulin-like growth factor 1 receptor, in patients with recurrent or refractory Ewing sarcoma family of tumors: results of a phase II Sarcoma Alliance for Research through Collaboration study." Journal of Clinical Oncology 29(34): 4541-4547.

Pinkerton, C. R., A. Bataillard, et al. (2001). "Treatment strategies for metastatic Ewing's sarcoma." European Journal of Cancer 37(11): 1338-1344.

Potratz, J. C., D. N. Saunders, et al. (2010). "Synthetic lethality screens reveal RPS6 and MST1R as modifiers of insulin-like growth factor-1 receptor inhibitor activity in childhood sarcomas." Cancer Research 70(21): 8770-8781.

Rosen, G., N. Wollner, et al. (1974). "Proceedings: Disease-free survival in children with Ewing's sarcoma treated with radiation therapy and adjuvant four-drug sequential chemotherapy." Cancer 33(2): 384-393.

Saylors, R. L., 3rd, K. C. Stine, et al. (2001). "Cyclophosphamide plus topotecan in children with recurrent or refractory solid tumors: a Pediatric Oncology Group phase II study." Journal of Clinical Oncology 19(15): 3463-3469.

Schwartz, G. K., W. D. Tap, et al. (2012). "A phase II multicenter study of the IGF-1 receptor antibody cixutumumab (A12) and the mTOR inhibitor temsirolimus (TEM) in patients (pts) with refractory IGF-1R positive (+) and negative (-) bone and soft tissue sarcomas (STS)." Journal of Clinical Oncology 30(15_suppl): 10003.

Scotlandi, K., S. Benini, et al. (1996). "Insulin-like growth factor I receptor-mediated circuit in Ewing's sarcoma/peripheral neuroectodermal tumor: a possible therapeutic target." Cancer Research 56(20): 4570-4574.

Scotlandi, K., M. C. Manara, et al. (2005). "Antitumor activity of the insulin-like growth factor-I receptor kinase inhibitor NVP-AEW541 in musculoskeletal tumors." Cancer Research 65(9): 3868-3876.

Sequist, L. V., D. W. Bell, et al. (2007). "Molecular predictors of response to epidermal growth factor receptor antagonists in non-small-cell lung cancer." Journal of Clinical Oncology 25(5): 587-595.

Stegmaier, K., J. S. Wong, et al. (2007). "Signature-based small molecule screening identifies cytosine arabinoside as an EWS/FLI modulator in Ewing sarcoma." PLoS Medicine 4(4): e122.

Subbiah, V., A. Naing, et al. (2011). "Targeted morphoproteomic profiling of Ewing's sarcoma treated with insulin-like growth factor 1 receptor (IGF1R) inhibitors: response/resistance signatures." PLoS one 6(4): e18424.

Takigami, I., T. Ohno, et al. (2011). "Synthetic siRNA targeting the breakpoint of EWS/Fli-1 inhibits growth of Ewing sarcoma xenografts in a mouse model." International Cournal of Cancer 128(1): 216-226.

Tap, W. D., G. Demetri, et al. (2012). "Phase II study of ganitumab, a fully human anti-type-1 insulin-like growth factor receptor antibody, in patients with metastatic Ewing family tumors or desmoplastic small round cell tumors." Journal of Clinical Oncology 30(15): 1849-1856.

Tolcher, A. W., J. Sarantopoulos, et al. (2009). "Phase I, pharmacokinetic, and pharmacodynamic study of AMG 479, a fully human monoclonal antibody to insulin-like growth factor receptor 1." Journal of Clinical Oncology 27(34): 5800-5807.

*Wagner, L. (2011). "Camptothecin-based regimens for treatment of ewing sarcoma: past studies and future directions." Sarcoma **2011**: 957957.*

*Wagner, L. M., N. McAllister, et al. (2007). "Temozolomide and intravenous irinotecan for treatment of advanced Ewing sarcoma." Pediatric Blood & Cancer **48**(2): 132-139.*

*Womer, R. B., D. C. West, et al. (2008). "Randomized comparison of every-two-week v. every-three-week chemotherapy in Ewing sarcoma family tumors (ESFT)." Journal of Clinical Oncology **26**(15_suppl): 10504.*

*Yeung, D. T. and T. P. Hughes (2012). "Therapeutic targeting of BCR-ABL: prognostic markers of response and resistance mechanism in chronic myeloid leukaemia." Critical Reviews in Oncogenesis **17**(1): 17-30.*

Animal Models of Cancer in Light of Evolutionary Biology and Complexity Science

Ray Greek

Americans For Medical Advancement

1   Survival Rates

David Scott, Director of Science Funding at Cancer Research UK, writing about the use animals in cancer research opened his article by stating: "More people are surviving cancer than ever before." (Scott 2011) He provided a link to the statistics on which he based the statement and went on todeclare: "Thanks to decades of research, survival from cancer has doubled in the last 40 years, giving thousands of people more time with their loved ones." He attributed this to using animals in cancer research stating that this progress "simply wouldn't have been possible without animal research …… In some areas there's simply no other way to get the information needed to make progress against the disease." As I will show, such statements supporting the importance of animal-based research and testing are not unique. However before addressing the use of animals in cancer research, I will clarify the actual survival rates for cancer and show that the above is very misleading and probably disingenuous.

When the War on Cancer began in 1971, less than 50% of people diagnosed with cancer lived for five years. Currently, the 5-year survival for all cancers is around 67% (American Cancer Society 2012). Moreover, the original cancer does not usually kill the patient, rather the metastatic component does. The mortality rate from metastatic disease is essentially unchanged from the 1970s. So why have the 5-year survival rates changed so dramatically? The answer lies in overdiagnosis in general and specifically over-diagnosis secondary to *lead-time bias* and *length bias*.

Figure 1 illustrates lead-time bias, which is the apparent increase in survival rate because the cancer was diagnosed earlier because of screening. The cancer patient actually dies exactly when he would have died without the screening but the time from diagnosis to death is longer because the cancer is detected earlier. This means the therapy had no effect in terms of lengthening life. Furthermore, it means that the mortality rate is unchanged. Because of very aggressive *screening*, many cancers are being diagnosed much earlier than they otherwise would have been. More pre-cancerous lesions are also being diagnosed and counted in statistics even though many would never have proceeded to cancer. This *overdiagnosis* also factors into lead-time bias. Many cancers that are now diagnosed would never have killed the individual but are now counted in survival rate calculations. Along related lines, because of the emphasis on screening, cancers are now being diagnosed in the elderly that would not have been diagnosed a few decades ago. The elderly do not usually succumb to these cancers, which is why they were not screened for them in the past, yet they are now counted as survivors.

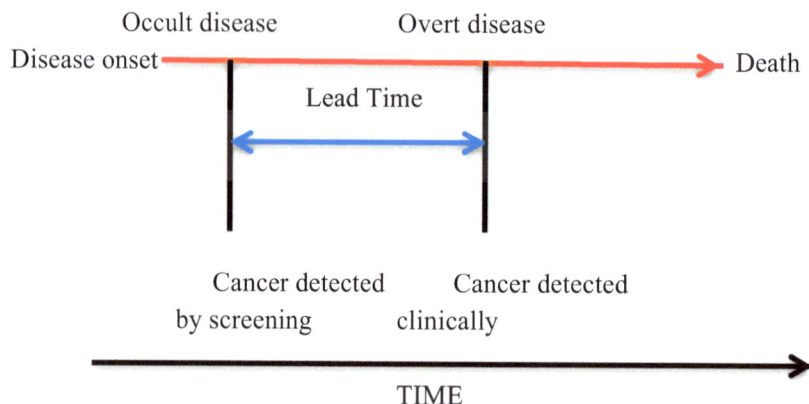

Figure 1: Lead-time bias

Length bias is similar to lead time bias in that it also allows an overestimate of survival because of faulty reasoning. Slowly progressing cancers are more likely to be detected by screens; they grow for a longer period of time hence there is a longer period of time in which to detect them. Rapidly growing cancers are less likely to be detected and more likely to result in death in a shorter period of time

There are other factors complicating the attempt to understand cancer survival rates. Cancer survival statistics are based on death certificates, which are very unreliable. The cause of death is usually given as the most proximate cause, for example pneumonia, when the actual cause, as well as the cause of the pneumonia, was the cancer. In part, the miscalculation of mortality and survival, including the reliance on death certificates, is due to the fact that autopsies are not performed with the same frequency they once were. Furthermore, the people receiving autopsies are disproportionately victims of non-disease, for example trauma patients, poisonings, and murder (Hendrick 2011). Without an autopsy, the actual cause of death may be missed or the more proximate cause may be listed as the primary cause.

This is not to say there are *no* chemotherapeutic agents that reliably treat cancer and extend life. Some of the leukemias have been treated successfully for decades and are no longer an automatic death sentence for the patient. Regardless of these advances in leukemia, the increase in survival rate referred to by David Scott in the opening paragraph is very misleading. There has been very little progress made in the War on Cancer. Statements such as Scott's are not uncommon among scientists and representatives of scientists who are engaged in research on cancer. I will now examine how animal models have been used during past five decades.

2 Prediction in Biomedical Science

Before examining the use of animal models specifically, I need to discuss prediction in biomedical science. Animals can be categorized into essentially nine areas of science and biomedical research (Table 1 (Greek & Shanks, 2009)). The two areas that concern cancer research and drug development for cancer are numbers 1 and 2, the use of animals as predictive models. Which leads us to the question of what the term *predict* means in science. *Predict* is used in basically two distinct ways in science. First, scientists generate hypotheses, which are then tested. The test usually involves a prediction about an unknown outcome and the hypothesis is strengthened or weakened, perhaps even falsified, by whether the prediction is found to be true. Thousands of predictions are generated by hypotheses and the validity or outcome of the prediction has no immediate meaning outside the specific context of the hypothesis.

This use of *predict* differs immensely from the way the word is used when judging the *predictive value* of a modality such as diagnostic test, research practice, medical intervention, or any practice that can be judged by realityor a gold standard (see Table 2). A modality, say a diagnostic test, is not being used to generate a hypothesis but rather to determine intervention. There are consequences to human health if the test does not do what the physician assumes it does. For example, if a chest x-ray reveals the absence of a pneumothorax (a collapsed lung) there is still a slight probability that the patient does in fact suffer from a pneumothorax. If the physician needs to be 100% certain that the patient does not have a pneumothorax, then a CT scan needs to be performed, as it is the gold standard for diagnosing the condition. All tests that might be useful in diagnosing a pneumothorax can be compared against the CT scan per table 2, because the CT scan is the gold standard.

1.	As predictive models for human disease
2.	As predictive models to evaluate human exposure safety in the context of pharmacology and toxicology (e.g., in drug testing)
3.	As sources of 'spare parts' (e.g., aortic valve replacements for humans)
4.	As bioreactors (e.g., as factories for the production of insulin, or monoclonal antibodies, or the fruits of genetic engineering)
5.	As sources of tissue in order to study basic physiological principles
6.	For dissection and study in education and medical training
7.	As heuristic devices to prompt new biological/biomedical hypotheses
8.	For the benefit of other nonhuman animals
9.	For the pursuit of scientific knowledge in and of itself

Table 1: Categories of animal use in science (Greek & Shanks 2009).

		Gold Standard	
		GS+	GS-
Test	T+	TP	FP
	T-	FN	TN
Sensitivity = TP/(TP+FN)			
Specificity = TN/(FP+TN)			
Positive Predictive Value = TP/(TP+FP)			
Negative Predictive Value = TN/(FN+TN)			
T- = Test negative			
T+ = Test positive			
FP = False positive			
TP = True positive			
FN = False negative			
TN = True negative			
GS- = Gold standard negative			
GS+ = Gold standard positive			

Table 2: Binary classification test. Allows calculations for determining how well a test or practice compares with reality or the gold standard.

When animal modelers claim that a model is predictive for humans be it for evaluating safety and efficacy or any other property of a drug, they are claiming that the positive predictive value (PPV) and negative predictive value (NPV) are high enough for the modality to be deemed predictive in biomedical science. The same applies when seeking to determine mechanisms of disease. When evaluating modalities in biomedical science and medical practice, PPVs and NPVs greater than 0.9 are needed if the modality is to be considered a predictive test, intervention, treatment, or practice. Ideally, NPVs and PPVs would be very close to 1.0. As we will see, animal models do not approach this standard and hence are not considered predictive for human response to drugs or disease, including cancer (Collins 2011; Cook *et al.* 2012; Dixit & Boelsterli 2007; Drake III *et al.* 2012; FDA 2006; Fletcher 1978; Greek & Greek 2010; Greek, Hansen, *et al.* 2011; Greek *et al.* 2012; Greek & Shanks 2009; Greek, Shanks, *et al.* 2011;

Heywood 1990; Horrobin 2003; Kola & Landis 2004; Lumley 1990; M.E. 2010; Markou *et al.* 2009; O'Collins *et al.* 2006; Shanks & Greek 2009; Shanks *et al.* 2009; Sharp & Langer 2011; Sietsema 1989; Suter 1990; Wall & Shani 2008; Weaver *et al.* 2003; Zielinska 2010).

3 Animal Models and Carcinogenesis

Over 400 chemicals had been discovered to cause cancer in animals (Gold *et al.* 1991; Ames & Gold 1990, 1990; Ames *et al.* 1996; Ashby & Paton 1993; Fung *et al.* 1993; McGregor *et al.* 1994) but only approximately 20-30 were shown to be definite carcinogens in humans as of the 1990s (Ennever *et al.* 1987; Stoloff 1992; Kleinman 1997). Performing the calculation for PPV, based on this data we find: 30 / (30 + 370) = 0.075. This is less than what one would expect from random chanceor just guessing which chemicals are carcinogens and is certainly unacceptable for a scientific modality. Other studies have been consistent with the 1990s datain that the PPV of animal models is far below what is acceptable in medical science (Coulston 1980; Abbott 2005; Anisimov *et al.* 2005; Salsburg 1983; Meijers *et al.* 1997; Dybing & Huitfeldt 1992; Dybing & Sanner 1999). Salsburg (1983) compared the predictive value of animal models for carcinogenesis to a coin toss. Granted, every chemical assessed in animal models does not have extensive epidemiological data proving the chemical is definitively *not* a human carcinogen. In light of intra-human differences, some of the chemicals probably could be carcinogens in some people at some time if given in high enough doses. However, this does not negate the fact that a vast majority of these chemicals are clearly not carcinogenic in a clinically significant manner or such would have been noted by physicians as well as individuals affected.

If all the chemicals that tested positive for carcinogenesis in animal models had been prevented from coming to the marketplace, society would have lost many valuable drugs as well as other chemicals. For example, isoniazid an anti-tuberculosis drug that has been used for decades, causes cancer in some animals (Clayson 1980; Shubick 1980). Phenobarbital, an anti-seizure medication, would not have been approved because it causes cancer in mice and rats (Clemmensen & Hjalgrim-Jensen 1980). Moreover, studies conducted on mice and rats revealed that 46% of chemicals discoveredto be carcinogens in rats were *not* carcinogensin mice, despite mice and rats being phylogenetically more closely related than rodents and humans (Di Carlo 1984). Di Carlo stated: "It is painfully clear that carcinogenesis in the mouse cannot now be predicted from positive data obtained from the rat and vice versa (Di Carlo 1984).

Studies like these led David Salsburg then-of Pfizer to state that the "lifetime feeding studies in mice or rats using maximum tolerated doses of the test compound" fail to meet the criteria for predicting human response and suggested that tossing a coin would have yielded better results (Salsburg 1983). The Centers for Disease Control and Prevention (CDC) stated: "Most of what we know about chemicals and cancer in humans comes from scientists' observation of workers. The most significant exposures to cancer-causing chemicals have occurred in workplaces where large amounts of toxic chemicals have been used regularly." (ATSDR 2002)

Intuitively, one would suspect that mice and rats would share more similarities with each other than either species would share with humans and that nonhuman primates would better predict human response. Beniashvili, writing in the book *Experimental Tumors In Monkeys*stated thatmonkeys are "highly resistant to certain blastogenic agents, carcinogenic for other animals" and that, "Spontaneous tumors in monkeys are very rare," as are lung tumors and tumors of the mediastinum and soft tissues. Beniashvili also noted that skin tumors rarely metastasize in nonhuman primates while they do so in humans (Beniashvili 1994). There are substantial inter-species differences in the genetics that lead to cancer. Human cancers appear to result from more alterations in genes that do rodent cancers (Hahn & Weinberg 2002; Rangarajan & Weinberg 2003). Multiple other inter-species differences in carcinogenesis have been described (Dybing & Sanner 1999; Ennever, Noonan, and Rosenkranz 1987; Habeck 2002; Marsoni *et al.* 1987; Corry 1952; Rohan *et al.* 2000; Editorial 2006; Kamb 2005).

The most infamous example of animal models failing to identify a carcinogen is cigarette smoking. Animal models were, and indeed still are, used by tobacco companies to cast doubt on whether their product causes cancer (Oreskes & Conway 2011). Eric Northrup, a journalists wrote in his 1957 book *Science Looks At Smoking*: "The failure of many investigators …… to induce experimental cancers [in animals], except in a handful of cases, during fifty years of trying, casts serious doubt on the validity of the cigarette-lung cancer theory." (Northrup, 1957, p.133) The introduction to the book was written by then-chairman of the Yale Department of Pathology, Dr. HSN Greene, who agreed with the statement. Even using current technologies, smoking simply does not cause cancer in a vast majority of lab animals (Chu *et al.* 1981). Utidjian states: "Surely, not even the most zealous toxicologist would deny that epidemiology, and epidemiology alone, has indicted and incriminated the cigarette as a potent carcinogenic agent, or would claim that experimental animal toxicology could ever have done the job with the same definition." (Utidjian 1988). Coulston and Shubick reinforce this stating: "For decades the clinical observation of an association between cigarette smoking and bronchial carcinoma was subject to unfounded doubt, suspicion, and outright opposition, largely because the disease had no counterpart in mice. There seemed no end of statisticians craving for more documentation, all resulting in the fateful delay of needed legislative initiative." (Clemmensen & Hjalgrim-Jensen 1980).

The use of animal models to cast doubt on the carcinogenicity of smoking continues. William Campbell, president and CEO of Phillip Morris was quoted in the *New York Times* December 6, 1993 as testifying under oath before the US Congress as follows:

Q: Does cigarette smoking cause cancer?

A: To my knowledge, it's not been proven that cigarette smoking causes cancer.

Q: What do you base that on?

A: I base that on the fact traditionally, there is, you know, in scientific terms, there are hurdles related to causation, and at this time there is no evidence that they have been able to reproduce cancer in animals from cigarette smoking.

Another notable failure for animal models was asbestos. It was not until the 1960s that researchers were able to reproduce *some* of the human effects of the asbestosis in animals. Asbestos had been linked to human cancer much earlier (Gardner 1938; Wagner 1963; Wagner *et al.* 1974; Enterline 1978; Smith *et al.* 1965; Enterline 1988). The *New York Academy of Sciences* assured people in 1965 that: "a large literature on experimental studies has failed to furnish any definitive evidence for induction of malignant tumors in animals exposed to various varieties and preparations of asbestos by inhalation or intratracheal injection." (Smith *et al.* 1965).

Casting doubt on the carcinogenicity of smoking and asbestos are not small indiscretions of a model. In terms of the number of deaths due to a failure of a model, these two examples might rank the highest. If a model fails this badly and continues to be used, one must question the motivation of the people using the model. The other side of the coin is the drugs and chemicals that society did not have access to secondary to false positives in animal models. For example, when saccharine first came on the market in the US, many people would not use it because it had caused cancer in rats. Rats have an enzyme in their bladder, which human lack, which interacts with the saccharine and causes cancer (Cohen & Ellwein 1990). Moreover, even female rats lack the enzyme. Cancer occurred only in male rats. As I will explain, there are simply too many differences between humans and animals for animal models to be used as surrogates for humans in carcinogenicity testing.

4 Animal Models and Antineoplastics

The idea behind using animal models in order to ultimately create new treatments for cancer can be summarized as follows: basic research using animal models of cancer will lead to the discovery of mechanisms that can then be targeted in the form of drugs. Targets for new drugs arise from basic research that usually involves animal models and the funding for this type of research has increased dramatically in recent decades. Despite this however, the number of new drugs being approved by the FDA is no greater than 50 years ago (Munos 2009). The above philosophy also assumes that inter-species extrapolation will be viable. In light of what I just discussed regarding animal models and carcinogenicity, and in light of the fact that evolution holds true for mechanisms related to treatments just as it does for mechanisms of carcinogenesis, we might expect treatments that were safe and efficacious in animals to fail in humans. As we will see, this is indeed the case. Yet, as late as 2011, Harold Varmus, Nobel laureate and then-director of the National Cancer Institute (NCI) confirmed that the NCI would continue to fund animal models and basic research (Wadman 2011). Varmus is not alone in this position. Nic Jones, the Chief Scientist for Cancer Research UK (CRUK), in 2011 also confirmed support from CRUK for basic research using animal models. When asked if such research might be the reason so little progress has been made in finding new treatments, he replied: "I would argue that we have been using the wrong mouse models." (Editors 2011)

The logic undergirding the above positions is problematic for empirical reasons in addition to evolutionary biology, however. The success rate for new drugs in all areas of development is dismal. Out of 5,000 – 10,000 chemicals that enter the drug development pipeline only one will enter the market (European Commission 2008; Hughes *et al.* 2011). Moreover, the major cost of drug development occurs during the clinical trials and the attrition rate during this stage is equally dreadful (Unknown 2002; Shaffer 2012; Paul *et al.* 2010; Schachter 2007). Drugs entering Phase I trials have approximately a 9% chance of coming to market (FDA 2004; Sarkar 2009; Editorial 2007; Paul *et al.* 2010). Of the drugs that advance to Phase III, less than 50% are marketed (Arrowsmith 2011). The failure rate for oncology drugs is even higher (Editorial 2011; Caponigro & Sellers 2011; Arrowsmith 2011; Begley & Ellis 2012). Only 5% of cancer drugs that have an Investigational New Drug Application (IND) eventually go to market (Kummar *et al.* 2007). Lack of safety or efficacy accounts for approximately 90% of drug failures during clinical trials. (Kola & Landis 2004; Arrowsmith 2011). Both safety and efficacy determinations rely on animal models. To complicate matters further, the pipeline in Pharma is drying up and fewer drugs, especially new chemical entities (NCEs) are being marketed (Editorial 2008; GBI Research 2011).

Why is the attrition rate so high? In large part: animal models. Björquist and Sartipy state: "Furthermore, the compound attrition rate is negatively affected by the inability to predict toxicity and efficacy in humans. These shortcomings are in turn caused by the use of experimental pre-clinical model systems that have a limited human clinical relevance ......" (Björquist & Sartipy 2007). Then U.S. Secretary of Health and Human Services Mike Leavitt stated in 2006: "Currently, nine out of ten experimental drugs fail in clinical studies because we cannot accurately predict how they will behave in people based on laboratory and animal studies." (FDA 2006). Johnson *et al.* (2001) found that out of 39 anticancer drugs tested on xenograft mice, only one mimicked the response in humans. Oncology drugs fail more frequently in clinical trials than most other categories (DiMasi & Grabowski 2007; DiMasi *et al.* 2010).

There have been many attempts to reproduce human cancers in mice. The nude mouse lacked the *FOX1* gene, the SCID mouse was created with a very deficient immune system, and there have been many more models. All have failed to predict human response and have misled researchers. Zielinska discusses mouse models of cancer stating they: "rarely predict how a human will respond to the same treatment." Zielinska then quotes Marks of the NCI, and who is also head of the Mouse Models of Human Cancers Consortium, as saying: "we had loads of models that were not predictive, that were [in fact] seriously misleading." (Zielinska 2010). The NCI had previously tested mice with 12 anti-cancer drugs being successfully used to treat humans. The mice were growing 48 different kinds of human cancers. The study revealed that 30 out of 48 times (63%) the drugs that were effective against human cancers were ineffective in the mice that were growing the human cancers. The NCI believes efficacious treatments for human cancers have been lost because of animal testing (Gura 1997).

The problem of animal models is well known to the drug development community. Cook *et al* state: "Over many years now there has been a poor correlation between preclinical therapeutic findings and the eventual efficacy of these [anti-cancer] compounds in clinical trials (Johnson *et al.* 2001; Suggitt & Bibby 2005). The development of antineoplastics is a large investment by the private and public sectors, however, the limited availability of predictive preclinical systems obscures our ability to select the therapeutics that might succeed or fail during clinical investigation." (Cook, Jodrell, and Tuveson 2012). Singh and Ferrara echo this, stating: "Over 90% of phase 3 clinical trials in oncology fail to meet their primary endpoints despite encouraging preclinical and even early-stage clinical data. This staggering and sobering figure underscores the limitations of existing animal models for the evaluation of potential anti-cancer agents. The paucity of models is especially apparent with the advent of drugs that target the tumor milieu, or microenvironment, such as anti-angiogenics ...... immunotherapies and compounds directed against tumor-associated fibroblasts." (Singh & Ferrara 2012).

Wittenburg and Gustafson agree, stating: "The current drug development pathway in oncology research has led to a large attrition rate for new drugs, in part due to a general lack of appropriate preclinical studies that are capable of accurately predicting efficacy and/or toxicity in the target population ...... One of the most serious challenges currently facing pharmaceutical research of novel anti-cancer therapeutics is the lack of translation of efficacy and safety from preclinical models to human clinical trials, leading to a large attrition rate of investigational compounds. For new oncology drugs, only about 5% of investigational new drug applications submitted progress beyond the investigational phase due to a general lack of preclinical systems that can accurately predict efficacy and toxicity of new agents." (Wittenburg & Gustafson 2011).

Animal models fail to predict safety as well as efficacy. Reviewers of Phase I trials conducted by the National Cancer Institute (NCI) from 1991-2002 discovered that 15% of participants undergoing single agent chemotherapy agents suffered serious side effects (Horstmann *et al.* 2005). Richard Klausner, then-director of the NCI said: "The history of cancer research has been a history of curing cancer in the mouse ...... We have cured mice of cancer for decades — and it simply didn't work in humans." (Cimons *et al.* 1998). In an editorial to two articles, *Nature Medicine* stated: "The complexity of human metastatic cancer is difficult to mimic in mouse models. As a consequence, seemingly successful studies in murine models do not translate into success in late phases of clinical trials, pouring money, time and people's hope down the drain." (Ellis & Fidler 2010; Van Dyke 2010). Caponigro and Sellers of the Novartis Institutes For BioMedical Research, Oncology Research and Oncology Translational Medicine stated in 2011: "Despite an improved understanding of the biology of cancer, and an unprecedented volume of new molecules in clinical trials, the number of highly efficacious drugs approved by the regulatory authorities remains disappointingly low. The significant attrition rate of drugs entering clinical trials comes at a high price. This price is paid primarily by the underserved patient and secondarily by the pharmaceutical and biotechnology community, which invests enormous resources perfecting a molecule only to watch it fail in humans ......" (Caponigro & Sellers 2011).

Cancer researcher Robert Weinberg, of Massachusetts Institute of Technology, was quoted by Leaf in *Fortune* magazine as saying: "And it's been well known for more than a decade, maybe two decades, that many of these preclinical human cancer models have very little predictive power in terms of how actual human beings — actual human tumors inside patients — will respond ...... preclinical models of human cancer, in large part, stink ...... hundreds of millions of dollars are being wasted every year by drug companies using these [animal] models." (Leaf 2004). Leaf also quotes Homer Pearce, "who once ran cancer research and clinical investigation at Eli Lilly and is now research fellow at the drug company" as saying: "...... that mouse models are 'woefully inadequate' for determining whether a drug will work in humans. 'If you look at the millions and millions and millions of mice that have been cured, and you compare that to the relative success, or lack thereof, that we've achieved in the treatment of metastatic disease clinically,' he says, 'you realize that there just has to be something wrong with those models.'" (Leaf 2004). Others have also pointed out the inadequacy of animal models of cancer, including genetically modified animal models (Frese & Tuveson 2007; Kerbel 2003; Singh *et al.* 2010; Talmadge *et al.* 2007; Peterson & Houghton 2004; Francia & Kerbel 2010; Johnson *et al.* 2001; Zielinska 2010; Wade 2009).

Tamoxifen is a good example of the shortcomings of animal models in general. Tamoxifen was originally touted as a birth control pill based on rat studies and was only later found to be an anticancer chemical. Moreover, it was ineffective as an oral contraceptive as it actually increased a woman's likelihood of becoming pregnant (Jordan & Robinson 1987). Tamoxifen acts by binding to the protein known as tubulin thus inhibiting cell division. After discovered to be effective against cancer, Tamoxifen was shown to causes liver tumors in some strains of rat, but not in mice or hamsters (Powles 1992). If this had been discovered in preclinical trials, the drug would not have come to market (Editorial 2003). According to D. N. Richardson of the Imperial Chemistries Industries PLC: "No laboratory tests for anti-tumour activity were carried out for Nolvadex [tamoxifen] until after the activity in human patients had been confirmed." (Richardson 1988). The most common side effect of Tamoxifen is nausea and vomiting, which was not seen in dogs, which are touted as the best species to use when looking for that side effect (Tucker *et al.* 1984).

Sadly, even the drugs that do come to market are too frequently not very effective against cancer. In the case of breast cancer, for instance, most women do not benefit from chemotherapy. As a general rule, one-third of women diagnosed with breast cancer would have improved without the chemotherapy and one-third would have died with or without it. Only one-third actually benefit from the treatment. Along the same lines, chemotherapies for cancer have decreased the size of the tumors but at the expense of an increase in frequency of secondary tumors and a very adversely affected lifestyle. Furthermore, most chemotherapy does not prolong life or result in a longer, high quality life (Bear 2003; Savage 2008; Mittra 2007).

5   Evolved Complex Systems

Medical science was very different in the 19th century when animals were first used as models for humans. The structure of DNA had not been elucidated, scientists thought the poliovirus entered via the nose (it enters through the gut) (Paul 1971), the notion of a *magic bullet* (that for every disease, or at least every infectious disease, a chemical existed that could interact with the single site causing the malady and thus cure the disease without harming the rest of the body) via Ehrlich and Salvarsan (Ehrlich & Hata 1910) was foremost in the minds of drug developers, the modern synthesis in evolution was brand new (Mayr 2002), and the creationist-based position of the influential animal modelers was that animals and humans seemed to be more or less the same except for humans having a soul (LaFollette & Shanks 1994; Bernard 1957; Elliot 1987). There were no organ transplants, infectious diseases were still a major killer in the developed world, the fields of cognitive ethology and animal cognition were unheard of, and differences between ethnic groups (Cheung *et al.* 1997; Couzin 2007; Gregor & Joffe 1978; Haiman *et al.* 2006; Spielman *et al.* 2007; Stamer & Stuber 2007; Wilke & Dolan 2011) and sexes (Holden 2005; Kaiser 2005; Simon 2005; Wald & Wu 2010; Willyard 2009) in terms of disease and drug reactions had not yet been discovered. Physics was just beginning to cast off the shackles of determinism and reductionism but chaos and complexity theory was still on the horizon. It was a different world. People in the 1800s are to be excused for thinking that animals and humans would react more or less the same to drugs and disease. I will now bring the reader into the current scientific environment as it relates to our topic (LaFollette & Shanks 1993; LaFollette & Shanks 1994, 1996; Shanks & Greek 2009; Shanks, Greek, and Greek 2009; Greek & Greek 2010; Greek, Shanks, and Rice 2011).

Two major advances in science, that are relevant to our topic, have occurred in the past three decades. First, the field of evolutionary biology has continued to develop. The new division of evolutionary biology known as evolutionary developmental biology, or evo devo, is one example of the important advances in the field of evolution. Evo devo arguably began in 1978, when Lewis (Lewis 1978) published his findings on the anterior–posterior layout of the fruit fly, *Drosophila*. In 1984, the homeobox genes were discovered by McGinnis *et al* (1984) The homeobox genes are responsible for the body plan of "bilaterian" organisms. Bilaterians, of which humans are an example, are symmetrical around two axes. The homeobox genes are responsible for the way the body is configured: the arms here, the thorax there and so on (Gellon & McGinnis 1998). The homeobox are active in early embryogenesis, organizing the cell and anterior–posterior body layout (Slack *et al.* 1993). While there are differences among species — for example, there are nine homeobox genes in flies contrasted with thirty-nine in mammals — the overall use of the homeobox is the same. Discoveries such as the homeobox allowed scientists to appreciate the fact that mammals, and animals in general, have much in common in terms of their genetic composition. The differences among species were not to be completely explained by different species having different genes.

The concepts learned from evo devo and evolutionary biology in general tie in closely with discoveries from the Human Genome Project (HGP) (McPherson *et al.* 2001; Venter *et al.* 2001) and other spin-off projects. Prior to the HGP, scientists thought the number of genes was proportional to the complexity of the organism. The number of genes in some organisms was known or approximated; therefore, the scientists involved in the HGP were looking for an estimated 100,000+ genes in humans. As the project advanced, it became clear that humans had nowhere near this many genes. This was perplexing.

Because of evo devo, the HGP and its spinoffs, and speculation by King and Wilson (King & Wilson 1975) in the 1970s, scientists now know the following. All mammals have more or less the same genes. Some species have a few genes that other species do not have, but one could more or less build any mammal using the genes from another. The differences among species lie, in large part, in the *regulation* and *expression* of the same genes. The genes that build the body are known as structural genes, while the genes that turn the structural gene on and off are called regulatory genes. Think of your genetic composition as the keys on a piano. Every piano has the same keys (structural genes). But each piano can be played so as to produce a variety of tunes. The reason for this is that the structure of the piano allows for keys to be pressed at various intervals and in various combinations. The sheet music dictates when and how to press the keys. Likewise, the regulatory genes (the sheet music) tell the structural genes (the keys) when to be active (expressed) and for how long. For example, humans and mice both have the gene that allows mice to grow a tail. In humans, this gene is not activated during embryogenesis, hence humans have no tail (Evidence for this is found in the fact that, very rarely, this gene will be turned on in humans and the baby will be born with a tail). Traits can be determined or modified based on how long a gene or set of genes is activated, for example allowing the thumb position to migrate down the hand or for the fingers to lengthen.

There are other differences among species and almost all are related to evolution. Different enzymes metabolize different drugs, metabolize the same drugs at different rates, and form different metabolites, all of which influence toxicity and dosing. There are also differences in how many copies of a drug-metabolizing gene various animals have. If species A has 10 copies and species B has one copy, then species A might metabolize a drug 10 times faster than species B. This also has significance for dosing and for toxicity. For example, trastuzumab (Herceptin), an anti-breast cancer drug, is prescribed for women who carry multiple copies of, or overexpress, the gene *HER-2/neu* (Gonzalez-Angulo *et al*. 2006).

Species, and even individual humans, can differ in genetic composition. For example, there may be differences in:

- The presence (or absence) of certain genes.

- The presence (or absence) of certain alleles.

- The background genes and modifier genes that influence the genes being perturbed by drugs or disease.

- The regulation and expression of genes.

- Gene networks.

- Alternative splicing, which allows one gene to form or be part of forming many different proteins.

- Proteins and protein–protein interactions.

- Gene–protein interactions.

- Old genes evolving to perform new functions.

- Horizontal gene transfer (HGT). HGT occurs when genes from one organism are incorporated into another organism without the recipient organisms being the offspring of the donor. For example, resistance to anti-bacterial drugs can occur through HGT.

- Epigenetics. Epigenetics is the relatively new field that studies changes in gene expression that can be inherited and that occur without changing the underlying DNA sequence. For example, because of environmental influences, a regulatory gene may be changed such that it is turned on or off thus allowing a disease to manifest.

- The presence of gene and chromosomal mutations such as single nucleotide polymorphisms (SNPs), copy number variants (CNVs), duplications, inversions, deletions, and insertions.

In response to a perturbation to the system, such as a drug or disease, even one of the above differences can result in life or death consequences. Furthermore, *convergent evolution* can result in the same trait being present but being mediated by very different pathways in different species. Different molecules can also perform the same function. *All* of these types of differences are present in every species.

There are, of course, similarities among species. Some of these similarities are referred to as *conserved processes*, which are basic functions of a cell that have been present since early evolutionary times. The homeobox, described above, is an example of a conserved process. Conserved processes occur in living complex systems that have differences like those outlined above. These differences result in the conserved process being influenced by various factors that are unique to each species and even each individual within each species. Importantly, we understand how modifications in the genome, like those mentioned above, have resulted in the evolution of different body types and indeed different species (Gellon & McGinnis 1998; Wagner *et al.* 2003; Amores *et al.* 1998; Garcia-Fernandez 2005). Therefore, even when animals and humans share genes and traits, they will most likely still react differently to diseases and drugs.

The second major change in science that is relevant to our discussion is the development of chaos and complexity science, replacing, in part, the deterministic paradigms. For centuries, physics, and science in general, saw the world through the eyes of Descartes and Newton. Newtonian physics is closely connected to reductionism and determinism. Reductionism maintains that everything can be reduced to its component parts, those parts examined and understood, and then the whole explained based on it being the sum of the parts. Determinism means that once for certain systems, once the initial conditions are known only one outcome is possible. Reductionism and determinism lead to a very linear process with A leading to B leading to C and so on. The Newtonian physics of inclined planes, velocities, forces, a point representing an object, and so forth explores simple systems amenable to reductionism and determinism. The early 20th century saw advances in science that challenged reductionism and determinism. For instance, relativity and quantum mechanics revolutions in physics could not be explained by reductionism. Later in the 20th century chaos and complexity science would be developed, thus changing the way reductionism and determinism were viewed by all of science.

Reductionism worked very well for science and still has a role to play. But some systems are not the simple systems that conform so well to study by reductionism. Some systems are *complex systems* and have rules and characteristics of their own. Complex systems are more than merely a sum of their component parts. Complexity is related to chaos theory. Chaos is perhaps best understood by examining the original experiments performed by Lorenz in 1961. While running weather simulations on a computer, Lorenz shortened a number in an equation from six decimal places to three. When he re-ran the program he found the results were very different from the original. Translating from computer-speak, what he found was that where it had been sunny on day 15, it now rained. Because of the extremely small change in the initial conditions of the program, the outcome was essentially the opposite from the original. This very small change in initial conditions is what phrases like "a butterfly flaps its wings in China and causes a tornado in Kansas" are referring to. Seemingly unimportant differences between two situations or systems can translate into major differences in outcomes. For example, you may eat chocolate but it can kill your dog. The reason for this is the fact that dogs lack the enzyme, or have the enzyme but only in very small quantities, that metabolizes a potentially toxic ingredient in chocolate known as theobromine. Something as simple as the presence or absence of an enzyme can have fatal consequences.

Lorenz's computer experiment, along with work done by other scientists including Poincaré, gave rise to chaos theory and complexity theory. A major difference between chaotic systems and complex systems is that chaotic systems are deterministic. Given enough computer power and knowledge of the system, outcomes could be predicted. This is not the case with complex systems because they exhibit, among other things, *emergent* properties. Emergence is the presence, in a system, of new properties that could not have been predicted even with total knowledge of the component parts from which the emergent property arose. Financial markets, the behavior of ant colonies, cells, and living organisms are examples of complex systems whereas the weather and the red spot on Jupiter are examples of chaotic systems.

Complex systems, including humans and other animals, have the following characteristics (Ahn *et al.* 2006; Alm & Arkin 2003; Cairns-Smith 1986; Csete & Doyle 2002; Goodwin 2001; Jura *et al.* 2006; Kauffman 1993; Kitano 2002, 2002; Monte *et al.* 2005; Morowitz 2002; Novikoff 1945; Ottino 2004; Sole & Goodwin 2002; Van Regenmortel 2004, 2004; Van Regenmortel & Hull 2002; Vicsek 2002; Woodger 1967).

1. The whole is greater than the sum of the parts. This is, in part, because of emergent properties. Because complex systems exhibit the characteristics of emergence and the whole being greater than the sum of its parts, they cannot be completely described via reductionism.

2. Different levels of organization exist and a perturbation to the system as a whole may affect each level differently.

3. There are a large number of components or parts and these can combine to form modules that interact with each other and the environment. Feedback loops also exist among the parts and modules.

4. The system displays robustness, meaning it is resistant to change, and redundancy, meaning that the loss of one part may be compensated for by another part.

5. Complex systems are best described by differential equations and are examples of nonlinearity. Nonlinearity means that a small perturbation may have no effect on the system or a very large effect. Cause does not give rise to effect in the linear way it does in a simple system.

6. The particular manifestations of complex systems and chaotic systems are both determined in part or in whole by initial conditions. For example, changing or deleting just one gene in a living complex system might result in death or in no noticeable change whatsoever. This has important implications as studies have demonstrated that deleting a gene in a mouse may result in the death of one strain but not another. Similarly, a gene may be required for human development but not the development of mice or other animals.

Other factors leading to complications for trans-species extrapolation, and even intra-species extrapolation, are the stochastic nature of mutations and theintrinsic fluctuations and environmental disturbances (noise) of the system (Chen & Lin 2011; Chen & Wang 2006). While addressing these concepts is beyond the scope of this chapter, they are nonetheless important factors and I refer the reader to Chen *et al* for more information.

Humans and animals are living complex systems that have different evolutionary trajectories. Therefore, animals and humans have very different initial conditions in the form of the genetic differences listed above. It follows that one species may respond to perturbations such as drugs and disease in a manner that cannot be predicted based on the response of a different species. Moreover, all of the characteristics of a complex system, and the differences between complex systems that have occurred because of evolution, have a major impact on inter-species extrapolation. This was not appreciated during the era of the Nuremberg trials. Predicting outcomes within a complex system is problematic; predicting an outcome for one complex system based on the outcome from another is virtually impossible. Nevertheless, this is exactly what scientists are attempting to do when they test a drug on a mouse or monkey in an attempt to ascertain what it will do to a human.

6   Personalized Medicine

Because humans are evolved complex systems it should not be surprising that even individual humans react differently to drugs and disease. Gabor Miklos writes: "There is enormous phenotypic variation in the extent of human cancer phenotypes, even among family members inheriting the same mutation in the adenomatous polyposis coli (APC) gene believed to be causal for colon cancer. In the experimental mouse knockout of the catalytic gamma subunit of the phosphatidyl-3-OH kinase, there can be a high incidence of colorectal carcinomas or no cancers at all, depending on the mouse strain in which the knockout is created, or into which the knockout is crossed ...... Thus, although a mutation-cataloging research megaproject may be a diverting occupation for sequencing centers and gene hunters, leading scientists should think carefully before they tout its therapeutic promise to patients and politicians. The simple truth is that the money would be much better spent if research priorities were reevaluated. A good place to start would be to dismiss the fallacious notion that single mutations in primary tumors are the optimal starting point for research that would lead to the discovery of new, more effective cancer drugs. The clinical reality is that it is not single genes, but rather the properties of aneuploid-based methylated networks that allow metastatic cancer cells to explore novel niches in different genetic backgrounds and to rapidly become resistant to drug-based therapies." (Miklos 2005).

Serrano *et al.* (2011) discussed the role of the gene *SULT1A1* and 33 alleles of the enzyme CYP2D6 and 3 of CYP2C19 in the metabolism of tamoxifen. They discovered that out of 182 patients, 8 were poor metabolizers of tamoxifen, 151 were extensive metabolizers, 17 were intermediate metabolizers and 3 were ultra metabolizers. Such intra-species differences alter treatment strategies.

Powell *et al.* (2012) examined circulating tumor cells (CTCs), cells that are circulating in the bloodstream that are derived from the original cancer. They discovered that the CTCs were genetically diverse. This is important but perhaps even more important some of the cells have genes turned on such that they can implant into other tissues easier. This also explains why patients respond so differently to treatments and why different treatments may be needed in the same patient. It also, again, supports the notion that animal models are never going to be predictive modalities for human response to drugs and disease.

Heng (2008), writing in *JAMA*, discussed the use of reductionism in biomedical research. Heng noted that approaching living systems like they were clockwork systems was rewarding in the early days of science. However, science is now studying human disease at the level where complexity science becomes important hence reductionism can be misleading. Heng: "Likewise, chemotherapy often initially reduces tumor size but also produces severe adverse effects leading to other complications, including the promotion of secondary tumors. Most important, little evidence exists that more aggressive chemotherapies prolong life for many patients. In fact, chemotherapies may have overall negative effects for some patients. One reason for this is what are classified as the same cancer can have different genetic profiles in addition to being caused by different genetic aberrations (Wood *et al.* 2007; Heng 2007; Heng *et al.* 2006). Complicating matters further, epigenetic factors that result in mutations in regulatory genes, can account for a high number of differences in response to chemotherapy (Brower 2011) (For more on personalized medicine see: Greek, Menache, and Rice, 2012).

7   Productive Areas of Research

There are many research modalities with a history of providing results that are applicable to humans and society should demand that biomedical researchers that use animal models switch to these methods. All of these methods are either human-based or come from the physical sciences. Nobel laureate Sydney Brenner, who was awarded the Prize for research on *Caenorhabditis elegans*, advocated for more research using *Homo sapiens* even referring to *Homo sapiens* as "the model organism." (Ledford 2008). Human-based research includes epidemiology, *in vitro* research with human tissues, clinical observation, post-mortem examinations, computer modeling based on human findings, genome-wide association studies, *enforced* post-marketing drug surveillance, microdosing, and research with human stem cells among other methods. The first chemotherapies were largely based on human observation, not mechanism-based. Lord and Ashworth state:"Clinicians will attest that cytotoxic chemotherapyregimens, developed with the limited biological information available at the time of their development, remain the mainstay of treatment for most cancers …… Following the discovery of chemotherapeutics, the next significant advance came in the 1960s with the straightforward notion of combining drugs. The rationale for thiscame from the treatment of tuberculosis, for which antibiotics, each with a different mechanism of action, were more effective when used in combination. For cancer, it was considered that the development of resistance to a battery of agents used concurrently, rather than a single drug, was less likely." (Lord & Ashworth 2010).

Brennan *et al.* (2010) also emphasize human-based research noting: "…… the cumulative adult death rate from cancer adjusted for the size and age of the population has improved by less than 5%." They contrast the mortality rate from adult cancers with mortality in the pediatric population, pointing out that the cure rate for pediatric cancer is approximately 80%, up from 30% in 1971. Why is this the case? Brennan *et al.* state: "Most of the progress in improving outcome for pediatric cancer has come from clinical research. Indeed, the majority (>90%) of pediatric cancer patients are enrolled on treatment protocols and there is now abundant evidence that research protocols have helped optimize treatment intensification, drug dosing and timing, chemotherapeutic drug combination, and the identification of prognostic features of disease in relation to treatment plans. In sharp contrast, only 3% of adult cancer patients are enrolled on research protocols. These numbers suggest that the advances in patient outcome for pediatric cancer since the beginning of the war on cancer can be attributed in part to the coordinated participation in clinical research protocols ……" Brennan *et al.* also opine state that inter-species extrapolation is "an incredible challenge." (Brennan, Federico, and Dyer 2010).

Human-based research also includes prevention and environmental factors. Former president of the American Cancer Society, Dileep G. Bal *et al.* state that two-thirds of cancer deaths in the US can be prevented by proper diet, proper weight, and avoiding known risk factors like smoking. They note that diet equals smoking in terms of prevention. Pan *et al* support this conclusion with their twenty-nine year study finding that: "Red meat consumption is associated with an increased risk of total, CVD, and cancer mortality." (Pan *et al*. 2012). The role of diet should be emphasized in light of the fact that "'Western cancers' [are] spreading to developing world." (Coghlan 2012; Bray *et al*. 2012). This is mainly secondary to the increasing standard of living with the concomitant increases in consumption of the Western diet and smoking.

8   Societal Concerns

The non-predictive and misleading nature of animal models must be placed into the context of societal concerns regarding the use of animals in research and testing. Giles writing in *Nature* states: "In the contentious world of animal research, one question surfaces time and again: how useful are animal experiments as a way to prepare for trials of medical treatments in humans? *The issue is crucial, as public opinion is behind animal research only if it helps develop better drugs.* Consequently, scientists defending animal experiments insist they are essential for safe clinical trials, whereas animal-rights activists vehemently maintain that they are useless." (Giles 2006) (Emphasis added.)

The Institute for Laboratory Animal Research (ILAR 2004) and other proponents of using animals in research (Frey 1983) have views similar to Giles. An editorial in *Nature* in 2009 reinforced the above stating: "Animal-research policies need to be guided by a moral compass—a consensus of what people find acceptable and unacceptable." (Editorial 2009). What does society find acceptable?

A survey conducted by YouGov in the UK, France, Germany, Italy, Sweden and the Czech Republic asked under what conditions should the use of dogs, cats, and primates in research be allowed.

- 81% of people surveyed agree or strongly agree the new law should prohibit all experiments causing pain or suffering to primates.

- 79% of people agree or strongly agree the new law should prohibit all experiments on animals which do not relate to serious or life-threatening human conditions.

- 84% of people surveyed agree or strongly agree the new law should prohibit all experiments causing severe pain or suffering to any animal.

- 73% of people disagree or strongly disagree that the new law should permit experiments causing pain or suffering to cats.

- 77% of people disagree or strongly disagree that the new law should permit experiments causing pain or suffering to dogs (ECEAE 2012).

The Pew Research Center and the American Association for the Advancement of Science (AAAS) revealed, in 2009, that only 52% of nonscientists supported the use of animals in general in scientific research (Pew/AAAS 2009). In 1999, MORI and*New Scientist* (Aldhous *et al*. May 22, 1999) asked people whether they favored using animals with 24% answering yes 64% answering no. The questions were then divided into several categories. Respondents were questioned about experiments in which mice would be subject to pain, illness or surgery, and 61% stated that they disapproved using mice in order to study how the sense of hearing works. That percentage dropped to 32% when the question concerned the use of mice to ensure a new drug to cure childhood leukemia was safe and effective. When monkeys were substituted for mice the disapproval went from 64% to 75% and 32% to 44%, respectively. As the previous sections reveal, animals cannot in fact be used to predict safety and efficacy and are in reality used for basic research, which The Organisation for Economic Cooperation and Development defined as: "Experimental or theoretical work undertaken primarily to acquire new knowledge of phenomena and observable facts without any particular application or use in view. It is usually undertaken by scientists who may set their own agenda and to a large extent organize their own work." (Organisation for Economic Cooperation and Development 1963).

While the above polls reveal variation in response the general message is clearly that society is uncomfortable with using animals in basic research. Since animal models are not predictive for human response to drugs and disease, including cancer, it would appear that, if society understood this, it would not approve of using animals in such a fashion (Greek & Greek 2010).

Contrast this entire chapter with the following statements.

From the American Medical Association's White paper: "Animal research holds the key for solutions to AIDS, cancer, heart disease, aging, and congenital defects." (American Medical Association 1992). Michael F. Jacobson, executive director of the *Center for Science in the Public Interest* stated in 2008: "We must test animals to determine whether a substance causes cancer." (CSPI 2008). Similarly, Huff *et al.* (2008) observe: "Chemical carcinogenesis bioassays in animals have long been recognized and accepted as valid predictors of potential cancer hazards to humans."

The Foundation for Biomedical Research (FBR) states: "Animal research has played a vital role in virtually every major medical advance of the last century, for both human and animal health. From the discovery of antibiotics, analgesics, anti-depressants, and anesthetics, to the successful development of organ transplants, bypass surgery, heart catheterization, and joint replacement, practically every present-day protocol for the prevention, control, and cure of disease is based on knowledge attained through research with laboratory animals. More than half of the Nobel Prizes in Physiology or Medicine have been given for research involving animals. Since 1900, modern medicine and public health have boosted the average lifespan in United States by almost 30 years. Much of this progress came from knowledge gained through animal research. Many diseases that once killed millions of people every year are now either preventable, treatable, or have been eradicated altogether. The survival rates for many other major diseases are at an all-time high thanks to the discovery of powerful new drugs, the development of new surgical procedures, and the design of sophisticated medical devices. Research with animals has played a critical role in nearly all of these advances." (FBR 2010).

Understanding Animal Research of the UK states: "As this [development of new treatments] is a relatively large area of research and testing, accounting for 18% of animal procedures in 2010, it is useful to split it into three main areas. Animals are vital in all three (Understanding Animal Research, 2011).

- research to find new vaccines and treatments
- developing new medicines and vaccines and improving existing ones
- testing potential new medicines to make sure they are effective and safe"

Botting and Morrison write: "In truth there are no basic differences between the physiology of laboratory animals and humans …… we can not think of an area of medical research that does not owe many of its most important advances to animal experiments." (Botting & Morrison 1997). Fomchenko and Holland state: "GEMs [genetically engineered mice] closely recapitulate the human disease and are used to predict human response to a therapy, treatment or radiation schedule …… GEMs that faithfully recapitulate human brain tumors and will likely result in high-quality clinical trials with satisfactory treatment outcomes and reduced drug toxicities. Additional use of GEMs to establish causal links between the presence of various genetic alterations and brain tumor initiation ......" (Fomchenko & Holland 2006). There appear to be reasons why animal models continue to be used that have nothing to do with the efficacy of the practice.

9   Summary

Animal models of cancer have failed both for carcinogenesis and chemotherapy. There has been empirical evidence for the failure of animal models for decades but only recently has a Theory been developed to place the evidence in context. Based on the fact that animals and humans are evolved complex systems, one species should not be expected to be predictive for another for responses to disease and drugs. A modality, be it a research modality or treatment modality, that fails to perform as needed should be abandoned just as bloodletting and trephination have been abandoned by physicians. The concern society has expressed for using sentient animals in research in general is cause for further concern regarding the continuation of a failed modality.

   Despite claims that research using animals to model human cancer has increased the life span of people with cancer, the use of animal models for developing new treatments for cancer has not been rewarding. In reality, it has been very misleading. In this chapter, I discussed the use of animal models for determining carcinogenesis and discovering chemotherapies. I also examine the empirical evidence pertaining to the predictive value of animal models for these purposes and placed this evidence into the context of scientific theory in the form of the Theory of Evolution and Complexity Theory. I then presented the position of society in general, as indicated by surveys as well as opinions from the scientific literature, regarding the use of animals in research and contrasted this stance with the actual benefits that result from animal models of cancer. I conclude that from a scientific perspective, animal models of cancer have failed and will continue to fail to predict the response of humans to carcinogens and antineoplastic therapies regardless of genetic modifications to animals or the use of chimeras. When this failure is placed in the context of what society demands in return for allowing scientists to use sentient animals, such as mammals, in such research, the continued use of animal models of cancer is difficult to justify.

Acknowledgements

The section on evolved complex systems was modified from the article: "The Nuremberg Code subverts human health and safety by requiring animal modeling" by Greek R, Pippus A, and Hansen LA. 2012. *BMC Med Ethics*. 13:16. 10.1186/1472-6939-13-16. http://www.ncbi.nlm.nih.gov/pubmed/22769234.

References

Abbott, A. 2005. *Animal testing: more than a cosmetic change. Nature 438 (7065):144-6.*

Ahn, A. C., M. Tewari, C. S. Poon, and R. S. Phillips. 2006. *The limits of reductionism in medicine: could systems biology offer an alternative? PLoS Med 3 (6):e208.*

Aldhous, Peter, Andy Coghlan, and Jon Copley. May 22, 1999. *Let the people speak. New Scientist (2187).*

Alm, E., and A. P. Arkin. 2003. Biological networks. Curr Opin Struct Biol 13 (2):193-202.

American Cancer Society. 2012. Cancer facts & Figures 2012. American Cancer Society 2012 [cited May 11 2012]. Available from http://www.cancer.org/acs/groups/content/@epidemiologysurveilance/documents/document/acspc-031941.pdf.

American Medical Association. 1992. White Paper on Animal Research: American Medical Association.

Ames, B. N., and L. S. Gold. 1990. Chemical carcinogenesis: too many rodent carcinogens. Proceedings of the National Academy of Sciences of the United States of America 87 (19):7772-6.

Repeated Author. 1990. Too many rodent carcinogens: mitogenesis increases mutagenesis. Science 249 (4972):970-1.

Ames, B. N., L. S. Gold, and M. K. Shigenaga. 1996. Cancer prevention, rodent high-dose cancer tests, and risk assessment. Risk analysis : an official publication of the Society for Risk Analysis 16 (5):613-7.

Amores, A., A. Force, Y. L. Yan, L. Joly, C. Amemiya, A. Fritz, R. K. Ho, J. Langeland, V. Prince, Y. L. Wang, M. Westerfield, M. Ekker, and J. H. Postlethwait. 1998. Zebrafish hox clusters and vertebrate genome evolution. Science 282 (5394):1711-4.

Anisimov, V. N., S. V. Ukraintseva, and A. I. Yashin. 2005. Cancer in rodents: does it tell us about cancer in humans? Nat Rev Cancer 5 (10):807-19.

Arrowsmith, John. 2011. Trial watch: Phase III and submission failures: 2008-2010. Nat Rev Drug Discov 10 (2):87-87.

Ashby, J., and D. Paton. 1993. The influence of chemical structure on the extent and sites of carcinogenesis for 522 rodent carcinogens and 55 different human carcinogen exposures. Mutation research 286 (1):3-74.

ATSDR. 2012. Cancer Fact Sheet. CDC. Agency for Toxic Substances & Disease Registry, August 30, 2002 2002 [cited May 22 2012]. Available from http://www.atsdr.cdc.gov/com/cancer-fs.html.

Bear, H. D. 2003. Earlier chemotherapy for breast cancer: perhaps too late but still useful. Annals of surgical oncology 10 (4):334-5.

Begley, C. Glenn, and Lee M. Ellis. 2012. Drug development: Raise standards for preclinical cancer research. Nature 483 (7391):531-533.

Beniashvili, Dzhemal Sh. 1994. Experimental Tumors in Monkeys: CRC Press.

Bernard, Claude. 1957. An Introduction to the Study of Experimental Medicine. 1865. Translated by H. C. Greene. New York: Dover.

Björquist, Petter, and Peter Sartipy. 2007. Raimund Strehl and Johan Hyllner. Human ES cell derived functional cells as tools in drug discovery. Drug Discovery World (Winter):17-24.

Botting, J. H., and A. R. Morrison. 1997. Animal research is vital to medicine. Sci Am 276 (2):83-5.

Bray, F., A. Jemal, N. Grey, J. Ferlay, and D. Forman. 2012. Global cancer transitions according to the Human Development Index (2008-2030): a population-based study. The lancet oncology 13 (8):790-801.

Brennan, R., S. Federico, and M. A. Dyer. 2010. The war on cancer: have we won the battle but lost the war? Oncotarget 1 (2):77-83.

Brower, Vicki. 2011. Epigenetics: Unravelling the cancer code. Nature 471 (7339):S12-S13.

Cairns-Smith, A G. 1986. Seven Clues to the Origin of Life: A Scientific Detective Story. Cambridge: Cambridge University Press.

Caponigro, G., and W. R. Sellers. 2011. Advances in the preclinical testing of cancer therapeutic hypotheses. Nat Rev Drug Discov 10 (3):179-87.

Chen, B. S., and Y. P. Lin. 2011. On the Interplay between the Evolvability and Network Robustness in an Evolutionary Biological Network: A Systems Biology Approach. Evolutionary bioinformatics online 7:201-33.

Chen, B. S., and Y. C. Wang. 2006. On the attenuation and amplification of molecular noise in genetic regulatory networks. BMC bioinformatics 7:52.

Cheung, D. S., M. L. Warman, and J. B. Mulliken. 1997. Hemangioma in twins. Ann Plast Surg 38 (3):269-74.

Chu, B. C., C. C. Fan, and S. B. Howell. 1981. Activity of free and carrier-bound methotrexate against transport-deficient and high dihydrofolate dehydrogenase-containing methotrexate-resistant L1210 cells. J Natl Cancer Inst 66 (1):121-4.

Cimons, Marlene, Josh Getlin, and Thomas H. Maugh_II. 2010. Cancer Drugs Face Long Road From Mice to Men 1998 [cited Nov 8 2010]. Available from http://articles.latimes.com/1998/may/06/news/mn-46795.

Clayson, DB. 1980. The carcinogenic action of drugs in man and animals. In Human Epidemiology and Animal Laboratory Correlations in Chemical Carcinogenesis edited by F. Coulston and P. Shubick: Ablex Pub.

Clemmensen, J, and S Hjalgrim-Jensen. 1980. On the absence of carcinogenicity to man of phenobarbital. In Human Epidemiology and Animal Laboratory Correlations in Chemical Carcinogenesis, edited by F. Coulston and S. Shubick: Alex Pub.

Coghlan, Andy. 2012. 'Western cancers' spreading to developing world. New Scientist, June 1 2012 [cited August 5 2012]. Available from http://www.newscientist.com/article/dn21874-western-cancers-spreading-to-developing-world.html.

Cohen, S. M., and L. B. Ellwein. 1990. Cell proliferation in carcinogenesis. Science 249 (4972):1007-11.

Collins, Francis S. 2011. Reengineering Translational Science: The Time Is Right. Science Translational Medicine 3 (90):90cm17.

Cook, Natalie, Duncan I. Jodrell, and David A. Tuveson. 2012. Predictive in vivo animal models and translation to clinical trials. Drug Discovery Today 17 (5/6):253-60.

Corry, D. C. 1952. Pain in carcinoma of the breast. Lancet 1 (6702):274-6.

Coulston, F. 1980. Final Discussion. In Human Epidemiology and Animal Laboratory Correlations in Chemical Carcinogenesis, edited by F. Coulston and P. Shubick: Ablex.

Couzin, J. 2007. Cancer research. Probing the roots of race and cancer. Science 315 (5812):592-4.

Csete, M. E., and J. C. Doyle. 2002. Reverse engineering of biological complexity. Science 295 (5560):1664-9.

CSPI. Longer Tests on Lab Animals Urged for Potential Carcinogens. CSPI 2008 [cited November 17. Available from http://www.cspinet.org/new/200811172.html.

Di Carlo, F. J. 1984. Carcinogenesis bioassay data: correlation by species and sex. Drug Metab Rev 15 (3):409-13.

DiMasi, J. A., L. Feldman, A. Seckler, and A. Wilson. 2010. Trends in risks associated with new drug development: success rates for investigational drugs. Clinical Pharmacology and Therapeutics 87 (3):272-7.

DiMasi, J. A., and H. G. Grabowski. 2007. Economics of new oncology drug development. Journal of clinical oncology : official journal of the American Society of Clinical Oncology 25 (2):209-16.

Dixit, R, and U Boelsterli. 2007. Healthy animals and animal models of human disease(s) in safety assessment of human pharmaceuticals, including therapeutic antibodies. Drug Discovery Today 12 (7-8):336-42.

Drake III, Donald R., Inderpal Singh, Michael N. Nguyen, Anatoly Kachurin, Vaughan Wittman, Robert Parkhill, Olga Kachurina, Janice M. Moser, Nicolas Burdin, Monique Moreau, Noelle Mistretta, Anthony M. Byers, Vipra Dhir, Tenekua M. Tapia, Charlotte Vernhes, Jyoti Gangur, T. Kamala, Nithya Swaminathan, and William L. Warren. 2012. In Vitro Biomimetic Model of the Human Immune System for Predictive Vaccine Assessments. Disruptive Science and Technology 1 (1):28-40.

Dybing, E., and H. S. Huitfeldt. 1992. Species differences in carcinogen metabolism and interspecies extrapolation. IARC Sci Publ (116):501-22.

Dybing, E., and T. Sanner. 1999. Species differences in chemical carcinogenesis of the thyroid gland, kidney and urinary bladder. IARC Sci Publ (147):15-32.

ECEAE. 2012. 12 Million Reasons. European Coalition to End Animal Experiments 2012 [cited August 4 2012]. Available from http://www.eceae.org/en/what-we-do/campaigns/12-million-reasons/public-opinion.

Editorial. 2003. Follow the yellow brick road. Nat Rev Drug Discov 2 (3):167.

Repeated Author. 2006. The end of the beginning? Nat Rev Drug Discov 5 (9):705.

Repeated Author. 2007. Same old story? Nat Rev Drug Discov 6 (2):97.

Repeated Author. 2008. Raising the game. Nature Biotechnology 26 (2):137.

Repeated Author. 2009. A slippery slope. Nature 462 (7274):699.

Repeated Author. 2011. A stronger role for science. Nature reviews. Drug discovery 10 (3):159.

Editors. 2011. Nic Jones. Nat Rev Drug Discov 10 (4):252-252.

Ehrlich, P, and S Hata. 1910. Die experimentalle Chemotherapie der Spirillosen. Berlin: Springer.

Elliot, P. 1987. Vivisection and the Emergence of Experimental Medicine in Nineteenth Century France. In Vivisection in Historical Perspective, edited by N. Rupke. New York: Croom Helm.

Ellis, L. M., and I. J. Fidler. 2010. Finding the tumor copycat. Therapy fails, patients don't. Nat Med 16 (9):974-5.

Ennever, F. K., T. J. Noonan, and H. S. Rosenkranz. 1987. The predictivity of animal bioassays and short-term genotoxicity tests for carcinogenicity and non-carcinogenicity to humans. Mutagenesis 2 (2):73-8.

Enterline, P. E. 1978. Asbestos and cancer: the international lag. The American review of respiratory disease 118 (6):975-8.

Enterline, PE. 1988. Asbestos and Cancer. In Epidemiology and Health Risk Assessment, edited by L. Gordis. New York: Oxford University Press.

European Commission. 2008. Innovative Medicines Initiative: better tools for better medicines. Luxembourg.

FBR. 2012. Animal Research Saves Lives. Foundation of Biomedical Research 2010 [cited August 5 2012]. Available from http://www.fbresearch.org/TwoColumnWireframe.aspx?pageid=122.

FDA. Innovation or Stagnation? Challenge and Opportunity on the Critical Path to New Medical Products 2004. Available from http://www.nipte.org/docs/Critical_Path.pdf.

Repeated Author. 2010. FDA Issues Advice to Make Earliest Stages Of Clinical Drug Development More Efficient. FDA, June 18, 2009 2006 [cited March 7 2010]. Available from http://www.fda.gov/NewsEvents/Newsroom/PressAnnouncements/2006/ucm108576.htm.

Fletcher, A. P. 1978. Drug safety tests and subsequent clinical experience. J R Soc Med 71 (9):693-6.

Fomchenko, E. I., and E. C. Holland. 2006. Mouse models of brain tumors and their applications in preclinical trials. Clin Cancer Res 12 (18):5288-97.

Francia, Giulio, and Robert S. Kerbel. 2010. Raising the bar for cancer therapy models. Nat Biotech 28 (6):561-562.

Frese, K. K., and D. A. Tuveson. 2007. Maximizing mouse cancer models. Nat. Rev. Cancer 7:645-658.

Frey, R. G. 1983. Vivisection, morals and medicine. J Med Ethics 9 (2):94-7.

Fung, V. A., J. Huff, E. K. Weisburger, and D. G. Hoel. 1993. Predictive strategies for selecting 379 NCI/NTP chemicals evaluated for carcinogenic potential: scientific and public health impact. Fundamental and applied toxicology : official journal of the Society of Toxicology 20 (4):413-36.

Garcia-Fernandez, J. 2005. Hox, ParaHox, ProtoHox: facts and guesses. Heredity 94 (2):145-52.

Gardner, Leroy U. 1938. Etiology of Pneumoconiosis. JAMA 111 (21):1925-1936.

GBI Research. 2011. Top R&D Drug Failures - Toxicity and Serious Adverse Events in Late Stage Drug Development are the Major Causes of Drug Failure. New York: GBI Research.

Gellon, G., and W. McGinnis. 1998. Shaping animal body plans in development and evolution by modulation of Hox expression patterns. Bioessays 20 (2):116-25.

Giles, J. 2006. Animal experiments under fire for poor design. Nature 444 (7122):981.

Gold, L. S., T. H. Slone, N. B. Manley, and L. Bernstein. 1991. Target organs in chronic bioassays of 533 chemical carcinogens. Environ Health Perspect 93:233-46.

Gonzalez-Angulo, Ana M., Gabriel N. Hortobagyi, and Francisco J. Esteva. 2006. Adjuvant Therapy with Trastuzumab for HER-2/neu-Positive Breast Cancer. The Oncologist 11 (8):857-867.

Goodwin, Brian. 2001. How the Leopard Changed Its Spots : The Evolution of Complexity. Princeton: Princeton University Press.

Greek, R., and J. Greek. 2010. Is the use of sentient animals in basic research justifiable? Philos Ethics Humanit Med 5:14.

Greek, Ray, Lawrence A Hansen, and Andre Menache. 2011. An analysis of the Bateson Review of research using nonhuman primates Medicolegal and Bioethics 1 (1):3-22.

Greek, Ray, Andre Menache, and Mark J. Rice. 2012. Animal models in an age of personalized medicine. Personalized Medicine 9 (1):47-64.

Greek, Ray, and Niall Shanks. 2009. FAQs About the Use of Animals in Science: A handbook for the scientifically perplexed. Lanham: University Press of America.

Greek, Ray, Niall Shanks, and Mark J Rice. 2011. The History and Implications of Testing Thalidomide on Animals. The Journal of Philosophy, Science & Law 11 (October 3).

Gregor, Z., and L. Joffe. 1978. Senile macular changes in the black African. Br J Ophthalmol 62 (8):547-50.

Gura, T. 1997. Cancer Models: Systems for identifying new drugs are often faulty. Science 278 (5340):1041-2.

Habeck, Martina. 2002. Of Mice and men, and cancer research. Drug Discovery Today 7 (19):981-2.

Hahn, W. C., and R. A. Weinberg. 2002. Modelling the molecular circuitry of cancer. Nat Rev Cancer 2 (5):331-41.

Haiman, C. A., D. O. Stram, L. R. Wilkens, M. C. Pike, L. N. Kolonel, B. E. Henderson, and L. Le Marchand. 2006. Ethnic and racial differences in the smoking-related risk of lung cancer. N Engl J Med 354 (4):333-42.

Hendrick, Bill. 2012. Steep Decline in Autopsy Rate Since 1970s. WebMD, August 4 2011 [cited May 11 2012]. Available from http://www.webmd.com/healthy-aging/news/20110804/autopsy-rate-shows-big-decline.

Heng, H. H. 2007. Cancer genome sequencing: the challenges ahead. BioEssays : news and reviews in molecular, cellular and developmental biology 29 (8):783-94.

Repeated Author. 2008. The conflict between complex systems and reductionism. JAMA : the journal of the American Medical Association 300 (13):1580-1.

Heng, H. H., J. B. Stevens, G. Liu, S. W. Bremer, K. J. Ye, P. V. Reddy, G. S. Wu, Y. A. Wang, M. A. Tainsky, and C. J. Ye. 2006. Stochastic cancer progression driven by non-clonal chromosome aberrations. Journal of cellular physiology 208 (2):461-72.

Heywood, R. 1990. Clinical Toxicity--Could it have been predicted? Post-marketing experience. In Animal Toxicity Studies: Their Relevance for Man, edited by CE Lumley and S. Walker. Lancaster: Quay.

Holden, C. 2005. Sex and the suffering brain. Science 308 (5728):1574.

Horrobin, D. F. 2003. Modern biomedical research: an internally self-consistent universe with little contact with medical reality? Nat Rev Drug Discov 2 (2):151-4.

Horstmann, E., M. S. McCabe, L. Grochow, S. Yamamoto, L. Rubinstein, T. Budd, D. Shoemaker, E. J. Emanuel, and C. Grady. 2005. Risks and benefits of phase 1 oncology trials, 1991 through 2002. The New England journal of medicine 352 (9):895-904.

Huff, J., M. F. Jacobson, and D. L. Davis. 2008. The limits of two-year bioassay exposure regimens for identifying chemical carcinogens. Environ Health Perspect 116 (11):1439-42.

Hughes, J. P., S. Rees, S. B. Kalindjian, and K. L. Philpott. 2011. Principles of early drug discovery. British Journal of Pharmacology 162 (6):1239-1249.

ILAR. 2004. Science, Medicine, and Animals: National Academies Press.

Johnson, J. I., S. Decker, D. Zaharevitz, L. V. Rubinstein, J. M. Venditti, S. Schepartz, S. Kalyandrug, M. Christian, S. Arbuck, M. Hollingshead, and E. A. Sausville. 2001. *Relationships between drug activity in NCI preclinical in vitro and in vivo models and early clinical trials. Br J Cancer 84 (10):1424-31.*

Jordan, V. C., and S. P. Robinson. 1987. *Species-specific pharmacology of antiestrogens: role of metabolism. Fed Proc 46 (5):1870-4.*

Jura, J., P. Wegrzyn, and A. Koj. 2006. *Regulatory mechanisms of gene expression: complexity with elements of deterministic chaos. Acta Biochim Pol 53 (1):1-10.*

Kaiser, J. 2005. *Gender in the pharmacy: does it matter? Science 308 (5728):1572.*

Kamb, A. 2005. *What's wrong with our cancer models? Nat Rev Drug Discov 4 (2):161-5.*

Kauffman, Stuart A. 1993. *The Origins of Order: Self-Organization and Selection in Evolution Oxford University Press.*

Kerbel, R. S. 2003. *Human tumor xenografts as predictive preclinical models for anticancer drug activity in humans: better than commonly perceived-but they can be improved. Cancer Biol. Ther. 2 (4 Suppl 1):S134-9.*

King, M. C., and A. C. Wilson. 1975. *Evolution at two levels in humans and chimpanzees. Science 188 (4184):107-16.*

Kitano, H. 2002. *Computational systems biology. Nature 420 (6912):206-10.*

Repeated Author. 2002. *Systems biology: a brief overview. Science 295 (5560):1662-4.*

Kleinman, Cindy. 2012. *Of Mice and Mandates. American Council on Science and health, 1997 1997 [cited October 2 2012]. Available from http://www.acsh.org/wp-content/uploads/2012/04/20040329_mice.pdf.*

Kola, I., and J. Landis. 2004. *Can the pharmaceutical industry reduce attrition rates? Nat Rev Drug Discov 3 (8):711-5.*

Kummar, S., R. Kinders, L. Rubinstein, R. E. Parchment, A. J. Murgo, J. Collins, O. Pickeral, J. Low, S. M. Steinberg, M. Gutierrez, S. Yang, L. Helman, R. Wiltrout, J. E. Tomaszewski, and J. H. Doroshow. 2007. *Compressing drug development timelines in oncology using phase '0' trials. Nature reviews. Cancer 7 (2):131-9.*

LaFollette, H, and N Shanks. 1993. *Animal models in biomedical research: some epistemological worries. Public Aff Q 7 (2):113-30.*

LaFollette, Hugh, and Niall Shanks. 1994. *Animal Experimentation: The Legacy of Claude Bernard. International Studies in the Philosophy of Science 8 (3):195-210.*

Repeated Author. 1996. *Brute Science: Dilemmas of animal experimentation. London and New York: Routledge.*

Leaf, C. 2004. *Why we are losing the war on cancer. Fortune (March 9):77-92.*

Ledford, H. 2008. *Translational research: the full cycle. Nature 453 (7197):843-5.*

Lewis, E. B. 1978. *A gene complex controlling segmentation in Drosophila. Nature 276 (5688):565-70.*

Lord, C. J., and A. Ashworth. 2010. *Biology-driven cancer drug development: back to the future. BMC Biol 8:38.*

Lumley, C. 1990. *Clinical toxicity: could it have been predicted? Premarketing experience. In Animal Toxicity Studies: Their Relevance for Man, edited by C. Lumley and S. Walker. London: Quay.*

M.E. 2010. *In This Issue. Models that better mimic human cancer. Nature Biotechnology 28 (1):vii.*

Markou, A., C. Chiamulera, M. A. Geyer, M. Tricklebank, and T. Steckler. 2009. *Removing obstacles in neuroscience drug discovery: the future path for animal models. Neuropsychopharmacology : official publication of the American College of Neuropsychopharmacology 34 (1):74-89.*

Marsoni, S., D. Hoth, R. Simon, B. Leyland-Jones, M. De Rosa, and R. E. Wittes. 1987. *Clinical drug development: an analysis of phase II trials, 1970-1985. Cancer Treat Rep 71 (1):71-80.*

Mayr, Ernst. 2002. *What evolution Is: Basic Books.*

McGinnis, W., C. P. Hart, W. J. Gehring, and F. H. Ruddle. 1984. *Molecular cloning and chromosome mapping of a mouse DNA sequence homologous to homeotic genes of Drosophila. Cell 38 (3):675-80.*

McGregor, D. B., J. Pangrekar, H. S. Rosenkranz, and G. Klopman. 1994. A reexamination of the low prevalence of carcinogens in an early carcinogen screen. Regulatory toxicology and pharmacology : RTP 19 (1):97-105.

McPherson, J. D., M. Marra, L. Hillier, R. H. Waterston, A. Chinwalla, J. Wallis, M. Sekhon, K. Wylie, E. R. Mardis, R. K. Wilson, R. Fulton, T. A. Kucaba, C. Wagner-McPherson, W. B. Barbazuk, S. G. Gregory, S. J. Humphray, L. French, R. S. Evans, G. Bethel, A. Whittaker, J. L. Holden, O. T. McCann, A. Dunham, C. Soderlund, C. E. Scott, D. R. Bentley, G. Schuler, H. C. Chen, W. Jang, E. D. Green, J. R. Idol, V. V. Maduro, K. T. Montgomery, E. Lee, A. Miller, S. Emerling, Kucherlapati, R. Gibbs, S. Scherer, J. H. Gorrell, E. Sodergren, K. Clerc-Blankenburg, P. Tabor, S. Naylor, D. Garcia, P. J. de Jong, J. J. Catanese, N. Nowak, K. Osoegawa, S. Qin, L. Rowen, A. Madan, M. Dors, L. Hood, B. Trask, C. Friedman, H. Massa, V. G. Cheung, I. R. Kirsch, T. Reid, R. Yonescu, J. Weissenbach, T. Bruls, R. Heilig, E. Branscomb, A. Olsen, N. Doggett, J. F. Cheng, T. Hawkins, R. M. Myers, J. Shang, L. Ramirez, J. Schmutz, O. Velasquez, K. Dixon, N. E. Stone, D. R. Cox, D. Haussler, W. J. Kent, T. Furey, S. Rogic, S. Kennedy, S. Jones, A. Rosenthal, G. Wen, M. Schilhabel, G. Gloeckner, G. Nyakatura, R. Siebert, B. Schlegelberger, J. Korenberg, X. N. Chen, A. Fujiyama, M. Hattori, A. Toyoda, T. Yada, H. S. Park, Y. Sakaki, N. Shimizu, S. Asakawa, K. Kawasaki, T. Sasaki, A. Shintani, A. Shimizu, K. Shibuya, J. Kudoh, S. Minoshima, J. Ramser, P. Seranski, C. Hoff, A. Poustka, R. Reinhardt, and H. Lehrach. 2001. A physical map of the human genome. Nature 409 (6822):934-41.

Meijers, J. M., G. M. Swaen, and L. J. Bloemen. 1997. The predictive value of animal data in human cancer risk assessment. Regul Toxicol Pharmacol 25 (2):94-102.

Miklos, G L Gabor. 2005. The human cancer genome project--one more misstep in the war on cancer. Nat Biotechnol 23 (5):535-7.

Mittra, I. 2007. The disconnection between tumor response and survival. Nature clinical practice. Oncology 4 (4):203.

Monte, Julio, Min Liu, Adam Sheya, and Toshimori Kitami. 2007. Definitions, Measures, and Models of Robustness in Gene Regulatory Network. Report of research work for CSSS05 2005 [cited March 30 2007]. Available from http://www.santafe.edu/education/csss/csss05/papers/monte_et_al._csssf05.pdf.

Morowitz, Harold J. 2002. The Emergence of Everything: How the World Became Complex. Oxford: Oxford University Press.

Munos, B. 2009. Lessons from 60 years of pharmaceutical innovation. Nature reviews. Drug discovery 8 (12):959-68.

Northrup, E. 1957. Science looks at smoking: A new inquiry into the effects of smoking on your health. . New York: Coward-McCann.

Novikoff, A. B. 1945. The Concept of Integrative Levels and Biology. Science 101 (2618):209-15.

O'Collins, V. E., M. R. Macleod, G. A. Donnan, L. L. Horky, B. H. van der Worp, and D. W. Howells. 2006. 1,026 experimental treatments in acute stroke. Ann Neurol 59 (3):467-77.

Oreskes, Naomi, and Erik M. M. Conway. 2011. Merchants of Doubt. How a Handful of Scientists Obscrued the Truth on Issues From Tobacco Smoke to Global Warming. New York: Bloomsbury Press.

Organisation for Economic Cooperation and Development. 1963. The Measurement of Scientific and Technical activities: Proposed Standard Practice for Surveys of Research and Development. Paris.

Ottino, J. M. 2004. Engineering complex systems. Nature 427 (6973):399.

Pan, An, Qi Sun, Adam M. Bernstein, Matthias B. Schulze, JoAnn E. Manson, Meir J. Stampfer, Walter C. Willett, and Frank B. Hu. 2012. Red Meat Consumption and Mortality: Results From 2 Prospective Cohort Studies. Arch Intern Med:archinternmed.2011.2287.

Paul, J R. 1971. A History of Poliomyelitis. New Haven: Yale University Press.

Paul, S. M., D. S. Mytelka, C. T. Dunwiddie, C. C. Persinger, B. H. Munos, S. R. Lindborg, and A. L. Schacht. 2010. How to improve R&D productivity: the pharmaceutical industry's grand challenge. Nat Rev Drug Discov 9 (3):203-14.

Peterson, J. K., and P. J. Houghton. 2004. Integrating pharmacology and in vivo cancer models in preclinical and clinical drug development. Eur. J. Cancer 40:837-844.

Pew/AAAS. 2009. Scientific Achievements Less Prominent Than a Decade Ago. Public praises science; scientists fault public, media. Pew Research Center 2009 [cited July 9 2009]. Available from http://people-press.org/report/528/.

Powell, Ashley A., AmirAli H. Talasaz, Haiyu Zhang, Marc A. Coram, Anupama Reddy, Glenn Deng, Melinda L. Telli, Ranjana H. Advani, Robert W. Carlson, Joseph A. Mollick, Shruti Sheth, Allison W. Kurian, James M. Ford, Frank E. Stockdale, Stephen R. Quake, R. Fabian Pease, Michael N. Mindrinos, Gyan Bhanot, Shanaz H. Dairkee, Ronald W. Davis, and Stefanie S. Jeffrey. 2012. Single Cell Profiling of Circulating Tumor Cells: Transcriptional Heterogeneity and Diversity from Breast Cancer Cell Lines. PLoS ONE 7 (5):e33788.

Powles, T. J. 1992. The case for clinical trials of tamoxifen for prevention of breast cancer. Lancet 340 (8828):1145-7.

Rangarajan, A., and R. A. Weinberg. 2003. Opinion: Comparative biology of mouse versus human cells: modelling human cancer in mice. Nat Rev Cancer 3 (12):952-9.

Richardson, D. N. 1988. The history of Nolvadex. Drug Des Deliv 3 (1):1-14.

Rohan, R. M., A. Fernandez, T. Udagawa, J. Yuan, and R. J. D'Amato. 2000. Genetic heterogeneity of angiogenesis in mice. FASEB J 14 (7):871-6.

Salsburg, D. 1983. The lifetime feeding study in mice and rats--an examination of its validity as a bioassay for human carcinogens. Fundam Appl Toxicol 3 (1):63-7.

Sarkar, Susanta K. 2009. Molecular imaging approaches. Drug Discovery World (Fall):33-38.

Savage, Liz. 2008. High-Intensity Chemotherapy Does Not Improve Survival in Small Cell Lung Cancer. Journal of the National Cancer Institute 100 (8):519.

Schachter, Asher D. 2007. Predictive Modelling in Drug Development. Innovations in Pharmaceutical Technology (April):20-24.

Scott, David. 2012. Animal research is helping us beat cancer. Cancer Research UK, June 21 2011 [cited May 11 2012]. Available from http://scienceblog.cancerresearchuk.org/2011/06/21/animal-research-is-helping-us-beat-cancer/.

Serrano, D., M. Lazzeroni, C. F. Zambon, D. Macis, P. Maisonneuve, H. Johansson, A. Guerrieri-Gonzaga, M. Plebani, D. Basso, J. Gjerde, G. Mellgren, N. Rotmensz, A. Decensi, and B. Bonanni. 2011. Efficacy of tamoxifen based on cytochrome P450 2D6, CYP2C19 and SULT1A1 genotype in the Italian Tamoxifen Prevention Trial. Pharmacogenomics J 11 (2):100-107.

Shaffer, Catherine. 2012. Safety Through Sequencing. Drug Discovery & Development January 1, 2012 2012 [cited January 30 2012]. Available from http://www.dddmag.com/article-Safety-Through-Sequencing-12412.aspx?et_cid=2450547&et_rid=45518461&linkid=http%3a%2f%2fwww.dddmag.com%2farticle-Safety-Through-Sequencing-12412.aspx.

Shanks, N, and R Greek. 2009. Animal Models in Light of Evolution. Boca Raton: Brown Walker.

Shanks, N., R. Greek, and J. Greek. 2009. Are animal models predictive for humans? Philos Ethics Humanit Med 4 (1):2.

Sharp, Phillip A., and Robert Langer. 2011. Promoting Convergence in Biomedical Science. Science 333 (6042):527.

Shubick, P. 1980. Statement of the Problem. In Human Epidemiology and Animal Laboratory Correlations in Chemical Carcinogenesis, edited by F. Coulston and P. Shubick: Ablex Pub. .

Sietsema, W. K. 1989. The absolute oral bioavailability of selected drugs. Int J Clin Pharmacol Ther Toxicol 27 (4):179-211.

Simon, V. 2005. Wanted: women in clinical trials. Science 308 (5728):1517.

Singh, M., and N. Ferrara. 2012. Modeling and predicting clinical efficacy for drugs targeting the tumor milieu. Nature Biotechnology 30 (7):648-657.

Singh, M., Anthony Lima, Rafael Molina, Patricia Hamilton, Anne C Clermont, Vidusha Devasthali, Jennifer D Thompson, Jason H Cheng, Hani Bou Reslan, Calvin C K Ho, Timothy C Cao, Chingwei V Lee, Michelle A Nannini, Germaine Fuh, Richard A D Carano, Hartmut Koeppen, Ron X Yu, William F Forrest, Gregory D Plowman, and Leisa Johnson.

2010. *Assessing therapeutic responses in Kras mutant cancers using genetically engineered mouse models. Nat. Biotechnol. 28:585-593.*

Slack, J. M., P. W. Holland, and C. F. Graham. 1993. *The zootype and the phylotypic stage. Nature 361 (6412):490-2.*

Smith, W. E., L. Miller, R. E. Elsasser, and D. D. Hubert. 1965. *Tests for carcinogenicity of asbestos. Annals of the New York Academy of Sciences 132 (1):456-88.*

Repeated Author. 1965. *Tests for carcinogenicity of asbestos. Ann N Y Acad Sci 132 (1):456-88.*

Sole, Richard, and Brian Goodwin. 2002. *Signs of Life: How Complexity Pervades Biology: Basic Books.*

Spielman, R. S., L. A. Bastone, J. T. Burdick, M. Morley, W. J. Ewens, and V. G. Cheung. 2007. *Common genetic variants account for differences in gene expression among ethnic groups. Nat Genet 39 (2):226-31.*

Stamer, U. M., and F. Stuber. 2007. *The pharmacogenetics of analgesia. Expert Opin Pharmacother 8 (14):2235-45.*

Stoloff, L. 1992. *An analysis of the 1987 list of IARC-identified human carcinogens and the correlated animal studies. Regulatory toxicology and pharmacology : RTP 15 (1):10-3.*

Suggitt, M., and M. C. Bibby. 2005. *50 years of preclinical anticancer drug screening: empirical to target-driven approaches. Clinical cancer research : an official journal of the American Association for Cancer Research 11 (3):971-81.*

Suter, KE. 1990. *What can be learned from case studies? The company approach. In Animal Toxicity Studies: Their Relevance for Man, edited by C. Lumley and S. Walker. Lancaster: Quay.*

Talmadge, J. E., R. K. Singh, I. J. Fidler, and A. Raz. 2007. *Murine Models to Evaluate Novel and Conventional Therapeutic Strategies for Cancer. Am. J. Pathol. 170:793-804.*

Tucker, MJ, HK Adam, and JS Patterson. 1984. *Tamoxifen. In Safety Testing of New Drugs Laboratory Predictions and Clinical Performance, edited by D. Laurence, A. McLean and M. Weatherall. London: Academic Press.*

Understanding Animal Research. 2012. *Development of new treatments. Understanding Animal Research 2011 [cited August 5 2012]. Available from http://www.understandinganimalresearch.org.uk/about_research/areas_of_research/development_of_new_treatments.*

Unknown. 2002. *Drug Discovery & Development (November):35.*

Utidjian, M. 1988. *The interaction between epidemiology and animal studies in industrial toxicology. In Perspectives in Basic and Applied Toxicology, edited by B. Ballantyne. London: Butterworth-Heinemann.*

Van Dyke, T. 2010. *Finding the tumor copycat: approximating a human cancer. Nat Med 16 (9):976-7.*

Van Regenmortel, Marc HV, and David L. Hull. 2002. *Promises and Limits of Reductionism in the Biomedical Sciences (Catalysts for Fine Chemical Synthesis). West Sussex: Wiley.*

van Regenmortel, MHV. 2004. *Biological complexity emerges from the ashes of genetic reductionism. Journal of Molecular Recognition 17 (3):145-148.*

Repeated Author. 2004. *Reductionism and complexity in molecular biology. Scientists now have the tools to unravel biological complexity and overcome the limitations of reductionism. EMBO Rep 5 (11):1016-20.*

Venter, J. C., M. D. Adams, E. W. Myers, P. W. Li, R. J. Mural, G. G. Sutton, H. O. Smith, M. Yandell, C. A. Evans, R. A. Holt, J. D. Gocayne, P. Amanatides, R. M. Ballew, D. H. Huson, J. R. Wortman, Q. Zhang, C. D. Kodira, X. H. Zheng, L. Chen, M. Skupski, G. Subramanian, P. D. Thomas, J. Zhang, G. L. Gabor Miklos, C. Nelson, S. Broder, A. G. Clark, J. Nadeau, V. A. McKusick, N. Zinder, A. J. Levine, R. J. Roberts, M. Simon, C. Slayman, M. Hunkapiller, R. Bolanos, A. Delcher, I. Dew, D. Fasulo, M. Flanigan, L. Florea, A. Halpern, S. Hannenhalli, S. Kravitz, S. Levy, C. Mobarry, K. Reinert, K. Remington, J. Abu-Threideh, E. Beasley, K. Biddick, V. Bonazzi, R. Brandon, M. Cargill, I. Chandramouliswaran, R. Charlab, K. Chaturvedi, Z. Deng, V. Di Francesco, P. Dunn, K. Eilbeck, C. Evangelista, A. E. Gabrielian, W. Gan, W. Ge, F. Gong, Z. Gu, P. Guan, T. J. Heiman, M. E. Higgins, R. R. Ji, Z. Ke, K. A. Ketchum, Z. Lai, Y. Lei, Z. Li, J. Li, Y. Liang, X. Lin, F. Lu, G. V. Merkulov, N. Milshina, H. M. Moore, A. K. Naik, V. A.

Narayan, B. Neelam, D. Nusskern, D. B. Rusch, S. Salzberg, W. Shao, B. Shue, J. Sun, Z. Wang, A. Wang, X. Wang, J. Wang, M. Wei, R. Wides, C. Xiao, C. Yan, A. Yao, J. Ye, M. Zhan, W. Zhang, H. Zhang, Q. Zhao, L. Zheng, F. Zhong, W. Zhong, S. Zhu, S. Zhao, D. Gilbert, S. Baumhueter, G. Spier, C. Carter, A. Cravchik, T. Woodage, F. Ali, H. An, A. Awe, D. Baldwin, H. Baden, M. Barnstead, I. Barrow, K. Beeson, D. Busam, A. Carver, A. Center, M. L. Cheng, L. Curry, S. Danaher, L. Davenport, R. Desilets, S. Dietz, K. Dodson, L. Doup, S. Ferriera, N. Garg, A. Glucksmann, B. Hart, J. Haynes, C. Haynes, C. Heiner, S. Hladun, D. Hostin, J. Houck, T. Howland, C. Ibegwam, J. Johnson, F. Kalush, L. Kline, S. Koduru, A. Love, F. Mann, D. May, S. McCawley, T. McIntosh, I. McMullen, M. Moy, L. Moy, B. Murphy, K. Nelson, C. Pfannkoch, E. Pratts, V. Puri, H. Qureshi, M. Reardon, R. Rodriguez, Y. H. Rogers, D. Romblad, B. Ruhfel, R. Scott, C. Sitter, M. Smallwood, E. Stewart, R. Strong, E. Suh, R. Thomas, N. N. Tint, S. Tse, C. Vech, G. Wang, J. Wetter, S. Williams, M. Williams, S. Windsor, E. Winn-Deen, K. Wolfe, J. Zaveri, K. Zaveri, J. F. Abril, R. Guigo, M. J. Campbell, K. V. Sjolander, B. Karlak, A. Kejariwal, H. Mi, B. Lazareva, T. Hatton, A. Narechania, K. Diemer, A. Muruganujan, N. Guo, S. Sato, V. Bafna, S. Istrail, R. Lippert, R. Schwartz, B. Walenz, S. Yooseph, D. Allen, A. Basu, J. Baxendale, L. Blick, M. Caminha, J. Carnes-Stine, P. Caulk, Y. H. Chiang, M. Coyne, C. Dahlke, A. Mays, M. Dombroski, M. Donnelly, D. Ely, S. Esparham, C. Fosler, H. Gire, S. Glanowski, K. Glasser, A. Glodek, M. Gorokhov, K. Graham, B. Gropman, M. Harris, J. Heil, S. Henderson, J. Hoover, D. Jennings, C. Jordan, J. Jordan, J. Kasha, L. Kagan, C. Kraft, A. Levitsky, M. Lewis, X. Liu, J. Lopez, D. Ma, W. Majoros, J. McDaniel, S. Murphy, M. Newman, T. Nguyen, N. Nguyen, M. Nodell, S. Pan, J. Peck, M. Peterson, W. Rowe, R. Sanders, J. Scott, M. Simpson, T. Smith, A. Sprague, T. Stockwell, R. Turner, E. Venter, M. Wang, M. Wen, D. Wu, M. Wu, A. Xia, A. Zandieh, and X. Zhu. 2001. The sequence of the human genome. Science 291 (5507):1304-51.

Vicsek, T. 2002. The bigger picture. Nature 418 (6894):131.

Wade, Nicholas. 2009. New Treatment for Cancer Shows Promise in Testing. New York Times, June 29.

Wadman, Meredith. 2011. News Q&A. NIH cancer chief wants more with less. Nature 475 (7354):18.

Wagner, G. P., C. Amemiya, and F. Ruddle. 2003. Hox cluster duplications and the opportunity for evolutionary novelties. Proc Natl Acad Sci U S A 100 (25):14603-6.

Wagner, J. C. 1963. Asbestosis in experimental animals. Br J Ind Med 20:1-12.

Wagner, J. C., G. Berry, J. W. Skidmore, and V. Timbrell. 1974. The effects of the inhalation of asbestos in rats. Br J Cancer 29 (3):252-69.

Wald, Chelsea, and Corinna Wu. 2010. Of Mice and Women: The Bias in Animal Models. Science 327 (5973):1571-2.

Wall, R. J., and M. Shani. 2008. Are animal models as good as we think? Theriogenology 69 (1):2-9.

Weaver, J. L., D. Staten, J. Swann, G. Armstrong, M. Bates, and K. L. Hastings. 2003. Detection of systemic hypersensitivity to drugs using standard guinea pig assays. Toxicology 193 (3):203-17.

Wilke, Russell A., and M. Eileen Dolan. 2011. Genetics and Variable Drug Response. JAMA: The Journal of the American Medical Association 306 (3):306-307.

Willyard, C. 2009. HIV gender clues emerge. Nat Med 15 (8):830.

Wittenburg, L. A., and D. L. Gustafson. 2011. Optimizing preclinical study design in oncology research. Chemico-biological interactions 190 (2-3):73-8.

Wood, L. D., D. W. Parsons, S. Jones, J. Lin, T. Sjoblom, R. J. Leary, D. Shen, S. M. Boca, T. Barber, J. Ptak, N. Silliman, S. Szabo, Z. Dezso, V. Ustyanksky, T. Nikolskaya, Y. Nikolsky, R. Karchin, P. A. Wilson, J. S. Kaminker, Z. Zhang, R. Croshaw, J. Willis, D. Dawson, M. Shipitsin, J. K. Willson, S. Sukumar, K. Polyak, B. H. Park, C. L. Pethiyagoda, P. V. Pant, D. G. Ballinger, A. B. Sparks, J. Hartigan, D. R. Smith, E. Suh, N. Papadopoulos, P. Buckhaults, S. D. Markowitz, G. Parmigiani, K. W. Kinzler, V. E. Velculescu, and B. Vogelstein. 2007. The genomic landscapes of human breast and colorectal cancers. Science 318 (5853):1108-13.

Woodger, J.H. 1967. Biological Principles. New York: Humanities Press.

Zielinska, Edyta. 2010. Building a better mouse. The Scientist 24 (4):34-38.

Cancer-preventive Mechanism from the Perspective of Effects of the *Astragalus* Polysaccharides on Mitochondrial Energy Metabolism Improvement

Xing-Tai Li
College of Life Science
Dalian Nationalities University, China

Jia Zhao
Norman Bethune College of Medicine
Jilin University, China

1 Introduction

Mitochondria are cellular organelles bounded by two distinct membranes. They hold about one tenth of the cellular proteins, their own DNA and comparing weight to weight, convert over 10,000 times more energy per second than the sun (Schatz, 2007). The Swiss anatomist Rudolf Albrecht von Koelliker first described mitochondria in 1857, calling them sarcosomes. In 1890, the German pathologist Richard Altman proposed that they were intracellular parasites and 8 years later the German microbiologist Carl Benda finally gave them the name "mitochondria". In 1945, the Belgian-American biochemist Albert Claude isolated them by centrifugation from disrupted cells and showed that they catalyzed respiration and since then mitochondria have been defined as the powerhouse of the cell. In the following decades, biochemists tracked down the different components of this powerhouse and characterized them (Slater, 1977; Slater, 2003). Among the forceful fruits of a very intense period during the first half of the 20th century were the uncovering of the electron transport chain (ETC) by Henrich Otto Weiland, David Keilin and Otto Warburg, the mechanism of complete oxidation of nutrients into carbon dioxide through the tricarboxylic acid (TCA) cycle by Hans Krebs, and the mechanism of oxidative phosphorylation (OXPHOS) by Peter Mitchell's chemiosmotic theory (Frezza & Gottlieb, 2009). One of the principal bioenergetic functions of mitochondria is to generate adenosine triphosphate (ATP) through the process of OXPHOS, which occurs in the inner mitochondrial membrane (IMM) (Verdin *et al.*, 2010).

The past decade has revealed a new role for the mitochondria in cell metabolism–regulation of cell death pathways (Gogvadze *et al.*, 2008), which occurs upon permeabilization of their membranes. Once mitochondrial membrane permeabilization (MMP) occurs, cells die either by apoptosis or necrosis (Armstrong, 2006). The impact of mitochondrial activities on cellular physiology is not restricted to ATP production for metabolic demands. Mitochondria also produce reactive oxygen species (ROS), which are involved in the regulation of many physiological processes, but which might also be harmful to the cell if produced excessively. Furthermore, mitochondria are crucial for the regulation of intracellular Ca^{2+} homeostasis, and they are key participants in the regulation of cell death pathways. Mitochondria play an important role in controlling the life and death of a cell. Consequently, mitochondrial dysfunction leads to a range of human diseases. Obviously, these functions are of crucial importance for tumor cell physiology, growth and survival (Gogvadze *et al.*, 2008).

Mitochondria are essential organelles and key integrators of metabolism, but they also play vital roles in cell signaling pathways critically influencing cell fate decisions (Wallace, 2005; Finkel & Holbrook, 2000; Ryan & Hoogenraad, 2007). In order to synthesize ATP through OXPHOS, mitochondria consume most of the cellular oxygen and produce the majority of ROS as by-products (Solaini & Harris, 2005). ROS have been implicated in the etiology of carcinogenesis via oxidative damage to cell macromolecules and through modulation of mitogenic signaling pathways (Samper *et al.*, 2009; Hervouet *et al.*, 2008). Proper mitochondrial function is crucial for maintenance of metabolic homeostasis and activation of appropriate stress responses. Not surprisingly, changes in mitochondrial number and activity are implicated in aging and age-related diseases, including diabetes, neurodegenerative diseases and cancer (Wallace, 2005). Despite the important link between mitochondrial dysfunction and human diseases, in most cases, the molecular causes for dysfunction have not been identified and remain poorly understood (Verdin *et al.*, 2010). How mitochondrial functions are associated with cancer is a crucial and complex issue in biomedicine that is still unravelled (Gogvadze *et al.*, 2008; Eng *et al.*, 2003), but it warrants an extraordinary importance since mitochondria play a major role not only as energy suppliers and ROS "regulators", but also because of their control on cellular life and death. This is of particular relevance since tumour cells can acquire resistance to apoptosis by a number of mechanisms, including mitochondrial dysfunction, the expression of anti-apoptotic proteins or by the down-regulation or mutation of proapoptotic proteins (Igney & Krammer, 2002). Mitochondria are vital for cellular bioenergetics and essential for maintaining cell life, and play a central role in determining the point-of-no-return of the apoptotic process. As a consequence, mitochondria exert a dual function in carcinogenesis (Galluzzi *et al.*, 2006).

Different alterations of mitochondrial activity such as the release of apoptogenic proteins from the intermembrane space, loss of mitochondrial membrane potential ($\Delta\psi_m$), stimulation of ROS production, inhibition of mitochondrial respiratory complexes, and decreases in ATP synthesis have been shown to be involved in, and possibly responsible for, the different manifestations of cell death (Bras *et al.*, 2005). Thus mitochondrial destabilization could be a promising step in stimulating tumor cell death (Gogvadze *et al.*, 2009). The recognition of the role that mitochondria play in human health and disease is evidenced by the emergence in recent decades of a whole new field of "Mitochondrial Medicine"(D'Souza *et al.*, 2011). The accumulation of huge numbers of abnormal mitochondria as seen by electron microscopy and immunohistochemistry is the hallmark of oncocytic cells regardless of the organ of origin (thyroid, parathyroid, kidney, salivary gland, etc.) and of the benign or malignant nature of the lesions (Máximo & Sobrinho-Simões, 2000a; Muller-Hocker, 1992; Muller-Hocker *et al.*, 1998; Muller-Hocker, 2000). Reviewing the evidence on record, Gottlieb and Tomlinson (Gottlieb & Tomlinson, 2005), advanced that mitochondrial dysfunction may lead to carcinogenesis through several mechanisms: decrease in apoptosis, increase in the production of ROS and activation of a hypoxia-like pathway (pseudo-hypoxia).

The mitochondria are at the crossroads of life sustaining and death inducing paths. As such, it is an attractive option to be targeted to restore normalcy in defective cells and abrogate progression to malignancy (Indran *et al.*, 2011). The morphological differences observed in the mitochondria vary between tumor cell lines in terms of size, shape and count. It has been noted that the mitochondria in rapidly growing tumors tend to be fewer in number and smaller and have fewer cristae than slow growing tumors, normal cells or well differentiated tumors (Máximo & Sobrinho-Simões, 2000a). In addition, differences in IMM composition have also been observed between normal and transformed cells (Pedersen, 1978). Alternatively, given the stark differences the mitochondria present in cancer cells, riding on its dysfunctions could help to select and sever the lifeline to these cancer cells (Indran *et al.*, 2011). However, in the early and mid future, we might expect the developing of therapeutic interventions based on controlling the mitochondrial pathway for apoptosis that seem very promising. In addition, mitochondrial targeting of ROS scavengers and compounds that interfere with the unique biochemistry in the mitochondria are under investigation as promising therapeutic attempts (Solaini *et al.*, 2011).

This chapter aims to provide a comprehensive overview of mitochondrial energy metabolism and cancer, analyze mitochondrial protection and energy metabolic improvement of Astragalus Polysaccharides (APS), find its cancer-preventive underlying mechanism, and provide a new way of thinking. The mechanism of APS on energy metabolism improvement will be explored from mitochondrial oxidative phosphorylation and intracellular adenylates levels.

2   Mitochondrial ATP Production and Its Regulation

2.1   Mitochondrial ATP Production

The main pathways of cellular energy generation in mammalian cells are described below. Briefly, nutrients such as glucose, amino acids and fatty acids are transformed by intermediary metabolism into their reduced equivalents (NADH, H^+ or $FADH_2$), which are further oxidized by the mitochondrion to generate ATP. Large amounts of ATP are used in muscle contraction, nerve impulse conduction, compound biosynthesis or other biological processes. Mitochondria of normal tissues typically oxidize combinations of these energy substrates (fatty acids, the glycolysis end product pyruvate and amino acids) to establish the electrochemical gradient of protons ($\Delta\mu_H^+$) used by the F_1F_o–ATP synthase to produce ATP. Pioneering studies of metabolic control analysis (MCA) in the late 1970s explained that the control of cellular energy fluxes is shared between all the enzymes of the metabolic pathway that were studied (e.g., glycolysis or OXPHOS). These enzymatic steps include the transport of energy metabolites (e.g., pyruvate carrier), substrate oxidation (e.g., pyruvate dehydrogenase complex) and ATP synthesis (e.g., mitochondrial complex V).

2.2   Central Mechanisms Regulating Cellular Energy Homeostasis

In mammalian cells, energy homeostasis requires a constant coordination between cell activity, nutrient availability and the regulation of energy transduction processes. This is obtained via a complex signaling system linking energy and nutrient sensing to cellular effectors that include kinases and transcription factors. While the intracellular energy status is mirrored by the respective concentrations of the adenine nucleotides ATP, ADP and AMP (as well as phosphocreatine/ creatine), nutrient availability is reflected more by the concentration of glucose and amino-acids. The S6 kinases (S6Ks) 1 and 2 and the AMP-activated protein kinases (AMPKs) intervene downstream of these sensors to modulate growth rate and energy metabolism (Um *et al.*, 2006). The AMPKs are activated by alterations in the cellular AMP/ATP ratio, which is dictated by the balance between energy supply (ATP production) and energy demand (ATP consumption). When activated by AMP, the AMPKs initiate a phosphorylation cascade to switch on the catabolic pathways that produce ATP (glycolysis and OXPHOS via the stimulation of mitochondrial biogenesis) and to switch-off the anabolic pathways that consume ATP (protein, fatty acid and cholesterol synthesis). AMPKs target numerous genes involved in lipid, carbohydrate and protein metabolism, as well as those involved in cell signaling, transcription and ion transport (Hardie, 2007). More recently, it was discovered in mouse skeletal muscle that AMPKs further regulate energy metabolism through the activation of the sirtuin SIRT1 (Canto *et al.*, 2009). This results in deacetylating and altering the activity of downstream SIRT1 targets. Accordingly, the AMPKs can be activated by cellular stress, exercise, and a wide range of hormones or pharmaceutical agents that affect cellular energy metabolism (e.g., metformin, thiazolidinediones, adiponectin, leptin, ghrelin/cannabinoids and resveratrol) (Zhang *et al.*, 2009). In addition to the master control exerted by the AMPKs and sirtuins, the regulation of cellular energy metabolism is also influenced by calcium and ROS (Benard *et al.*, 2010).

2.3   Regulatory Mechanisms of Mitochondrial ATP Production

Cellular adaptation to environmental and physiological constraints necessitates that the control of mitochondrial respiration be fine tuned in its response to changes in energy demand and substrate delivery. This is accomplished by regulatory events which modulate OXPHOS, both structurally and functionally. Accordingly, different tissues exhibit large differences in the composition of the OXPHOS machinery and in the organization of mitochondria, and these differences could reflect their unique physiological activity. In addition, mitochondria also participate in fundamental cell signaling and apoptotic processes, the regulation of which might also lead to changes in organellar content, composition and functionality.

Yet, the regulation of mitochondrial energy production is concerted and dispersed. There are five different levels of OXPHOS regulation. (1) The first level includes the direct modulation of respiratory chain kinetic parameters via the expression of rapid or slow isoforms of complex IV (Capaldi *et al.*, 1988), the biochemical modulation of complex IV catalytic activity by $\Delta\psi_m$ (Piccoli *et al.*, 2006; Dalmonte *et al.*, 2009), numerous regulations of all ETC complexes by post-translational modifications including phosphorylation or nitrosylation (Carroll *et al.*, 2005; Das *et al.*, 1998). (2) The intrinsic efficiency of OXPHOS can be regulated by changes in the basal proton conductance or the induced proton conductance (Parker *et al.*, 2009), by changes in the P/O ratio, which is notably linked to oxygen levels (Gnaiger *et al.*, 2000), or by changes in the channeling of respiratory chain intermediate substrates (via differences in the organization and content of supercomplexes (D'Aurelio *et al.*, 2006; Bianchi *et al.*, 2004). (3) OXPHOS capacity may also depend on the morphological state of the mitochondrial compartment (networked or fragmented) in living mammalian cells (Benard *et al.*, 2007), which relies on highly regulated fusion and fission events, mitochondrial motility and changes in organellar membrane lipid composition (Choi *et al.*, 2006; Furt & Moreau, 2009) as well as the osmotic phenomena of mitochondrial swelling or shrinking (Hackenbrock, 1968; Hackenbrock *et al.*, 1971). (4) An upper level of mitochondrial-energetics regulation consists of the modulation of mitochondrial biogenesis and degradation, including the determination of cellular mitochondrial DNA (mtDNA) content by peroxisome proliferator-activated receptor-γ coactivator 1 alpha (PGC1α) and sirtuins (Canto *et al.,* 2009; Arany *et al.*, 2005; Ventura-Clapier *et al.*, 2008). (5) Cell biology has revealed the heterogeneity of mitochondrial function within the cell, such that energy production can be further regulated *in situ* by the cellular and mitochondrial microenvironment, including the availability of energy substrates (NADH, H^+/NAD^+, ADP/ATP, oxygen gradients, glucose and glutamine) and their delivery at the Q-junction (Gnaiger, 2009), interactions with other organelles (ER, Golgi, plasma membrane) (Koziel *et al.*, 2009; de Brito & Scorrano, 2008), the concerted regulation of OXPHOS with other functions (apoptosis and calcium signaling) and the impact of various chemicals (environmental drugs or medicine).

Lastly, mitochondria can also generate feedback signals via metabolites in the cytosol, such as ATP/ADP, ROS, Ca^{2+} or $NADH/NAD^+$, which participate in the regulation of energy production. The field of mitochondrial bioenergetics is examining the possible regulation of mitochondrial ATP production by organellar dynamics and motility, in concert with the regulation of other mitochondrial functions including cell death execution (Benard *et al.*, 2010).

3   Production of ROS by Mitochondria and the Damage to Mitochondria

In recent years, cellular oxidation and reduction (redox) environment has gained significant attention as a critical regulator of human health and disease. Cellular redox environment is a balance between the production of ROS and their removal by antioxidants. ROS are oxygen containing molecules that are highly reactive in redox reactions. ROS are primarily produced intracellularly by two metabolic sources: the mitochondrial ETC and oxygen metabolizing enzymatic reactions. Approximately 98–99% of all mitochondrial oxygen consumption is efficiently reduced by Complex IV. Despite this high efficiency, the 1-electron reduction of oxygen at Complexes I and III is known to generate superoxide. Once formed, superoxide is rapidly converted to hydrogen peroxide via the spontaneous ($10^5 \ mol^{-1} \ sec^{-1}$) or enzymatic ($10^9 \ mol^{-1} \ sec^{-1}$) driven dismutation reaction. Hydrogen peroxide is neutralized both by catalase and glutathione peroxidase. Hydrogen peroxide reacts with transition metal ions (e.g. cuprous and ferrous ions) through Fenton and Haber-Weiss chemistry generating the highly reactive hydroxyl radical that is well known to cause damage to cellular macromolecules (Goswami, 2009). ROS, if not detoxified, oxidize cellular proteins, lipids, and nucleic acids and, by doing so, cause cell dysfunction or death. A cascade of water and lipid soluble antioxidants and antioxidant enzymes suppresses the harmful ROS activity. An imbalance that favors the production of ROS over antioxidant defenses, defined as oxidative stress, is implicated in a wide variety of pathologies, including malignant diseases (Gogvadze *et al.*, 2008).

ROS impair mitochondrial function. The hypoxic environment of proliferating tumor tissue facilitates ROS production. However, ROS levels can also be increased by hypoxia, when electron transport complexes are in the reduced state (Guzy & Schumacker, 2006). Therefore, under hypoxic conditions and, in particular, after normalization of oxygen supply, production of ROS in tumor cells can be enhanced to an extent that might induce damage to vital cellular components, including mtDNA. This might trigger a vicious cycle (i.e. hypoxia, ROS production, mtDNA mutations, malfunction of the mitochondrial respiratory chain, further stimulation of ROS production etc.), thus impairing mitochondrial function and causing a shift to glycolytic ATP production (Gogvadze *et al.*, 2008). It should be mentioned that mitochondria are not only a major source of ROS but also a sensitive target for the damaging effects of oxygen radicals. ROS produced by mitochondria can oxidize proteins and induce lipid peroxidation, compromising the barrier properties of biological membranes. One of the targets of ROS is mtDNA, which encodes several proteins essential for the function of the mitochondrial respiratory chain and, hence, for ATP synthesis by OXPHOS. Oxidative damage induced by ROS is probably a major source of mitochondrial genomic instability leading to respiratory dysfunction (Gogvadze *et al.*, 2008).

One characteristic feature of tumor cells is an elevated level of ROS (Pelicano *et al.*, 2004). They are generated continuously in cells and play important roles in a variety of cellular processes (Storz, 2005). Another reason for the enhanced ROS production in cancer cells could be the hyperpolarized mitochondria. It is known that the formation of ROS intensifies when the $\Delta\psi_m$ increases (Brand *et al.*, 2004). Many tumor cells demonstrate an elevated $\Delta\psi_m$ due to its decreased utilization for ATP synthesis, and this could be one reason for the elevated ROS production in cancer cells (Derdak *et al.*, 2008). ROS stimulate cell proliferation and cellular migration. Uncontrolled production of ROS might lead to genetic lesions, tumorigenicity and tumor progression (Storz, 2005). ROS appear to play a major role in the metastatic potential, since pre-treatment with ROS scavengers abolished metastasis formation (Ishikawa *et al.*, 2008).

4   Mitochondrial Energy Metabolic Changes of Cancer Cells

4.1 Warburg Effect

Cell death is an essential part of the normal development and maturation cycle (Jacobson *et al.*, 1997), and a homeostatic balance between the rates of cell proliferation and cell death is critical for maintaining normal physiological processes. Alterations or defiance against these natural death mechanisms can lead to diseases such as AIDS, diabetes mellitus, neurodegenerative diseases and cancer, many of which are now, also known to be ROS-mediated (Indran *et al.*, 2011). Cancer is a disease of aberrant proliferation. Cancer is an extremely complex, chimeric new growth, a sort of highly regulated, successful, invasive clone of our own tissues (Máximo *et al.*, 2009). Cancer is not an invader in our bodies like a virus or bacterial infection, nor is it a genetic distortion determined to kill us. Cancer is the body, at the cellular level, attempting to allow the injured tissue or organ to survive by reverting to a primitive survival mechanism

(Peskin, 2009). In their millennium review Hanahan and Weinberg described six essential alterations in cell physiology that collectively might dictate malignant growth: self-sufficiency in growth signals, insensitivity to growth-inhibitory (antigrowth) signals, limitless replicative potential, sustained angiogenesis, tissue invasion and metastasis, and evasion of programmed cell death (apoptosis) (Hanahan &Weinberg, 2000). Accumulating evidence now suggests that, in addition to these alterations, another feature of tumor cells, i.e. their dependence on glycolysis for ATP generation, might be added to this list.

The possible role of mitochondrial function and carcinogenesis was first proposed by the German scientist Otto Warburg in 1926 as a shift in cancer cell energy production from respiration to aerobic glycolysis, even in the presence of abundant oxygen. A prominent metabolic alteration in cancer cells is that they exhibit a substantial increase in aerobic glycolysis and seem to rely more on this non-oxidative glucose metabolism for generation of ATP (which causes local acidification owing to lactate production) and for production of other molecules for cell growth and proliferation. This phenomenon, known as the Warburg effect, has been observed in a variety of cancer types including solid tumors and leukemia (Wanga et al.,2010). Cancer cells frequently reprogram cellular metabolism in parallel with activation of cell cycle progression to support the demands of rapid cell growth and mitogenesis. The benefits of altered metabolism for cancer cells are not fully understood, but include rapid ATP production, increased production of macromolecular building blocks for the synthesis of nucleotides (via the pentose phosphate pathway) and amino and fatty acids (from intermediates formed in the glycolytic and TCA cycle), and increased survival in oxygen-limiting conditions. What is clear, however, is that metabolic reprogramming renders cancer cells hypersensitive to interruptions in the availability or the metabolism of glucose (Khatri & Plas, 2009). In order to favour the production of biomass, proliferating cells are commonly prone to satisfy the energy requirement utilizing substrates other than the complete oxidation of glucose (to CO_2 and H_2O). More precisely, only part [40 to 75%, according to (Mathupala et al., 2010)] of the cells need of ATP is obtained through the scarcely efficient catabolism of glucose to pyruvate/lactate in the cytoplasm and the rest of the ATP need is synthesized in the mitochondria through both the TCA cycle (one ATP produced each acetyl moiety oxidized) and the associated OXPHOS that regenerates nicotinamide- and flavin-dinucleotides in their oxidized state (NAD^+ and FAD) (Solaini et al., 2011).

Warburg hypothesize that cancer cells derive most of their energy from glycolysis even under aerobic conditions, and that cancer is an outcome of defective mitochondrial energy metabolism (i.e., a decrease in mitochondrial energy metabolism might lead to development of cancer) (Gogvadze et al., 2008). Warburg's hypothesis profoundly influenced the present perception of cancer metabolism (Frezza & Gottlieb, 2009). A comparison of multiple cancer cell lines revealed that they rely on glycolysis for ATP production to different extents, and typically, the more "glycolytic" tumor cells were shown to be the most aggressive ones (Simonnet et al., 2002).

4.2   OXPHOS Peculiarities in Cancer Cells — the Potential Underlying Mechanism for the Warburg Effect

Although the underlying mechanisms responsible for the Warburg effect remain to be defined, it has been postulated that mitochondrial dysfunction (respiration injury) may be a key event that compromises the cancer cell's ability to generate ATP through OXPHOS, and thus forces them to increase glucose fermentation to compensate the energy supply (Warburg et al., 1956). Many studies in the last decade indicate that mitochondrial dysfunction is one of the more recurrent features of cancer cells, as reported at microscopic, molecular, biochemical, and genetic level (Hervouet et al., 2008; Genova et al., 2008; Smolková et al., 2010). Although cancer cells under several conditions, including hypoxia, oncogene activation, and mDNA mutation, may substantially differ in their ability to use oxygen, only few reports have been able to identify a strict association between metabolic changes and mitochondrial respiratory chain complexes composition and activity. In renal oncocytomas (Simonnet *et al.*, 2003) and in lung epidermoid carcinoma (Bellance *et al.*, 2009), the NADH dehydrogenase activity and protein content of Complex I were found to be strongly depressed; subsequently, in a thyroid oncocytoma cell line (Bonora *et al.*, 2006) a similar decrease of Complex I activity was ascribed to a specific mutation in the ND1 gene of mtDNA (Solaini *et al.*, 2011). Mitochondrial mutations, oncogenic signals, and metabolic stress are possible factors that can lead to mitochondrial dysfunction (Chen & Pervaiz, 2010).

Moreover, some studies showed that cancer cells have increased mitochondrial transmembrane potential (Bernal *et al.*, 1982; Johnson *et al.*, 1981). In addition, increased ROS generation in cancer cells may reflect an increased leakage of electrons from the transport complexes (complex I and complex III). Thus, elevated ROS generation in cancer cells may be considered as an indication of mitochondrial dysfunction (Wanga *et al.*, 2010). In addition to having to adopt the aerobic glycolysis, many cancer cells present a number of other metabolic changes that in the mitochondria include: decreased oxidation of substrates (mostly NADH-linked), altered expression and activity of respiratory chain subunits, overproduction of ROS, mtDNA mutations, impaired both respiratory chain complexes and ATP synthase organization within the inner mitochondrial membrane, and altered control of apoptosis. All these reasons locate mitochondria at central stage to understanding the molecular basis of tumour growth and to seeking for novel therapeutical approaches (Solaini *et al.*, 2011).

In addition to the increased glycolysis, the altered bioenergetics observed in many human carcinomas has been highly correlated with the downregulation of the catalytic subunit of the mitochondrial H^+-ATP synthase (β-F_1-ATPase) (Cuezva *et al.*, 2002). Remarkably, the expression level of the β-F1-ATPase protein correlated inversely with the rate of aerobic glycolysis. Furthermore, inhibition of OXPHOS by oligomycin in lung carcinoma was shown to trigger a rapid increase in aerobic glycolysis. This finding demonstrated that tumor cells can become glycolytic as a result of suppression of mitochondrial energy production. Similarly, inhibition of respiration in some human lung cancer cell lines was found to significantly upregulate glycolysis. However, when glycolysis was suppressed, tumor cells were unable to sufficiently upregulate mitochondrial OXPHOS, indicating partial mitochondrial impairment (Wu, 2007). From a clinical perspective it is important to note that the degree of glycolysis correlates with tumour prognosis. A biochemical analysis of different types of cancer showed that tumour aggressiveness can be defined by a bioenergetic index calculated as the ratio between the activities of the mitochondrial enzyme ATP synthase and the glycolytic enzyme glyceraldehyde-3-phosphate dehydrogenase. One can therefore consider that mitochondrial function in cancer cells, even if not damaged, might be inhibited by low oxygen levels, changes in metabolic fluxes and gene expression reprogramming (Moreno-Sánchez *et al.*, 2007; Cuezva *et al.*, 2004). Analysis of mitochondrial and glycolytic phenotypes in cancer cells and normal cells has also resulted in a bioenergetic signature, consistent across several types of human carcinomas including breast, colon and stomach. In this regard, Cuezva *et al.* defined a bioenergetic index based on the levels of a bioenergetic marker of mitochondria relative to a cellular glycolytic marker (Cuezva *et al.*, 2004). Their observations demonstrated that bioenergetic index served as a reliable indicator along with the expression of β-F1-ATPase in breast, gastric, lung and esophageal cancers (Indran *et al.*, 2011).

In the years following the postulation of the Warburg's hypothesis, the discovery of numerous critical cancer regulators, such as the p53 protein and other tumor suppressors or oncogenes have shifted the focus of cancer research away from studies of energy metabolism to other areas. In the last decade however, a renewed interest has returned to the role of mitochondria and energy metabolism in cancer (Gogvadze *et al.*, 2008; Indran *et al.*, 2011). Today, we are witnessing a renaissance of Warburg's fundamental observation. Studies during the past decade have shed light on some of the peculiarities of mitochondrial function in cancer cells, and suggest that the Warburg effect is more closely related to alterations in signaling pathways that govern glucose uptake and utilization than to mitochondrial defects *per se* (Gogvadze *et al.*, 2008).

This metabolic shift may be due to defects in OXPHOS that force cancer cells towards glycolysis. Genetic evidence for OXPHOS defects has been provided, during the past 10 years, with the identification of mutations in mtDNA-encoded OXPHOS genes in most types of human cancers (Máximo *et al.*, 2009). Conceptually, any alteration that disrupts either the OXPHOS system or the Krebs cycle will have a direct effect on the cell's metabolism: If ATP production through OXPHOS is no longer viable, glycolysis remains the only way to obtain energy. There are two consequences of this metabolic shift that constitute important advantages to tumour cells: overproduction of lactic acid and acidification of the media with concomitant injury to "normal" cells, as well as oxygen-independent growth and survival (Máximo *et al.*, 2009). In this way, OXPHOS inactivation would be an initial step in tumour development conferring tumourigenic potential to the cells. Biochemical analyses of oncocytic thyroid tumours revealed that the ATP synthesis in the tumour cells is impaired, suggesting an inactivation of the OXPHOS system (Savagner *et al.*, 2001).

However, further studies challenged this idea and revealed that tumor mitochondria do respire and produce ATP (Weinhouse, 1976), subsequent studies revealed that tumor mitochondria could function normally with regards to the oxidation of respiratory substrates and maintenance of P/O and respiratory control ratios (Nakashima *et al.,* 1984). Whether mitochondrial respiration is low or not, there is now general agreement that cancer cells do exhibit high rates of glycolysis—aerobic or anaerobic. In fact, the extensive glucose utilization by malignant cells is widely used nowadays for the visualization of tumors by positron emission tomography, emphasizing the importance of Warburg's original observation (Gogvadze *et al.*, 2009).

4.3 The Crabtree Effect and Its Induction

Today, the Warburg effect is regarded as the phenomenon of increased glycolysis in cancer cells even in the presence of oxygen, without a corresponding increase in OXPHOS. However, the original hypothesis claimed that impaired mitochondrial function caused the glycolytic phenotype and the formation of cancer (Warburg, 1956). This *tout court* statement was immediately criticized by Sydney Weinhouse (Weinhouse, 1956) who demonstrated that mitochondrial function in cancer tissues was normal, and strongly stood against the emerging picture of impaired mitochondria as a cause of cancer. Weinhouse wrote: "no substantial evidence has been found that would indicate a respiratory defect, either in the machinery of electron transport or in the coupling of respiration with ATP formation, or in the unique presence or absence of mitochondrial enzymes or cofactors involved in electron transport"(Weinhouse, 1976).

The switch between glycolysis and OXPHOS is controlled by the relative activities of two enzymes, pyruvate dehydrogenase (PDH) and lactate dehydrogenase (LDH). Several recent studies have confirmed that restricting glycolysis or diverting pyruvate into the mitochondria, can significantly induce respiration in cancer cells (Fantin *et al.*, 2006; Bonnet *et al.*, 2007). These studies confirmed that the fate of pyruvate (either reduction in the cytosol by LDH or oxidation in the mitochondria by PDH) determines the direction of tumour metabolism. The inhibition of LDH or the activation of PDH [via the inhibition of pyruvate dehydrogenase kinase (PDK)], can induce tumour cells to oxidize pyruvate in the TCA cycle and stimulate mitochondrial respiration (Fantin *et al.*, 2006). Hypoxia-induced factor 1 (HIF-1) was shown to induce PDK1 and thereby inactivate PDH and, as a result, to suppress the Krebs cycle and mitochondrial respiration. This indicates that mitochondrial activity is not fundamentally impaired in cancer cells. More recent data showed that for most, but not all, cancer cells glycolysis accounts for about 60% of ATP production (Busk *et al.*, 2008). In other words, most cancer cells appear capable of performing respiration, but the rate of OXPHOS is reduced by a dramatic increase in glycolysis and lactate production.

Warburg's hypothesis was, at the time, a conceptual leap and it resulted in a new understanding of tumor metabolic behavior. However, almost a century later, the metabolic transformation of cancer is still a riddle. While it is clear today that many, if not most, tumor cells are capable of performing OXPHOS when forced to, glucose metabolism is increased dramatically in most tumors. Increased glucose metabolism may reflect the need for rapid-production of ATP and/or for anabolic metabolites. Notably, there are examples of tumor cell lines that exhibit inherent decreased mitochondrial functions caused by mutations in either the mtDNA itself or in nuclear-encoded mitochondrial proteins. In other tumors, decreased OXPHOS could be a consequence of accelerated glycolysis and lactate production due to genetic or environmental alterations (Frezza & Gottlieb, 2009). Therefore, owing to the heterogeneity of tumor cells, the OXPHOS capacity of each particular tumor should be evaluated to determine whether the enhanced glycolysis is indeed a consequence of impaired mitochondrial functions.

Two distinct scenarios were presented, in which mitochondria play a key role in tumorigenesis: mitochondrial dysfunction as the driving cause of tumorigenesis and mitochondrial dysfunction as a 'second hit' in the process of cancer metabolic transformation. In the latter, mitochondria impairment can be the outcome of accelerated glycolysis brought about by the loss of tumor suppressors or the activation of oncogenes. In both cases however, metabolic reprogramming increases the cancer cells' survival and proliferation advantage by increasing ATP production in an oxygen independent manner and providing building blocks for macromolecule biosynthesis, two parameters which are critically required when excessive growth limits nutrient and oxygen supplies. However, it is medically important that regardless of the cause of metabolic transformation, it may render cancer cells dependent on distinctive metabolic pathways and/or isoenzymes. Identifying and targeting these could take the metabolic transformation process from the realm of intriguing phenomena to the platform of cancer therapeutics (Frezza & Gottlieb, 2009).

Back in the 1920s, Herbert Crabtree observed that increased glycolysis in cancer and normal proliferating cells inhibits respiration, an observation is now known as the 'Crabtree effect'(Crabtree, 1929). He further suggested that this observation is sufficient to explain the decrease in OXPHOS-derived ATP in cancer, arguing against Warburg's initial hypothesis that defects in respiration are the cause for increased glycolysis. Years later it was suggested that respiration inhibition by glycolysis was caused by glycolysis competing with OXPHOS for Pi and ADP (Ibsen, 1961). However, the Crabtree effect does not provide an explanation for the actual cause of the observed increased aerobic glycolysis in cancer.

Some cancer cells, in spite of possessing functional mitochondria, can switch between glycolytic and oxidative metabolism in a reversible fashion (Díaz-Ruiz *et al.*, 2009). Regarding the novel therapies based on the inhibition of tumor cell energy metabolism, the sole inhibition of glycolysis would not be sufficient to eliminate all malignant cells some of them may easily overcome the inhibition of the fermentative metabolism. This would bring as a consequence the incomplete elimination of cancer cells and it also would increase the probability of reoccurrence after treatment. Because of this, it is important to precisely know the Crabtree effect and its underlying causes in order to properly target the cancer cells.

The mechanism by which the Crabtree effect is triggered is unknown. Moreover, it is probable that its induction may be due to a combination of several factors (Rodríguez-Enriquez *et al.*, 2001). The most accepted hypothesis is that the glycolysis enzymes (phosphoglycerate kinase and pyruvate kinase) and mitochondria compete for free cytoplasmic ADP (Weinhouse, 1972; Gatt & Racker, 1959). If glycolysis is overactive it could, in theory, override mitochondria regarding ADP uptake. As the latter is one of the substrates of OXPHOS, this would limit one of the substrates of the ATP synthase and consequently respiration would be decreased. Nonetheless, it is unlikely that this could occur *in vivo* as the Km for the mitochondrial ANT is almost 100-times lower than that of the glycolysis enzymes (Veech *et al.*, 1979). This implies that mitochondria would still use the cytosolic ADP even if the glycolysis enzymes increase their activity.

Nonetheless, there is a considerable body of evidence that challenges the paradigm of the purely "glycolytic" cancer cell (Moreno-Sánchez *et al.*, 2007). It has been demonstrated that some glioma, hepatoma and breast cancer cell lines possess functional mitochondria and that they obtain their ATP mainly from OXPHOS (Rodríguez-Enríquez *et al.*, 2006; Pasdois *et al.*, 2003). Moreover, it has been demonstrated that some cancer cells can reversibly switch between fermentation and oxidative metabolism, depending on the absence or the presence of glucose and the environmental conditions (Rodríguez-Enríquez *et al.*, 2008; Smolková *et al.*, 2010). Interestingly, a recent model proposed that "glycolytic" cells could establish a metabolic symbiosis with the "oxidative" ones through lactate shuttling (Sonveaux *et al.*, 2008). This points out that the metabolic plasticity observed *in vitro* may have an impact on tumor physiology *in vivo*. Therefore, it is crucial to understand the mechanisms by which cancer cells can reversibly regulate their energy metabolism. Regarding this, a well-defined feature of some cancer cells is the glucose-induced suppression of respiration and OXPHOS (Crabtree, 1929; Díaz-Ruiz *et al.*, 2009). This is a short-term and reversible event and is referred to as the "Crabtree effect". This reversible shift might represent an advantage of cancer cells *in vivo*, as it would allow them to adapt their metabolism to the rather heterogeneous microenvironments in malignant solid overgrowths.

Recently, cancer cell energy metabolism has been suggested as a possible target in therapy (Rodríguez-Enríquez *et al.*, 2006; Díaz-Ruiz *et al.*, 2009) and much of the actual research in the field is being addressed to this particular issue. It is therefore crucial to clearly understand the long-term metabolic reprogramming of cancer cells (the Warburg effect) and the short-term adaptation mechanisms (the Crabtree effect) as the targeting of both would lead to much more effective therapeutic strategies.

Another interesting feature of cancer cell energy metabolism is their extensive consumption of glutamine. Glutamine is a crucial amino acid in cancer cell metabolism, it is the most abundant free amino acid in plasma and cancer patients have increased glutamine plasma levels (Ko *et al.*, 2011). Glutamine is consumed at high rates by many cancer and proliferating cells in order to support bioenergetics. Glutamine also contributes carbon and nitrogen to biosynthetic processes and can impact signal transduction. Increased glutaminolysis is now recognized as a key feature of the metabolic profile of cancer cells, along with increased aerobic glycolysis (the Warburg effect) (Daye & Wellen, 2012). Glutamine's involvement in oxidative mitochondrial metabolism in cancer cells was reported as early as the 1970s (Kovacevic & Morris, 1972), and recent investigation has greatly expanded our understanding of the role and regulation of glutamine metabolism in cancer. Glutamine contributes to bioenergetics (ATP production) and biosynthesis through reactions that use its α-nitrogen, γ-nitrogen or carbon skeleton. The final major fate of glutamine, following its conversion to glutamate and then glutamate's conversion to α-ketoglutarate (α-KG), is the oxidation of its carbon backbone in the mitochondria leading to energy production (Daye & Wellen, 2012). Some cancer cells produce more than 50% of their ATP by oxidizing glutamine-derived α-KG in the mitochondria (Rajagopalan & DeBerardinis, 2011). Glutaminolysis contributes to production of mitochondrial NADH, which is used to support ATP production by OXPHOS. Glutamine metabolism also contributes to production of NADPH and lipid and amino acid biosynthesis. The TCA cycle metabolite citrate can also exit the mitochondria to be used for generation of cytoplasmic acetyl-CoA, a precursor for fatty acid biosynthesis. Recent estimates indicate that 10–25% of acetyl-CoA used for *de novo* lipogenesis comes from glutamine under normoxic conditions, and that up to 80% of acetyl-CoA for lipogenesis may come from glutamine in hypoxia. Glutamine metabolism produces oxaloacetate (OAA) and also supplements the pyruvate pool, which is predominantly formed from glucose (DeBerardinis & Cheng, 2010). Similarly, malate produced in the TCA cycle can exit the mitochondria and contribute to pyruvate and lactate production.

5   Hypoxia and Mitochondrial OXPHOS in Cancer Cells

One of the main characteristics of tumor cells is their fast proliferation. Due to the high growth rate, tumor tissue easily becomes hypoxic because of the inability of the local vasculature to supply an adequate amount of oxygen. Similar conditions are often lethal to non-malignant cells due to hypoxia-induced, p53-mediated apoptosis (Hammond & Giaccia, 2005), but tumor cells can successfully escape hypoxia-mediated death due to mutations, or lowered expression, of p53 (Moll &Schramm, 1998). The inability of mitochondria to provide enough ATP for cell survival under hypoxic conditions, results in upregulation of the glycolytic pathway. This occurs by induction of HIF-1, which not only stimulates key steps of glycolysis, but also regulates genes that control angiogenesis, as well as cell survival and invasion (Wang & Semenza, 1993). The role of HIF-1 is not restricted to upregulation of the enzymes stimulating glucose utilization. Recent findings demonstrate that, in addition, HIF-1 suppresses mitochondrial function in tumor cells, suggesting that it modulates the reciprocal relationship between glycolysis and OXPHOS (Gogvadze *et al.*, 2009). These findings demonstrate that a switch to glycolysis might also result from suppression of mitochondrial OXPHOS.

Over 80 years ago, medical physicist, physiologist, and Nobel Prize-winner Otto Warburg, proved that a 35% reduction in oxygen causes any cell to either die or turn cancerous. Cancers live and ultimately thrive on the energy from glycolysis, and that is why they need such large vascular networks providing tremendous amounts of carbohydrates. Glycolysis is also a much simpler biochemical process, compared with cellular respiration (OXPHOS). In the presence of oxygen deficiency, cells that can't obtain enough energy through glycolysis perish. But the cells that succeed in utilizing glycolysis exhibit their innate will to survive; these are the ones that don't die from the oxygen deficiency. But there is a huge price to be paid for lack of oxygen: lack of cellular intelligence – these cells have the intelligence of "dumb yeast." In essence, cancer is the "idiot cell" that can survive but do little more than reproduce more "idiot cells" with no fully functional mitochondria (Peskin, 2009). Many physicians approach cancer as a localized issue, meaning that they focus only on the affected tissue as the problem because the genes have been ruined there. While this concept has been advocated in the past, the most recent noteworthy research suggests that the cancerous tissue is the most oxygen-deprived tissue; that's why that particular tissue became cancerous (Peskin & Carter, 2008). Cancer is a systemic problem – not just a local one. Once the cell is chronically oxygen deprived, the genetic material does change, but that is solely a consequence, not a cause. You've got much more to worry about than one cancerous area, since many tissues are oxygen deprived along with the cancerous ones. They just haven't reached the critical 35% cellular oxygen deficiency threshold yet (Peskin, 2009).

Molecular oxygen (O_2) is the ultimate electron acceptor of the mitochondrial ETC. It is consumed at complex IV (cytochrome c oxidase, COX) where it is reduced to water. The affinity of COX to oxygen is high considering the available oxygen levels in well-oxygenated (normoxic) tissues (Brahimi-Horn & Pouyssegur, 2007). However, it is clear that many tumor regions are deeply hypoxic, with oxygen concentrations approaching 0 mm Hg (Braun et al., 2001). Thus, it can be argued that in large regions of solid tumors, OXPHOS is effectively limited leaving glycolysis as the main energy-generating pathway (the Pasteur Effect). It is important to mention that phosphofructokinase-1 (PFK1), a key regulatory enzyme of glycolysis, is negatively regulated by ATP. Therefore, when OXPHOS is inhibited due to lack of oxygen and ATP levels decrease, glycolysis can be enhanced to compensate for ATP loss. However, the pathological influence of hypoxia on mitochondrial respiration in solid tumors is still unclear.

There is also emerging evidence suggesting that mitochondrial dysfunction may lead to the activation of HIF 1-alpha (HIF-1α), therefore triggering the hypoxia pathway in the tumourigenic process. The activation of this pathway would result in the transcription of a number of genes known to be associated with human tumourigenesis, such as those involved in glucose metabolism, angiogenesis, extra-cellular matrix modification, motility and survival (Pouyssegur et al., 2006; Bristow & Hill, 2008; Chiang & Massague, 2008). Mitochondria can also promote HIF-1α stabilization if the TCA flux is severely inhibited with release of intermediate molecules like succinate and fumarate into the cytosol. On the other hand, HIF-1 can modulate mitochondrial functions through different mechanisms, that besides metabolic reprogramming (Hervouet et al., 2008; Solaini et al., 2010), include alteration of mitochondrial structure and dynamics (Chiche et al., 2010), induction of microRNA-210 that decreases COX activity by inhibiting the gene expression of the assembly protein COX10, that also increases ROS generation. Moreover, these stress conditions could induce the anti-apoptotic protein Bcl-2, which has also been reported to regulate COX activity and mitochondrial respiration (Chen & Pervaiz, 2010), conferring resistance to cells death in tumors. This effect might be further enhanced upon severe hypoxia conditions, since COX is also inhibited by NO, the product of activated nitric oxide synthases (Hagen et al., 2003). The reduced respiration rate occurring in hypoxia favors the release of ROS also by Complex III, which contribute to HIF stabilization and induction of Bcl-2 (Bell et al., 2007). In addition, hypoxia reduces OXPHOS by inhibiting the ATP synthase complex through its natural protein inhibitor IF1, which contributes to the enhancement of the "aerobic glycolysis", all signatures of cancer transformation. Considering the protumoral effect of hypoxia, some research groups have investigated whether hyperoxia may be useful in cancer therapy. These very preliminary investigations seem interesting, but much more has to be known in order to attempt therapeutic treatments of tumors by this approach.

6   The Mitochondrial Membrane Potential Alteration in Cancer Cells

As high-energy electrons derived from glucose, amino acids or fatty acids are passed through a series of protein complexes (I–IV), their energy is used to pump protons from the mitochondrial matrix through the inner membrane into the intermembrane space, generating a proton gradient known as $\Delta\psi_m$ (Wallace, 2005). Interestingly, studies have also shown that the $\Delta\psi_m$ is approximately 60 mV higher in carcinomas as compared to their normal controls (Modica-Napolitano & Aprille, 2001). Critical mitochondrial functions, including ATP synthesis, ion homeostasis, metabolites transport, ROS production, and cell death are highly dependent on $\Delta\psi_m$ (Solaini *et al.*, 2007). In normal cells, under normoxic conditions, $\Delta\psi_m$ is build up by the respiratory chain and is mainly used to drive ATP synthesis, whereas in anoxia or severe hypoxia it is generated by the hydrolytic activity of the ATP synthase complex and by the electrogenic transport of ATP in exchange for ADP from the cytosol to the matrix, operated by ANT (Shaw& Cantley, 2006). In addition, an increase in $\Delta\psi_m$, whether caused by impaired OXPHOS or by an overabundance of nutrients relative to ADP, will result in aberrant electron migration in the ETC and elevated ROS production (Wallace, 2005). Dissipation of $\Delta\psi_m$ (proton leak) causes uncoupling of the respiratory chain electron transport from ADP phosphorylation by the ATP synthase complex. Proton leak functions as a regulator of mitochondrial ROS production and its modulation by uncoupling proteins (UCP) may be involved in pathophysiology, including tumors. In addition, $\Delta\psi_m$ plays a role in the control of mitochondria permeability transition pore (MPTP), that might be critical in determining reduced sensitivity to stress stimuli that were described in neoplastic transformation (Klöhn *et al.*, 2003), implying that dysregulation of pore opening might be a strategy used by tumor cells to escape death.

7   Targeting the Mitochondria as a Novel Strategy for Cancer Therapy

7.1   Mitochondrial Targets for Cancer Therapy

Why cancers are highly resistant to treatment once they return? Oncologists already know that when cancer returns, chemotherapy often won't work again. The reason for the returning cancer's virulence requires understanding that chemotherapy and radiation kill both respiring (normal) and cancerous (fermenting) cells (Peskin, 2009). Conventional chemotherapy using cytotoxic agents tends to damage both tumor and normal cells and cause significant toxic side effects, which compromise the therapeutic outcomes. The emergence of targeted therapy which is based on the concept of specifically targeting critical molecules unique to cancer cells may provide promising means of selectively killing malignant cells. However, cancer may be caused by multiple genetic alterations and environmental factors. As such, there are many potential targets in cancer cells but no single critical target can be readily identified in most cancer types. A comprehensive understanding of mitochondrial biology in cancer cells and the interaction between cellular metabolism and drug action is essential in developing mitochondrial-targeted agents for cancer treatment.

Targeting mitochondria as a cancer therapeutic strategy has gained momentum in the recent years. The signaling pathways that govern mitochondrial function, apoptosis and molecules that affect mitochondrial integrity and cell viability have been important topics of the recent review in the literature (Wanga *et al.*, 2010). Mitochondria are known to play a key role in the complex apoptotic mechanism and trigger cell death via several mechanisms that include disrupting electron transport and energy metabolism, releasing or activating proteins that mediate apoptosis and altering cellular redox potential (Gulbins *et al.*, 2003). Therefore this organelle is increasingly described as a "prime target" for pharmacological intervention (Szewczyk & Wojtczak, 2002) and there is a growing interest in the study of the molecular interactions of xenobiotics with cellular components located on or inside the mitochondrion. Research by several groups has identified various mitochondria associated molecular targets for bioactive molecules (Dias& Bailly, 2005; Hail, 2005). These targets include mtDNA, the mitochondrial respiratory chain, the permeability transition pore complex (PTPC), potassium channels on the mitochondria and the various mitochondria associated anti and proapoptotic factors (Szewczyk & Wojtczak, 2002; Dias & Bailly, 2005; Bouchier-Hayes *et al.*, 2005).

The possible sites and functions of mitochondria as potential targets for anti-cancer therapy are summarized below. (1) Certain compound, often with positive charge, may preferentially accumulate in the mitochondria of cancer cells due to the elevated $\Delta\psi_m$, with the inner surface of the IMM being highly negatively-charged. As discussed, one current chemotherapeutic strategy utilizes a selection of lipophilic cations that target cancer cell mitochondria due to their increased $\Delta\psi_m$ and the possibility of linking these agents to a variety of thiol crosslinking agents to eradicate Bcl-2 overexpressing cells exists (Armstrong, 2006). (2) An alternative strategy may be to use the mitochondrial protein-import machinery to deliver toxic macromolecules to mitochondria while drugs targeting mtDNA such as dithercalinium may also offer unique opportunities for use in cancer therapy (Armstrong, 2006). Due to the important role of respiratory chain in mitochondrial ATP generation, compounds that target mtDNA are likely to significantly affect cellular energy metabolism and cell viability (Wanga *et al.*, 2010). (3) Inhibition of mitochondrial respiration through targeting the electron transport complexes has been shown to elevate ROS production, deplete ATP and induce apoptosis. (4) Targeting the mitochondria permeability transition pore (MPTP) may alter $\Delta\psi_m$, induce change in membrane permeability, and result in a release of apoptotic factors. (5) Enzymes of the glycolytic pathways are often found elevated in cancer cells with mitochondrial dysfunction, likely being a mechanism to compensate energy supply and provide metabolic intermediates for cell growth and proliferation. Inhibition of glycolytic enzymes has been shown to preferentially kill cancer cells, especially those with significant mitochondrial dysfunction or under hypoxic conditions (Wanga *et al.*, 2010).

7.2 Targeting Mitochondria – A Tool for Tumor Cell Elimination

Drug discovery studies must include approaches aimed at conferring selective accumulation on molecules with promising selective action. Direct conjugation to ligands that mediate the desired tumor and subcellular accumulation has been used effectively and therefore offer significant promise. Pharmaceutical nanocarriers offer much promise for tumor-specific delivery and have also recently been explored for sub-cellular delivery. We expect that an ideal approach to mitochondrial targeting in cancer therapy might therefore be represented by the identification of a molecule with a high level of selective action on the mitochondrial target. The molecule may then be conjugated with a mitochondria-specific ligand and then loaded into a tumor cell targeting nanocarrier, thus conferring in one composite system, all the required levels of selective accumulation and selective action to constitute a truly targeted approach.

Though targeting the inherent adaptive anti-apoptotic strategies enhance sensitization of cancer cells to therapeutic regimes, the rise of resistance in cancer cells poses a challenge for scientists and physicians. In this regard, numerous anticancer agents target pathways that lie upstream of the mitochondria, which then converge onto the intrinsic death pathway. However, the deregulation of several master switch proteins such as HIF1, hexokinase (HK) II, c-Myc and P53, leads to resistance in these cells. Thus, directly targeting the mitochondria may allow us to overcome the problem of resistance that arises from engaging the upstream pathways (Fulda *et al.*, 2010). Therefore a better understanding of the key pathophysiological differences between mitochondria in cancer cells and in their non-cancer surrounding tissue is crucial to the finding of tools interfering with these peculiar tumor mitochondrial functions and will disclose novel approaches for the prevention and treatment of malignant diseases. Here, we review the peculiarity of tumor mitochondrial bioenergetics and the mode it is linked to the cell metabolism, providing a short overview of the evidence accumulated so far, but highlighting the more recent advances.

7.2.1   Inhibition of Glycolysis in Tumor Cells

Cancer-specific mitochondrial alterations and bioenergetics may be taken advantage for the development of two novel classes of antineoplastic agents. A first approach would target glycolysis and/or reverse the Warburg phenomenon, whereas a second approach would aim at inducing apoptosis by targeting mito-chondrial proteins and membranes. Since tumor cells rely on the glycolytic pathway of ATP production, much more than non-malignant cells, exploitation of the Warburg effect could represent an approach to overcome some of the current limitations of radio- and chemotherapies. Thus, drugs able to perturb can-cer cell metabolism, specifically at the level of glycolysis, might display beneficial therapeutic effects in cancer. The antitumor effect of these glycolytic inhibitors is based predominantly on ATP depletion, but also involves diminution of multi-drug resistance and reduced hypoxia-linked tumor cell resistance (Sca-tena *et al.*, 2008). It is conceivable to inhibit glycolysis for therapeutic purposes, either by targeting gly-colytic enzymes or by attempting to release hexokinase from its mitochondrial receptor, voltage depend-ent anion channel (VDAC). Inhibitors of glycolytic enzymes that have been successfully used to slow down the growth in human tumors transplanted to mice include 3-bromopyruvate (an inhibitor of hexoki-nase) and oxythiamine (an inhibitor of the transketolase-like enzyme). Some glycolytic inhibitors are be-ing evaluated in clinical trials. This applies to 2-deoxyglucose (an inhibitor of the initial steps of glycoly-sis) as well as to lonidamine (LND), an inhibitor of glycolysis that also has direct pro-apoptotic proper-ties. LND, which is derived from indazole-3-carboxylic acid, has been shown to block aerobic glycolysis in cancer cells, possibly by inhibiting hexokinase. LND disrupts energy metabolism in cells resulting in ATP depletion, and in addition, leads to an accumulation of lactate in the cells (Floridi *et al.*, 1981). This drug is now being used in combination therapy to sensitize cancer cells to conventional chemotherapeutic drugs such as cisplatin at lower doses (Fliss *et al.*, 2000; De Lena *et al.*, 2001). Its prospects are also be-ing reviewed in Phase III clinical trials (Gatzemeier *et al.*, 1991).

7.2.2   Induction of Mitochondrial Permeability Transition (MPT)

The induction of MPT was described some thirty years ago by Haworth and Hunter (Hunter & Haworth, 1979), who found that Ca^{2+} uptake by mitochondria stimulates drastic changes in mitochondrial morphol-ogy and functional activity due to the opening of a non-specific pore in the IMM, commonly known as the MPT pore (MPTP). Traditionally, the MPTP has been regarded as a multimeric complex, composed of VDAC located in the outer mitochondrial membrane (OMM), the adenine nucleotide translocase (ANT), an integral protein of the IMM, and a matrix protein, cyclophilin D (CyP-D). In addition, other proteins may bind to the pore complex, particularly kinases (e.g., hexokinase, creatine kinase) (Cromp-ton, 2000). The pore is thought to form at contact sites between the mitochondrial inner and outer mem-branes. MPT was shown to be a key event in necrotic as well as in some experimental models of apoptot-ic cell death. If permeability transition and subsequent uncoupling of mitochondria occur in a large sub-population of the organelles, this would lead to destructive consequences for the cell.

The MPT refers to an abrupt transition in mitochondrial permeability that occurs when mitochon-dria *in vitro* are treated with calcium and reagents that increase oxidative stress (Haworth & Hunter, 1979; Crompton, 1999). Opening of the MPTP can be facilitated by inorganic phosphate, oxidation of NAD(P)H, ATP depletion, low pH, and ROS (Crompton, 1999). In addition, the levels of peripheral ben-zodiazepine receptor (PBR), hexokinase II (HK II) and mitochondrial creatine kinase have also been found upregulated in some tumors (Dang& Semenza, 1999; Katabi *et al.*, 1999), and they can bind to the pore complex and modulate its permeability (Crompton, 2000). MPT is followed by the influx of water and ions into the matrix, causing mitochondrial swelling, rupture of the OMM, and the release of inter-membrane space proteins such as cytochrome c into the cytosol. Mitochondria from tumor cells are relatively less susceptible to Ca^{2+}-induced MPT (Gogvadze et al., 2008). Thus, comparison of Ca^{2+} accumulation by mitochondria from liver and hepatoma revealed that hepatoma mitochondria were able to accumulate from two to five times more Ca^{2+} than rat liver mitochondria before the permeability transition was induced (Gogvadze et al., 2009). Thus drugs that can disturb permeability transition pore complex (PTPC) would allow for direct targeting of the mitochondria and help circumvent the problem of apoptosis resistance upstream of the intrinsic mitochondrial pathway.

MPTP can depolarize the mitochondrial potential by its opening. Abnormal opening of MPTP may result in the collapse of $\Delta\psi_m$ and the release of apoptotic factors from the mitochondria to cytosol, leading to cell death. Several compounds have been shown to effectively induce changes in mitochondrial membrane permeability and exhibit anti-cancer activity. Extracted from *Magnolia officinals*, honokiol has been used for the treatment of thrombotic stroke, anxiety and gastrointestinal diseases for a long time. Honokiol can induce not only cancer cell death through caspase-dependent and independent apoptosis but also necrosis through MPTP (Filomeni et al., 2007; Ishitsuka et al., 2005). Mechanistically, honokiol was able to cause a decrease in $\Delta\psi_m$, which could be inhibited by pretreatment with cyclosporine A, suggesting that the cyclosporine-sensitive MPTP is a possible target of Honokiol. Other strategies include the use of specific peptides that are toxic by their disruption of mitochondrial membranes and $\Delta\psi_m$, while a selection of drugs, including betulinic acid and LND target MPT (Armstrong, 2006).

The anticancer effect of multiple conventional treatments (e.g., ionizing radiation, etoposide and arsenates) is based on their ability to stimulate production of ROS—key factors facilitating MPT induction. Anticancer drug-induced MPT may thus result from ROS-mediated modification of components of the MPTP. Arsenic trioxide (As_2O_3) has long been used in traditional Chinese medicine to treat a variety of diseases. In the 1970s, As_2O_3 was introduced for the treatment of acute promyelocytic leukemia and showed a striking therapeutic effectiveness (Shen et al., 1997). Several studies showed As_2O_3 caused generation of superoxide and hydrogen peroxide, leading to oxidative modification of thiol groups in ANT and subsequent release of cytochrome c through MPT induction, and a decrease of $\Delta\psi_m$ and apoptosis (Chen et al., 1998; Iwama et al., 2001; Wang et al., 1996). In leukemia cells, As_2O_3 was capable of inhibiting mitochondrial respiration, resulting in a substantial decrease of oxygen consumption as early as 3 h, concurrent with the increase of ROS generation. It appears that by interfering with electron transport in the mitochondria, As_2O_3 may cause an increase in electron leakage and therefore promotes ROS generation (Pelicano et al., 2003). High metabolic rates and mitochondrial dysfunction has been shown to lead to elevated intracellular ROS levels in cancer cells. Thus anticancer compounds that push the cellular ROS levels past the threshold for cancer cells are potent inducers of apoptosis.

7.2.3   Modulation of Mitochondrial Respiratory Chain Activity

Since cancer cells display a high energy demand, drugs that can directly perturb mitochondrial respiration and glycolysis could lead to an extensive depletion of ATP, sensitizing cancer cells to death. Similar to that observed in embryos or neonates, mitochondria in tumor cells seem to maintain a low electron transfer activity at approximately 20–30% of that seen in normal quiescent organelles (Galli et al., 2003). The relatively lower mitochondrial ETC activity in cancer cells seems to reflect dysfunction of OXPHOS of cancer mitochondria. Because the ETC is a major site of ROS generation due to capture of electrons by molecular oxygen, compounds that interfere with the respiratory chain may promote leakage of electrons and thus, increase the production of ROS, leading to mitochondrial damage and activation of apoptosis in cancer cells. The killing of cancer cells by ROS-mediated mechanisms is considered to have therapeutic selectivity against malignant cells due to their intrinsic high ROS generation (Trachootham *et al.*, 2009).

Various attempts have been performed to stimulate tumor cell death by modulation of mitochondrial respiratory chain activity. Thus, inhibitors of the mitochondrial respiratory chain, rotenone or antimycin A, and an inhibitor of mitochondrial ATP synthase, oligomycin, were shown to induce apoptotic cell death in cultured human lymphoblastoid and other mammalian cells within 12–18 h (Wolvetang *et al.,* 1994). No signs of apoptosis were detected in cells lacking mtDNA, indicating that cell death was a result of a direct effect on mitochondrial ETC activity or on mitochondrial ATP synthase. Inhibitors of the mitochondrial ETC were also shown to enhance cell susceptibility towards other apoptotic stimuli (Gogvadze *et al.*, 2009). Inhibition of the mitochondrial ETC can induce other forms of cell death as well. Thus, inhibitors of complex I (rotenone) and complex II (TTFA) caused autophagic cell death, in the transformed cell line HEK 293 and in cancer cell lines U87 and HeLa (Chen *et al.*, 2007). These results indicate that inhibitors of respiratory chain complexes I and II can selectively induce autophagic cell death via a ROS-mediated mechanism.

Resveratrol (3,5,40-trihydroxystilbene) is a natural compound found in certain fruits, particularly in some grapes and blueberries, and has been suggested to have cancer chemopreventive properties. This compound seems to inhibit cellular events associated with tumor initiation, promotion, and progression (Jang *et al.*, 1997). It was found that the mitochondrial respiratory chain (complexes I-III) was inhibited by resveratrol in mice. By competing with UbQ, resveratrol decreased complex III activity and lowered ROS levels (Zini *et al.*, 1999). Though considered as an antioxidant, resveratrol was shown to induce apoptosis through the mitochondrial pathway (Juan *et al.*, 2008; Vetvicka *et al.,* 2007). Sahra *et al.* demonstrated that treatment with 2-deoxyglucose (2DG), a potent inhibitor of glucose metabolism via the inhibition of hexokinase and metformin, a widely used anti diabetic agent that inhibits OXPHOS, induced massive reduction in cell viability in LNCaP prostate cancer cells as compared to normal prostate epithelial cells by depletion of cellular ATP (Ben Sahra *et al.*, 2010).

Elesclomol [N-malonyl-bis(N′-methyl-N′-thiobenzoylhydrazide)], previously designated as STA-4783, is a first-in-class investigational drug currently undergoing clinical evaluation as a novel cancer therapeutic and a novel small-molecule oxidative stress inducer that has been granted Orphan Drug and Fast Track designation from the United States Food and Drug Administration for the treatment of metastatic melanoma. It is also being actively pursued for clinical evaluation in other solid tumors (Qu *et al.*, 2010). Elesclomol leads to mitochondria-induced apoptosis by increasing oxidative stress in cancer cells. The induction of oxidative stress by elesclomol exploits this unique characteristic of cancer cells by increasing ROS levels beyond a threshold that triggers cell death (Kirshner *et al.*, 2008). Elesclomol does not work through a specific cellular protein target. Instead, it targets a biologically coherent set of processes occurring in the mitochondrion. Specifically, elesclomol, driven by its redox chemistry, interacts with mitochondrial ETC to generate high levels of ROS within the organelle and consequently cell death (Blackman *et al.*, 2012).

Lamellarin D (Lam D), a marine pyrrole alkaloid initially isolated from a prosobranch mollusk of the genus *Lamellaria* (Kluza *et al.*, 2006), exhibits a potent cytotoxicity against many different tumors. At doses in the micromolar range, Lam D exhibits high apoptotic activities in leukemia cell lines characterized by the dissipation of the $\Delta\psi_m$, the release of cytochrome c from mitochondria, and caspase-3 activation (Ballot *et al.*, 2009). MPT triggered by Lam D is a result of an indirect effect on mitochondrial bioenergetics (Ballot *et al.*, 2010). MPT, as a process used by mitochondria to activate cell death, is accompanied by severe alterations of mitochondrial bioenergetics such as reduction of $\Delta\psi_m$, uncoupling of mitochondrial electron transport and ATP synthesis (Crompton, 1999). In isolated mitochondria, it is well established that the opening of MPT pore results in uncoupling of respiratory chain and ROS production (Zoratti & Szabo, 1995). Conversely, Gallego *et al.* observed a global reduction of the mitochondrial respiration upon Lam D exposure. Additionally, unlike most of the direct MPT inducers, Lam D had little or no effect on mitochondrial ROS production in cancer cells (Gallego *et al.*, 2008). Lam D reduces mitochondrial respiration by interfering with the ETC. The partial decrease in mitochondrial respiration by Lam D resulted in low $\Delta\psi_m$ and low ATP production through inhibition of the complex III, conditions known to favor MPT (Zoratti & Szabo, 1995). MPT triggers mitochondrial matrix swelling leading to OMM rupture and subsequent cell death. Thus, Lam D appears to have unique mitochondrial mechanisms of action, leading to cancer cell death (Ballot *et al.*, 2010).

8   Summary on Metabolic Changes of Cancer Cells

In normal cells, glucose is phosphorylated by HK, then the major part is degraded via glycolysis to pyruvate, which prevalently enters the mitochondria, it is decarboxylated and oxidized by PDH to acetyl-CoA, which enters the TCA cycle where the two carbons of acetyl are completely oxidized to CO_2 whereas hydrogen atoms reduce NAD^+ and FAD, which feed the respiratory chain. Minor part of glycolytic Glucose-6-P is diverted to produce ribose-5-P and NADPH via pentose phosphate pathway, will be used to synthesize nucleotides, whereas triose phosphates in minimal part will be used to synthesize lipids and phospholipids with the contribution of NADPH and acetyl-CoA. Amino acids, including glutamine will follow the physiological turnover of the proteins, in minimal part will be used to synthesize the nucleotides bases, and the excess after deamination will be used to produce energy. In the IMM are located the respiratory chain complexes and the ATP synthase, which phosphorylates ADP releasing ATP, that in turn is carried to the cytosol by ANT in exchange for ADP. About 1–2% O_2 uptaken by the mitochondria is reduced to superoxide anion radical and other ROS. In any cell, the majority of ROS are by-products of mitochondrial respiration. The mitochondrial ETC contains several redox centers (e.g. in complex I and III) that can leak electrons to molecular oxygen, serving as the primary source of superoxide production in most tissues. One major targets of ROS is mtDNA, owing to its close proximity to the ETC and the lack of protective histones, which encodes 13 proteins essential for the function of the ETC and, hence, for ATP synthesis by OXPHOS (Figure 1).

In cancer cells, anabolism is enhanced, both glucose and glutamine, are important carbon sources which are metabolized for the generation of energy and anabolic precursors, heavily consumed by cancercells, are early precursors of non-essential amino acids (Figure 1). This process predominates in cancer cells rendering glutamine an essential amino acid and the source of TCA cycle-derived anabolic metabolites. Mitochondrial dysfunction may lead to the activation of HIF-1, therefore triggering the hypoxia pathway in the tumourigenic process. The inability of mitochondria to provide enough ATP for cellsurvival under hypoxic conditions, results in upregulation of the glycolytic pathway. This occurs by induction of HIF-1, which not only stimulates key steps of glycolysis but also suppresses mitochondrial function in tumor cells, suggesting that it modulates the reciprocal relationship between glycolysis and OXPHOS. Normally, the switch between glycolysis and OXPHOS is controlled by the relative activities of two enzymes, PDH and LDH. HIF-1 inactivates PDH through PDK1 induction, resulting in suppression of the Krebs cycle and mitochondrial respiration. In addition, HIF-1 stimulates the expression of lactate dehydrogenase A, which facilitates the conversion of pyruvate to lactate. As a result, mitochondrial

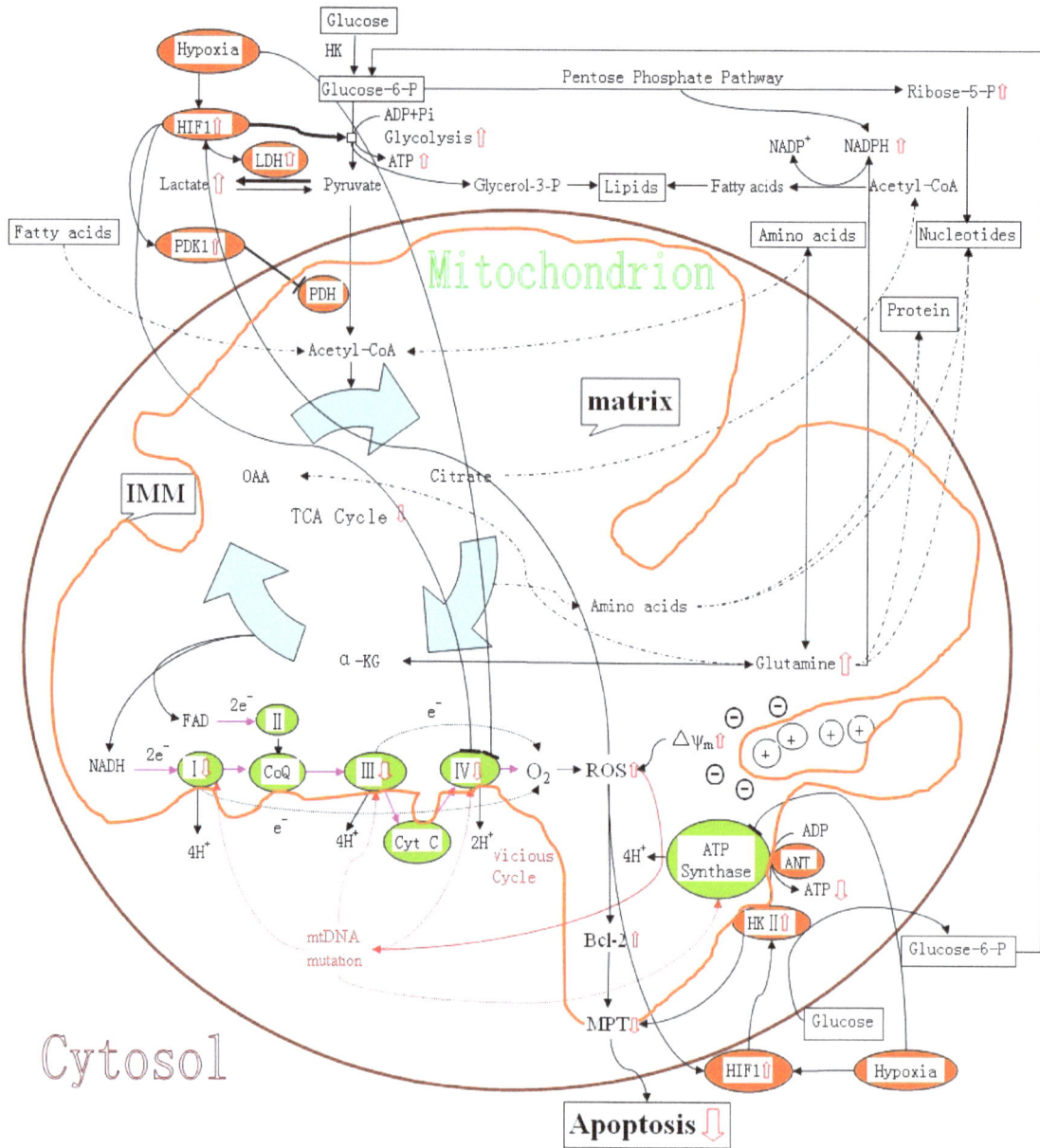

Figure 1: Schematic illustration of metabolic reprogramming frequently occurring in cancer cells compared with mitochondrial metabolism in normal cells. Cancer cells showed increased glycolysis, pentose phosphate pathway, glutamine consumed, anabolism, $\Delta\psi_m$ and ROS generation; and reduced TCA cycle flux, respiratory complex activities, MPT and apoptosis.

contribution to ATP synthesis declines, although the mitochondria might remain functionally intact.

Glucose is mostly phosphorylated by HK II in cancer cells, which is up-regulated being its gene promoter sensitive to typical tumor markers such as HIF-1and has an easy access to ATP being more strictly bound to the mitochondria. It plays a pivotal role in both the bioenergetic metabolism and the biosynthesis of required molecules for cancer cells proliferation. HK II phosphorylates glucose using ATP synthesized by the mitochondrial OXPHOS and it releases the product ADP in close proximity of the ANT to favor ATP re-synthesis within the matrix. Its product, Glucose-6-P, is only in part oxidized to pyruvate. This, in turn, is mostly reduced to lactate being both LDH and PDK1 up-regulated. A significant part of Glucose-6-P is used to synthesize nucleotides that also require amino acids and glutamine. Glutaminolysis (breaking down glutamine into α-KG) generates malate which, through the malic enzyme, will give rise to NADPH that can be used to fuel lipid biosynthesis, and OAA, which will generate citrate, which is necessary for lipid biosynthesis. Citrate in part is diverted from the TCA cycle to the cytosol, where it is a substrate of citrate lyase, which supplies acetyl-CoA for lipid and phospholipid synthesis that also requires NADPH. The reprogramming of mitochondrial metabolism in many cancer cells comprises reduced pyruvate oxidation by PDH followed by the TCA cycle, increased anaplerotic feeding of the same cycle, mostly from glutamine, whose entry in the mitochondrial matrixis facilitated by UCP2 up-regulation. This increases also the free fatty acids uptake by mitochondria, therefore β-oxidation is pushed to produce acetyl-CoA, whose oxidation contributes to ATP production. In cancer cells many signals can converge on the mitochondrion to decrease the MPT, which may respond by elevating the MPT pore threshold, with consequent enhancement of apoptosis resistance. ROS belong to this class of molecules since it can enhance Bcl-2 and may induce mtDNA mutations. As indicated, ROS in many cancer cells are over produced. Interestingly, studies have also shown that the $\Delta\psi_m$ is approximately 60 mV higher in carcinomas as compared to their normal controls, which also contribute to the increased ROS (Figure 1).

The differences in mitochondrial function between normal cells and cancer cells may offer a unique potential for the design of anticancer agents that deliver mitochondrial targeting drugs to selectively kill cancer cells. The long process that has led from the discovery of cancer-related mitochondrial abnormalities to the clinical exploration of novel anticancer therapies illustrates how the slow accumulation of fundamental knowledge eventually generates medically exploitable information. The success of an anticancer attack must be based on the concerted modulation of cellular energy metabolism, mitochondrial stability, and other mechanisms responsible for the resistance of tumor cells to death stimuli.

9   Research Idea on Cancer-preventive Mechanism – Mitochondrial Energy Metabolism Improvement Perspective

Astragalus membranaceus (AM) is the most popular for Qi-invigorating herbal medicines in traditional Chinese medicine (TCM) and is often used as an immunostimulant and a supplementary medicine during cancer therapy (Zheng, 2005). AM is often used in formulas for deficiency of Qi characterized by limb weakness, fatigue, lack of appetite, and dizziness. AM has various bioactivities, such as anti-aging (Wang *et al.*, 2003), hepatoprotective, antibacterial, inducing cancer cell apoptosis (Cheng *et al.*, 2004), and preventing apoptosis in cultured neonatal cardiomyocytes (Luo *et al.*, 2009). AM inhibited mitochondrial oxygen consumption and malondialdehyde (MDA) production (Hong *et al.,* 1994). As an important bioactive component of AM, Astragalus polysaccharides (APS) have immunoregulatory, antiviral, antioxidant, and anti-tumor properties (Shao *et al.*, 2004; Yin *et al.*, 2010; Mao *et al.*, 2009; Chen *et al.*, 2011). Therefore, APS have been applied in the treatment of tumor in Chinese medicine. APS therapy ameliorated vacuolar degeneration of mitochondria and fragmentation of mitochondrial cristae of hepatocytes in insulin-resistance mice, which indicates the mitochondrial dysfunction coupled with the increased metabolic stress and the protective effect of APS (Mao *et al.*, 2009). Our preliminary studies indicate that APS can protect mitochondria by scavenging ROS, inhibiting lipid peroxidation and mitochondrial swelling, and increasing the activities of antioxidant enzymes (Li *et al.*, 2012). We proposed that APS ameliorate mitochondrial dysfunction perhaps ultimately by improving energy metabolism; this may be the hypothetical anticancer and cancer-preventive mechanism of APS.

Although aerobic glycolysis has now been generally accepted as a metabolic hallmark of cancer, its cause and its causal relationship with cancer progression are still unclear. A comparison of multiple cancer cell lines revealed that they rely on glycolysis for ATP production to different extents, and typically, the more "glycolytic" tumor cells were shown to be the most aggressive ones. Some cancer cells can switch between glycolytic and oxidative metabolism in a reversible fashion. Silencing of mitochondria, a characteristic feature of most tumor cells, might thus be one reason for their evasion of cell death. This is because apoptosis is dependent on mitochondrial energy metabolism (Gogvadze *et al.*, 2009). Recent findings demonstrate that stimulation of mitochondrial activity and restoration of the mechanisms of ATP generation characteristic of non-malignant cells might be an efficient tool in anticancer strategy. In particular, shifting cellular metabolism towards mitochondrial ATP production might overcome the effects of HIF-1-mediated upregulation of the glycolytic pathway (Gogvadze *et al.*, 2008). This would reverse the suppressed mitochondrial apoptosis pathway in cancer and result in inhibition of tumor growth. Apparently, the ultimate fate of the cancer cell will depend on how efficiently mitochondrial OXPHOS can substitute for the inhibited glycolysis in providing the ATP needed for cellular demands. In the last decade, a renewed interest has returned to the role of mitochondria and energy metabolism in cancer, while, how to enhance mitochondrial energy metabolism to avoid the occurrence of cancer?

According to TCM theory, all kinds of diseases and ailments are born from Qi, Qi is the subtle substance with a strong vitality which constitutes the human body and maintain the activities of human life. Qi is fundamental to our body, both life and death of human all depend on Qi. Qi is often described in the West as energy, or vital energy. Here are Chinese people from all walks of life as they seek relief, through a rebalancing of their Qi for ailments from colds to cancer. And from the Chinese perspective, Qi is the origin of true strength and power as well as genuine health—body, mind, and spirit. In order to have good health you must have sufficient Qi. If there isn't enough Qi (Qi deficiency), one or more organs can become imbalanced and develop energy function disorders. Impaired mitochondrial ATP formation may be the key characteristic of Qi deficiency. The author found that Qi deficiency led to a marked fall in cellular ATP, and a rise in cellular AMP. Qi deficiency is the common cause of a variety of diseases and can lead to mitochondrial energy metabolism dysfunction, and Qi-invigoration is the basic principle for treatment of Qi deficiency (Li, 2012). As ATP, an energy-rich biomolecule, is universally used for energizing cellular activities, the "Qi-invigorating" action may be mediated by the enhancement of mitochondrial ATP generation. In this regard, our previous studies show that all the four widely used Qi-invigorating herbal medcines (QIHM) (including ginseng, astragalus root, pilose asiabell root, white atractylodes rhizome) can increase ATP levels of liver cells *in vivo*. We propose a hypothesis that Qi is closely related to bioenergy (Li & Zhao, 2012). Based on our findings that Qi-invigorating representative prescription Sijunzi decoction (Li, 2012) and QIHM can enhance the mitochondrial ATP generation capacity, and they have a good effect for treatment of cancer. It is plausible that cancer prevention involves an improvement of cellular energy status which can be accomplished by Qi-invigoration. We believed that the up-regulation of cellular activities by "Qi-invigoration" in Chinese medicine requires an increased supply of ATP, which is in turn largely supported by mitochondrial OXPHOS.

Deeper and more integrated knowledge of mitochondrial mechanisms and cancer-specific mitochondrial modulating means are expected for reducing tumorigenicity and/or preventing cancer at the mitochondrial level. With the extraordinary progress of mitochondrial science and cell biology, novel biochemical pathways have emerged as strategic points of bioenergetic regulation and control. However, there has been no report on mitochondrial energy metabolism improvement and cancer preventive mechanism of APS so far. As the 'hubs' for cellular metabolism, mitochondria are crucial for both life and death of eukaryotic cells, and are the main switch of cell apoptosis. It is conceivable that impairment of mitochondrial ATP production and the resulting energy depletion can lead to apoptosis. Lower ATP levels can decrease the efficiency of energy-dependent processes and ATP-mediated signal transductions. Inadequate ATP availability would initiate and accentuate the adverse consequences of energy-dependent pathways. Based on the above analysis and research results, we performed the following experiments.

TCM pay more attention to the prevention than treatment of diseases. The prevention of cancer is of particular important due to the unsatisfactory treatment effect. In the present study, the mechanism underlying cancer prevention of APS were investigated and evaluated by mitochondrial energy metabolism improvement. One of the main characteristics of tumor cells is their fast proliferation. Due to the high growth rate, tumor tissue easily becomes hypoxic because of the inability of the local vasculature to supply an adequate amount of oxygen. The inability of mitochondria to provide enough ATP for cell survival under hypoxic conditions, results in upregulation of the glycolytic pathway. Warburg proved that a 35% reduction in oxygen causes any cell to either die or turn cancerous. Since early carcinogenesis is thought to occur in a hypoxic microenvironment and the pro-tumoral effect of hypoxia, the chronic hypoxia model was set up. OXPHOS inactivation would be an initial step in tumour development conferring tumourigenic potential to the cells. The effects of APS on the hepatic mitochondrial OXPHOS were observed *in vivo*. While the intracellular energy status is mirrored by the respective concentrations of the adenine nucleotides ATP, ADP and AMP, whose levels in liver cells were determined by high performance liquid chromatography.

9.1 Materials and Methods

9.1.1 Animals and Materials

Male BALB/c mice, weighing 22 ± 2.0 g, were purchased from the Experimental Animal Center, Dalian Medical University. All mice were cared according to the Guiding Principles in the Care and Use of Animals. The experiment was approved by Animal Care Committee of Dalian Medical University (China) in accordance with the Chinese Council on Animal Care Guidelines. Rodent laboratory chow and tap water were available *ad libitum* during the period.

Spherisorb C_{18} reversed-phase chromatographic column (4.6 mm×250 mm, 5 μm particle size) was produced by Dalian Institute of Chemistry and Physics, Chinese Academy of Sciences. Adenosine triphosphate (ATP), adenosine diphosphate (ADP), adenosine monophosphate (AMP), L-glutamic acid, and DL-malate were from Sigma Chemical (St Louis, MO, USA). N-2-Hydroxyethylpiperazine-N'-2-ethane sulfonic acid (HEPES) was from Merck (Darmstadt, Germany). Coomassie Brilliant Blue G-250 (CBBG-250) was purchased from Fluka (Bushs SG, Switzerland). Bovine serum albumin (BSA) was from Boehringer Mannheim Corp. (Indianapolis, IN, USA). Tris(hydroxymethyl)aminomethane (Tris) was from Gibco BRL (GrandIsland, NY, USA). All other chemicals and solvents used in the study were of analytical grade made in China. Astragali Radix was collected in the primitive forest of Daxing'anling region in Heilongjiang Province of China, which was authenticated by professor Haixue Kuang as the roots of *Astragalus membranaceus* (Fisch.) Bunge var. *mongholicus* (Bunge) Hsiao (AM), and its voucher specimen was deposited in the Herbarium of Chinese Herbal Medicines, College of Pharmacy, Heilongjiang University of Chinese Medicine.

9.1.2   Preparation of the Astragalus Polysaccharides

The collected AM was washed, dried, pulverized, then immersed in distilled water (the ratio of AM and distilled water was 1:15) for 24 h and extracted thrice with distilled water for 1 h each in a boiling water bath. The filtrate was collected after filtration with gauze, mixed and condensed to 1 g crude drug/mL by rotary evaporation. Sevage reagents (ratio of chloroform and n-butanol was 4:1) were used to remove all protein constituents. The resultant liquor was precipitated with 3 times volume of 95% ethanol. Precipitation of polysaccharides proceeded at 4 °C for 24 h and the precipitate which was collected by centrifugation at $5000 \times g$ for 10 min was dissolved in distilled water, ethanol was added to final concentration of 25% to settle. The precipitate was discarded and the supernatant was added with 95% ethanol to final concentration of 75% and stood at 4 °C for 24 h after centrifugation at $5000 \times g$ for 10 min. The resultant precipitate was washed with 95% ethanol and water-free ethanol respectively after suction and lyophilized *in vacuo*. The polysaccharides content (91.6%) in extracts was determined using the phenol-sulfuric acid method (Dubois *et al.*, 1956).

9.1.3   Chronic Hypoxia Model

Forty mice were randomly divided into four groups: Normal group, model group, APS low dose group (APSL, 200 mg/kg/day) and APS high dose group (APSH, 300 mg/kg/day). Model group and APS group mice were exposed to hypoxia (10.5% O_2, 89.5% N_2) for 10 days in specially constructed plastic cages. The cages were sealed at the top by plastic covers. Small openings were made in the top covers to allow inflow and outflow of gases and to accommodate water bottles. The oxygen content in the chambers was monitored using a Clark O_2 electrode inserted through an opening in the top cover. Total gas flow was set at about 1.5 L/min to maintain 10.5% O_2 in the cage and prevent excessive accumulation of moisture and ammonia. Soda lime was put into the chambers to absorb the CO_2 which was breathed out by mice. Cages were opened daily to change bedding and food, a APS group mouse was administered a dose of APS (200, 300 mg/kg/day) by oral gavage and a model group mouse an equivalent volume of normal saline. Normal group mice were housed in standard open cages (21% O_2) and given normal saline. All the mice were maintained with free access to food and drinking water.

9.1.4   Isolation of Liver Mitochondria

Mitochondria were isolated by differential centrifugation using a modified protocol of Fink *et al.*(2005). Mice were dislocated, the livers were excised immediately, placed in precooled normal saline to wash the blood on the surface, then placed in an ice-cold isolation medium (containing 0.25 M sucrose, 0.5 mM EDTA and 3 mM HEPES, pH 7.4) and were homogenized with a motor-driven Teflon pestle in wet ice. Following homogenization, samples were centrifuged at $1,000 \times g$ for 10 min. A Beckman JA-25.50 rotor and Beckman Coulter Avanti J-E centrifuge were used in this and all other centrifugation steps at 4 °C. Supernatants were removed and centrifuged at $10,000 \times g$ for 10 min. The pellets were washed twice in the isolation medium, and respun at $10,000 \times g$ for 10 min each. After the final wash, mitochondria were resuspended in the same medium and stored in ice until use. Protein determinations were carried out by Bradford method using BSA as a standard (Bradford, 1976).

9.1.5 Measurement of ATP, ADP, and AMP in Liver Cells by HPLC

Briefly, determination of ATP, ADP, and AMP in liver cells, which was carried out with our previous method (Li *et al.*, 2009), by gradient RP-HPLC (reversed-phase high performance liquid chromatography) with ultraviolet detector at room temperature and with mobile phase at a rate of 0.8 mL/min. Mobile phases used for the gradient system were buffer A (0.05 M KH_2PO_4-K_2HPO_4, pH 6.0) and buffer B, consisting of buffer A plus 10% methanol (*v/v*). Gradient elution procedure: buffer A was used as mobile phase between 0 and 3 min, buffer A was changed from 100% to 0% and buffer B from 0% to 100% between 3 and 6 min, buffer B was mobile phase between 6 and 9 min, then changed to buffer A after 9 min, all the running time was 12 min, the detection wavelength was set at 254 nm. ATP, ADP and AMP contents in liver cells was calculated by computing the peak area of standard solutions of nucleotides with known concentrations. Total adenylate pool (TAP) and adenylate energy charge (AEC) were calculated by the following formulas respectively: TAP = [ATP] + [ADP] + [AMP], AEC = ([ATP] + 0.5[ADP])/TAP.

9.1.6 Measurement of Liver Mitochondrial Respiratory Function

Respiratory function of liver mitochondria was measured using the method described by Estabrook (Estabrook, 1967). Oxygen consumption was measured at 30°C in a closed, stirred, and thermostatted glass vessel equipped with a Clark-type oxygen electrode in 2.0 mL respiration buffer (pH 7.4), which consisted of sucrose 225 mM, EDTA 1 mM, $MgCl_2$ 5 mM, KCl 15 mM, KH_2PO_4 15 mM, Tris 50 mM, L-glutamic acid 5 mM, DL-malate 10 mM, and mitochondrial protein 5 mg/mL. Respiratory state 3 was the oxygen (O_2) consumption by mitochondria in the presence of substrate after the addition of 0.25 mM ADP (a potent stimulator of mitochondrial respiration). Respiratory state 4 was the oxygen consumption when all the ADP has been phosphorylated. state 3 and 4 can be calculated according to the OXPHOS curve. Respiration rates were expressed in nanomoles atom O per minute per milligram of protein. Respiratory control ratio (RCR) was the ratio of state 3 to state 4 respiration. P/O ratio is the number of ADP molecules phosphorylated per oxygen atom reduced.

9.1.7 Statistical Analysis

Data were expressed as means ± SD and statistical differences between groups were analyzed by one-way analysis of variance (ANOVA) followed by least significant difference (LSD) *post hoc* multiple comparisons test using the statistical software package SPSS 16.0 for Windows (SPSS Inc., Chicago, Illinois, USA). Results were considered statistically significant at the probability (*P*) values < 0.05 level.

9.2 Results and Discussion

9.2.1 Effects of APS on Energy State of Mice Hepatocyte under Chronic Hypoxia *in vivo*.

We found that hypoxia led to a marked fall in cellular ATP and ADP, and a rise in cellular AMP associated with decreases in TAP, AEC, ATP/ADP and ATP/AMP ratios compared to the normal group. Hypoxia affects structure, dynamics, and function of the mitochondria, and in particular it has a significant inhibitory effect on the OXPHOS machinery, which is the main energy supplier of cells. Considering the pro-tumoral effect of hypoxia, hypoxia reduces OXPHOS by inhibiting the ATP synthase complex, which contributes to the enhancement of the "aerobic glycolysis", all signatures of cancer transformation. The changes in ATP/ADP ratio might significantly influence $\Delta\psi_m$ (Kann & Kovács, 2007). Through the action of adenylate kinase (AK), any decrease in the cellular ATP/ADP ratio is converted into a decrease in the ATP/AMP ratio (Shetty *et al.*, 1993). Hypoxia elicits a marked decrease in the ATP/AMP ratio. The cellular AMP/ATP ratio was monitored as an index of metabolic stress (Salt *et al.*, 1998). The ATP/AMP ratio reduced from 9.86 of normal group to 3.44 under hypoxia conditions which indicated oxidative stress occurred, whereas the ATP/ADP ratio reduced from 1.45 to 1.17. The cellular energy state has been altered under the hypoxic condition. The hypoxic environment of proliferating tumor tissue facilitates ROS production. However, ROS levels can also be increased by hypoxia, when electron transport complexes are in the reduced state (Guzy & Schumacker, 2006). ROS impair mitochondrial function, and appear to play a major role in the metastatic potential, since pre-treatment with ROS scavengers abolished metastasis formation (Ishikawa *et al.*, 2008). The AMPK are activated by alterations in the cellular ATP/AMP ratio, which is dictated by the balance between energy supply (ATP production) and energy demand (ATP consumption). When activated by AMP, the AMPK initiate a phosphorylation cascade to switch on the catabolic pathways that produce ATP and to switch-off the anabolic pathways that consume ATP (Hardie, 2007).

Adenylate energy charge (AEC) represents a linear measure of the metabolic energy stored in the adenine nucleotide system. Energy metabolism would be regulated by the relative amount of ATP available, as described by AEC. The metabolic pathway of ATP generation was inhibited by high AEC, and that of ATP consumption was enhanced by high AEC. TAP is a measure of the cell energy status. TAP levels and AEC in liver cells of model group were decreased compared with normal group. The AMP level in model group remained near doubled than that for normal group. APS treatment (APSH) could increase ATP, ADP, TAP levels and ATP/ADP, ATP/AMP ratio, AEC in liver cells of hypoxic mice, and there is no significant difference between APSH and normal group. ATP/AMP ratio in APSH group increased over twofold than in model group (Table 1). The hypoxic mice are initially restless, then characterized by lassitude of the limbs and poor appetite etc. The TCM therapeutic approach of invigorating Qi by APS can improve the mitochondrial energy metabolism of liver cells as well as the hypoxic symptoms of experimental animals, and reduce oxidative stress. This is consistent with our recent investigations that APS can scavenge ROS, inhibit lipid peroxidation, and increase the activities of antioxidant enzymes (Li *et al.*, 2012).

Group	Dose (mg/kg/d)	ATP (mM)	ADP (mM)	AMP (mM)	TAP (mM)	AEC	ATP/ADP	ATP/AMP
Model	-	0.73 ± 0.29^f	0.62 ± 0.18^e	0.21 ± 0.13^e	1.56 ± 0.26^f	0.66 ± 0.06^f	1.17 ± 0.16^e	3.44 ± 1.32^g
Normal	-	1.19 ± 0.32^b	0.81 ± 0.24^a	0.12 ± 0.07^a	2.12 ± 0.39^b	0.75 ± 0.08^b	1.45 ± 0.25^a	9.86 ± 2.83^c
APSL	200	0.96 ± 0.26^a	0.74 ± 0.22	0.14 ± 0.05	1.84 ± 0.42	0.72 ± 0.05^a	1.31 ± 0.22	6.77 ± 2.46^{be}
APSH	300	1.12 ± 0.31^a	0.80 ± 0.23^a	0.11 ± 0.06^a	2.03 ± 0.51^a	0.75 ± 0.07^a	1.41 ± 0.26^a	9.98 ± 2.33^c

Table 1: Effects of APS on adenylates level in liver cells of mice *in vivo*. All values are mean±SD (n=10). [a]$P < 0.05$, [b]$P < 0.01$, [c]$P < 0.001$ compared to model group; [e]$P < 0.05$, [f]$P < 0.01$, [g]$P < 0.001$ compared to normal group. Each value expressed in mM (ATP, ADP, AMP, TAP) or as a ratio (AEC, ATP/ADP, ATP/AMP). APSL: APS low dose group; APSH: APS high dose group; ATP: adenosine triphosphate; ADP: adenosine diphosphate; AMP: adenosine monophosphate; TAP: total adenylate pool; AEC: adenylate energy charge.

At steady-state, the cellular energy production is dictated by the energy demand, the energy supply, and the capacity of the energy transformation systems. Cellular adaptation to environmental and physiological constraints necessitates that the control of mitochondrial respiration be fine tuned in its response to changes in energy demand and substrate delivery (Benard *et al.*, 2010). The intracellular energy status is mirrored by the respective concentrations of the adenine nucleotides ATP, ADP and AMP. ATP is the energy currency of cells and a high ratio of ATP/ADP is produced primarily by the oxidation of glucose (Indran *et al.*, 2011). Polysaccharides from the functional fractions of Astragalus have received much attention in the research community. Due to all the QIHM contain large amounts of water soluble polysaccharides, we deduced that polysaccharides are the active components that invigorating Qi (by improving mitochondrial energy metabolism), and were demonstrated by *Panax ginseng* polysaccharides (Li *et al.*, 2009). It has been shown that the bioactivities of polysaccharides are most closely related to their chemical composition and configuration. One kind of APS from *A. membranaceus* contained one single α-D-glucose at the C-6 position of every nine residue, with a molecular weight of approximately 3.6×10^4 Da, was an α-(1→4)-D-glucan with α-(1→6)-linked branches attached to the O-6 of branch points (Li *et al.*, 2009); APS from *A. membranaceus* (Fisch.) Bunge var. *mongholicus* were mainly composed of glucose, and a small amount of arabinose and xylose. Their main chains mainly composed of major α-(1→3) glucose and a few α-(1→4), α-(1→6) glucoses, while the side chain contained arabinoses and xyloses. The research suggested that the anti-tumor activities of APS may be related to their structures (Zhu *et al.*, 2011). Therefore, APS increase ATP levels and ATP/ADP, ATP/AMP ratio in liver cells maybe closely related to their high glucose content and configuration.

The cytosolic ratio of ATP/ADP reflects the cellular energy state, as indicated by the level of AMP produced from ADP. In situations of high energy demand (low ATP/ADP), the adenylate kinase produces AMP which activates the AMPK that initiate cascades of phosphorylation and stimulates the expression of genes involved in ATP production, while reducing that of genes involved in ATP consumption (Benard *et al.*, 2010). Recently, a second mechanism of respiratory control has been found in eukaryotes. This control is based on the intramitochondrial ATP/ADP ratio, with a high ratio inhibiting oxidative phosphorylation through allosteric binding of ATP to a subunit of Complex IV. This inhibition is reversed when the concentration of ADP increases (Horton *et al.*, 2002). Energy metabolism would be regulated by AEC. In this study, we found that hypoxia leads to a marked fall in cellular ATP and ADP, and a rise in cellular AMP, while APS could improve mitochondrial energy metabolism by increasing levels of ATP, TAP and AEC in liver cells of hypoxic mice. Cellular ATP levels are closely linked to mitochondrial function, which is regulated perhaps by AEC. APS was able to regulate AEC, possibly linked to mitochondrial ATP production. Data showed APS to be an enhancer of ATP production under hypoxia. ATP levels were drastically lowered by hypoxia but APS stimulated an increased output of ATP.

9.2.2   The Effects of APS on Liver Mitochondrial Respiratory Function *in vivo*

Control of OXPHOS allows a cell to produce only the precise amount of ATP required to sustain its activities. Recall that under normal circumstances, electron transport and ATP synthesis are tightly coupled. The value of P/O ratio (the number of moles of Pi consumed or ATP produced for each oxygen atom reduced to H_2O) reflects the degree of coupling observed between electron transport and ATP synthesis (Mckee & Mckee, 1999). Oxygen consumption increase dramatically when ADP is supplied. The control of aerobic respiration by ADP is referred to as respiratory control. Substrate oxidation accelerates only when an increase in the concentration of ADP signals that the ATP pool needs to be replenished. This regulation matches the rates of phosphorylation of ADP and of cellular oxidations via glycolysis, the citric acid cycle, and the electron transport chain to the requirement for ATP (Horton *et al.*, 2002). The intrinsic efficiency of OXPHOS can be regulated by changes in the P/O ratio, which is notably linked to oxygen levels (Gnaiger *et al.*, 2000). Cell biology has revealed the heterogeneity of mitochondrial function within the cell, such that energy production can be further regulated *in situ* by the cellular and mitochondrial microenvironment, including the availability of energy substrates (NADH/NAD$^+$, ATP/ADP, oxygen gradients, glucose and glutamine) (Gnaiger, 2009).

Liver plays important role in metabolism to maintain energy level and structural stability of body (Hodgson, 2004). The state 3 respiration (oxygen consumption), the respiratory control ratio (RCR) values and P/O ratio of liver mitochondria from model mice driven by complex I substrates were all significantly decreased compared with the normal; liver mitochondria isolated from APS (300 mg/kg/day) treated rats showed significant decrease in state 3 respiration, RCR and P/O ratio, compared to the rates in mitochondria from models (Table 2), but mitochondria from APS (200 mg/kg/day) treated rats didn't. State 4 respiration was not significantly altered in APS treated rats. It showed that the rate of ATP production via ADP phosphorylation was decreased. Hypoxia allows tissues to minimize their energy needs. In perfectly coupled mitochondria, there would be no proton leak across the inner mitochondrial membrane, and the entire gradient generated by the respiratory chain would be used to generate ATP (Boudina & Dale Abel, 2006).

APS can further decrease state 3 respiration, RCR, and P/O ratio of liver mitochondria compared to normal group, we consider this is the result of feedback inhibition by improving mitochondrial energy metabolism and bioenergetic level (Figure 2). The mitochondrial energy state can retro-regulate the nuclear-encoded energy genes. The changes in mitochondrial respiratory chain activity are followed by changes in "energy-state messengers" which include ROS (such as the diffusive H_2O_2), mitochondrial and cytosolic calcium, NADH/NAD$^+$, ATP/ADP, GTP, AMP, cyclic AMP (cAMP), $\Delta\psi_m$ and ΔpH (Benard *et al.*, 2010). Another mechanism by which the mitochondrial energy state imparts feedback regulation on OXPHOS was recently proposed (Acin-Perez *et al.*, 2009), where soluble adenylyl-cyclase (Mito-SAC) plays a determinant role in the generation of cAMP (produced from the OXPHOS-synthesized ATP) inside the mitochondrion, which activates the mitochondrial protein kinase A (PKA), and triggers the reversible phosphorylation of mitochondrial proteins.

Group	Dose (mg/kg/day)	State 3 (nmol/min/mg)[d]	State 4 (nmol/min/mg)[d]	RCR	P/O ratio
Model	-	63±11[f]	18.1±2.3	3.5±0.6[e]	2.11±0.29[e]
Normal	-	78±13[b]	18.9±2.5	4.1±0.5[a]	2.53±0.26[a]
APSL	200	59±16[e]	18.5±2.4	3.2±0.8[f]	1.92±0.27[g]
APSH	300	54±10[af]	17.9±2.3	3.0±0.5[ag]	1.85±0.23[ag]

Table 2: Effects of APS on liver mitochondrial respiratory function *in vivo*.[d] nanomole O_2 per minute per milligram protein (nmol $O_2 \cdot$ min$^{-1} \cdot$ mg protein^{-1}). All values are mean±SD ($n = 10$). [a]$P < 0.05$, [b]$P < 0.01$ compared to model group; [e]$P < 0.05$, [f]$P < 0.01$, [g]$P < 0.001$ compared to normal group. RCR: respiratory control ratio; APSL: APS low dose group; APSH: APS high dose group.

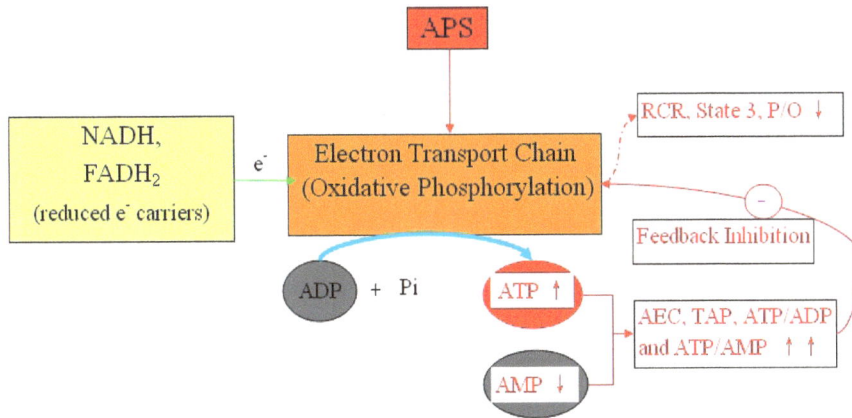

Figure 2: The feedback regulation of APS on OXPHOS. APS treatment could increase ATP and TAP, decrease AMP levels and increase ATP/ADP, ATP/AMP ratio, AEC in hypoxic liver cells which feedback inhibit OXPHOS by decreasing RCR, state 3 respiration and P/O ratio of liver mitochondria. This is the result of improved mitochondrial energy metabolism and bioenergetic level and the potential cancer-preventive mechanism of APS.

10   Conclusion

Warburg hypothesize that cancer is an outcome of defective mitochondrial energy metabolism (i.e., a decrease in mitochondrial energy metabolism might lead to development of cancer). Warburg's hypothesis profoundly influenced the present perception of cancer metabolism. Although the underlying mechanisms responsible for the Warburg effect remain to be defined, it has been postulated that mitochondrial dysfunction (respiration injury) may be a key event that compromises the cancer cell's ability to generate ATP through OXPHOS. Many studies in the last decade indicate that mitochondrial dysfunction is one of the more recurrent features of cancer cells. Therefore, if mitochondrial dysfunction was prevented, the cancer metastatic potential would be prevented, in this regard, we proposed that mitochondrial protection and mitochondrial energy metabolism improvement are the key mechanism for cancer prevention. Based on our previous research results, that mitochondrial protection and mitochondrial energy metabolism improvement can be achieved by Qi-invigoration. We designed this experiment, and demonstrated that APS could protect mitochondria and enhance mitochondrial bioenergetics. An explanation of the protective effects of APS on mitochondria is based on the improvement of energy status. APS can decrease state 3 respiration and RCR of liver mitochondria, we consider this is the result of improved mitochondrial energy metabolism and bioenergetic level.

Mitochondria produce significant amounts of cellular ROS via aberrant O_2 reaction during electron transport. The rate of mitochondrial respiration and ROS formation is largely influenced by the coupling state of the mitochondria. APS decrease oxygen consuming rate and RCR of liver mitochondria, therefore, reduce mitochondrial ROS production. We consider this is appearance of lowering standard metabolic rate and is a kind of protective adaptation. Cancer patients need nutritional supplements, adequate rest, and should reduce energy consumption, APS can just achieve this goal.

In conclusion, APS would have a beneficial effect on protecting mitochondria while maintaining efficient cellular metabolism. APS was able to improve mitochondrial function by enhancing cellular bioenergetics and had the pharmaceutical activities of mitochondrial protection. Lastly, mitochondria can also generate feedback signals via bioenergy level or metabolites in the cytosol, such as ATP, ADP, TAP levels, ATP/ADP and ATP/AMP ratio, AEC, or ROS, which participate in the regulation of energy production. The study provides scientific evidence for the mechanism of APS ameliorate mitochondrial dysfunction which is achieved by improving mitochondrial energy metabolism, and this may be the hypothetical cancer-preventive mechanism of APS. In summary, APS was able to improve mitochondrial function by enhancing cellular bioenergetics and had the pharmaceutical activities of mitochondrial protection by scavenging ROS, inhibiting lipid peroxidation, and increasing the activities of antioxidant enzymes. The study provides scientific evidence for the mechanism of cancer prevention which is achieved by improving mitochondrial energy metabolism.

Acknowledgments

This work was supported by the Fundamental Research Funds for the Central Universities in China (No. DC12010210); Dalian Municipal Science and Technology Project (No.2013E15SF131); the Post-doctoral Research Station of Daxing'anling Beiqishen Green Industry Group, Doctoral Research Center of Heilongjiang University of Chinese Medicine (No.LRB10-316); and the Talents Project of Dalian Nationalities University (No.20116126).

References

Acin-Perez, R., Salazar, E., Kamenetsky, M., Buck, J., Levin, L.R. & Manfredi, G. (2009). Cyclic AMP produced inside mitochondria regulates oxidative phosphorylation. Cell Metab., 9, 265–276.

Arany, Z., He, H., Lin, J., Hoyer, K., Handschin, C., Toka, O., Ahmad, F., Matsui, T., Chin, S., Wu, P.H., Rybkin, I.I., Shelton, J.M., Manieri, M., Cinti, S., Schoen, F.J., Bassel-Duby, R., Rosenzweig, A., Ingwall, J.S. & Spiegelman, B.M. (2005). Transcriptional coactivator PGC-1 alpha controls the energy state and contractile function of cardiac muscle. Cell Metab., 1, 259–271.

Armstrong, J.S. (2006). Mitochondria: a target for cancer therapy. Br. J. Pharmacol.,147, 239–248.

Ballot, C., Kluza, J., Martoriati, A., Nyman, U., Formstecher, P., Joseph, B., Bailly, C. & Marchetti, P. (2009). Essential role of mitochondria in apoptosis of cancer cells induced by the marine alkaloid Lamellarin D. Mol. Cancer Ther., 8, 3307–3317.

Bell, E.L., Klimova, T.A., Eisenbart, J., Moraes, C.T., Murphy, M.P., Budinger, G.R. & Chandel, N.S. (2007). The Qo site of the mitochondrial complex III is required for the transduction of hypoxic signaling via reactive oxygen species production. J. Cell Biol., 177, 1029–1036.

Bellance, N., Benard, G., Furt, F., Begueret, H., Smolková, K., Passerieux, E., Delage, J.P., Baste, J.M., Moreau, P. & Rossignol, R. (2009). Bioenergetics of lung tumors: alteration of mitochondrial biogenesis and respiratory capacity. Int. J. Biochem. Cell Biol., 41, 2566–2577.

Ben Sahra, I., Laurent, K., Giuliano, S., Larbret, F., Ponzio, G., Gounon, P., Le Marchand-Brustel, Y., Giorgetti-Peraldi, S., Cormont, M., Bertolotto, C., Deckert, M., Auberger, P., Tanti, J.F. & Bost, F. (2010). Targeting cancer cell metabolism: the combination of metformin and 2-deoxyglucose induces p53-dependent apoptosis in prostate cancer cells. Cancer Res., 70, 2465–2475.

Benard, G., Bellance, N., James, D., Parrone, P., Fernandez, H., Letellier, T. & Rossignol, R. (2007). Mitochondrial bio-energetics and structural network organization. J. Cell Sci., 120, 838–848.

Benard, G., Bellance, N., Jose, C., Melser, S., Nouette-Gaulain, K. & Rossignol, R. (2010). Multi-site control and regulation of mitochondrial energy production. Biochim. Biophys. Acta, 1797, 698–709.

Bernal, S.D., Lampidis, T.J., Summerhayes, I.C. & Chen, L.B. (1982). Rhodamine-123 selectively reduces clonal growth of carcinoma cells in vitro. Science, 218, 1117–1119.

Bianchi,C., Genova, M.L. & Parenti Castelli, G., Lenaz, G. (2004). The mitochondrial respiratory chain is partially organized in a supercomplex assembly: kinetic evidence using flux control analysis. J. Biol. Chem., 279, 36562–36569.

Blackman, R.K., Cheung-Ong, K., Gebbia, M., Proia, D.A., He, S., Kepros, J., Jonneaux, A., Marchetti, P., Kluza, J., Rao, P.E., Wada, Y., Giaever, G. & Nislow, C. (2012). Mitochondrial electron transport is the cellular target of the oncology drug elesclomol. PLoS ONE 7(1): e29798. doi:10.1371/journal.pone.0029798.

Bonnet, S., Archer, S.L., Allalunis-Turner, J., Haromy, A., Beaulieu, C., Thompson, R., Lee, C.T., Lopaschuk, G.D., Puttagunta, L., Bonnet, S., Harry, G., Hashimoto, K., Porter, C.J., Andrade, M.A., Thebaud, B. & Michelakis, E.D. (2007). A mitochondria-K$^+$ channel axis is suppressed in cancer and its normalization promotes apoptosis and inhibits cancer growth. Cancer Cell, 11, 37–51.

Bonora, E., Porcelli, A.M., Gasparre, G., Biondi, A., Ghelli, A., Carelli, V., Baracca, A., Tallini, G., Martinuzzi, A., Lenaz, G., Rugolo, M. & Romeo, G. (2006). Defective oxidative phosphorylation in thyroid oncocytic carcinoma is associated with pathogenic mitochondrial DNA mutations affecting complexes I and III. Cancer Res., 66, 6087–6096.

Bouchier-Hayes, L., Lartigue, L. & Newmeyer, D.D. (2005). Mitochondria: pharmacological manipulation of cell death. J. Clin. Invest., 115, 2640–2647.

Boudina, S. & Dale Abel, E. (2006). Mitochondrial uncoupling: A key contributor to reduced cardiac efficiency in diabetes. Physiology, 21, 250–258.

Bradford, M.M. (1976). A rapid and sensitive method for the quantation of microgram quantities of protein utilizing the principle of protein-dye binding. Anal. Biochem., 72, 248–254.

Brahimi-Horn, M.C. & Pouyssegur, J. (2007). Oxygen, a source of life and stress. FEBS Lett., 581, 3582–3591.

Brand, M.D., Affourtit, C., Esteves, T.C., Green, K.,Lambert, A.J. & Miwa, S. (2004). Mitochondrial superoxide: production, biological effects, and activation of uncouplingproteins. Free Radic. Biol. Med., 37, 755–767.

Bras, M., Queenan, B. & Susin, S.A. (2005). Programmed cell death via mitochondria: different modes of dying. Biochemistry (Mosc), 70, 231–239.

Braun, R.D., Lanzen, J.L., Snyder, S.A. & Dewhirst, M.W. (2001). Comparison of tumor and normal tissue oxygen tension measurements using OxyLite or microelectrodes in rodents. Am. J. Physiol. Heart Circ. Physiol., 280, H2533–2544.

Bristow, R.G. & Hill, R.P. (2008). Hypoxia and metabolism. Hypoxia, DNA repair and genetic instability. Nat. Rev. Cancer, 8, 180–192.

Busk, M., Horsman, M.R., Kristjansen, P.E., van der Kogel, A.J., Bussink, J. & Overgaard, J. (2008). Aerobic glycolysis in cancers: implications for the usability of oxygenresponsivegenes and fluorodeoxyglucose-PET as markers of tissue hypoxia. Int. J. Cancer, 122, 2726–2734.

Canto, C., Gerhart-Hines, Z., Feige, J.N., Lagouge, M., Noriega, L., Milne, J.C., Elliott, P.J., Puigserver, P. & Auwerx, J. (2009). AMPK regulates energy expenditure by modulating NAD$^+$ metabolism and SIRT1 activity. Nature, 458, 1056–1060.

Capaldi, R.A., Halphen, D.G., Zhang, Y.Z. & Yanamura, W. (1988). Complexity and tissue specificity of the mitochondrial respiratory chain. J. Bioenerg. Biomembr., 20, 291–311.

Carroll, J., Fearnley, I.M., Skehel, J.M., Runswick, M.J., Shannon, R.J., Hirst, J. & Walker, J.E. (2005). The posttranslational modifications of the nuclear encoded subunits of complex I from bovine heart mitochondria. Mol. Cell. Proteomics, 4, 693–699.

Chen, R., Shao H., Lin, S., Zhang, J.J. & Xu, K.Q. (2011). *Treatment with Astragalus membranaceus produces antioxidative effects and attenuates intestinal mucosa injury induced by intestinal ischemia-reperfusion in rats. Am. J. Chin. Med., 39, 879–887.*

Chen, Y.C., Lin-Shiau, S.Y. & Lin, J.K. (1998). *Involvement of reactive oxygen species and caspase 3 activation in arsenite-induced apoptosis. J. Cell Physiol., 177, 324–333.*

Chen, Y., McMillan-Ward, E., Kong, J., Israels, S.J. & Gibson, S.B. (2007). *Mitochondrial electrontransport-chain inhibitors of complexes I and II induce autophagic cell death mediated by reactive oxygen species. J. Cell Sci., 120, 4155–4166.*

Chen, Z.X. & Pervaiz, S. (2010). *Involvement of cytochrome c oxidase subunits Va and Vb in the regulation of cancer cell metabolism by Bcl-2. Cell Death Differ., 17, 408–420.*

Cheng, X.D., Hou, C.H., Zhang, X.J., Xie, H.Y., Zhou, W.Y., Yang, L., Zhang, S.B. & Qian, R.L. (2004). *Effects of Huangqi (Hex) on inducing cell differentiation and cell death in K562 and HEL cells. Acta Biochim. Biophys. Sin., 36, 211–217.*

Chiang, A.C. & Massague, J. (2008). *Molecular basis of metastasis. N. Engl. J. Med., 359, 2814–2823.*

Chiche, J., Rouleau, M., Gounon, P., Brahimi-Horn, M.C., Pouysségur, J. & Mazure, N.M. (2010). *Hypoxic enlarged mitochondria protect cancer cells from apoptotic stimuli. J. Cell. Physiol., 222, 648–657.*

Choi, S.Y., Huang, P., Jenkins, G.M., Chan, D.C., Schiller, J. & Frohman, M.A. (2006). *A common lipid links Mfn-mediated mitochondrial fusion and SNARE-regulated exocytosis. Nat. Cell Biol., 1255–1262.*

Crabtree, H.G. (1929). *Observations on the carbohydrate metabolism of tumors. Biochem. J., 23, 536–545.*

Crompton, M. (1999). *The mitochondrial permeability transition pore and its role in cell death. Biochem. J., 341, 233–249.*

Crompton, M. (2000). *Mitochondrial intermembrane junctional complexes and their role in cell death. J. Physiol., 529, 11–21.*

Cuezva, J.M., Chen, G., Alonso, A.M., Isidoro, A., Misek, D.E., Hanash, S.M. & Beer, D.G. (2004). *The bioenergetic signature of lung adenocarcinomas is a molecular marker of cancer diagnosis and prognosis. Carcinogenesis, 25, 1157–1163.*

Cuezva, J.M., Krajewska, M., de Heredia, M.L., Krajewski, S., Santamaria, G., Kim, H., Zapata, J.M., Marusawa, H., Chamorro, M. & Reed, J.C. (2002). *The bioenergetic signature of cancer: a marker of tumor progression. Cancer Res., 62, 6674–6681.*

Dalmonte, M.E., Forte, E., Genova, M.L., Giuffre, A., Sarti, P. & Lenaz, G. (2009). *Control of respiration by cytochrome c oxidase in intact cells: role of the membrane potential. J. Biol. Chem., 284, 32331–32335.*

Dang, C.V. & Semenza, G.L. (1999). *Oncogenic alterations of metabolism. Trends Biochem. Sci., 24, 68–72.*

Das, T.K., Pecoraro, C., Tomson, F.L., Gennis, R.B. & Rousseau, D.L. (1998). *The post-translational modification in cytochrome c oxidase is required to establish a functional environment of the catalytic site. Biochemistry, 37, 14471–14476.*

D'Aurelio, M., Gajewski, C.D., Lenaz, G. & Manfredi, G. (2006). *Respiratory chain super complexes set the threshold for respiration defects in human mtDNA mutant cybrids. Hum. Mol. Genet., 15, 2157–2169.*

Daye, D. & Wellen, K. E. (2012). *Cancer cell metabolism & notch signaling metabolic reprogramming in cancer: Unraveling the role of glutamine in tumorigenesis. Cell Dev. Biol., 23, 362–369.*

de Brito, O.M. & Scorrano, L. (2008). *Mitofusin 2 tethers endoplasmic reticulum to mitochondria. Nature, 456, 605–610.*

De Lena, M., Lorusso, V., Latorre, A., Fanizza, G., Gargano, G., Caporusso, L., Guida, M., Catino, A., Crucitta, E., Sambiasi, D. & Mazzei, A. (2001). *Paclitaxel, cisplatin and lonidamine in advanced ovarian cancer. A phase II study. Eur. J. Cancer, 37, 364–368.*

DeBerardinis, R.J. & Cheng, T. (2010). *Q's next: the diverse functions of glutamine in metabolism, cell biology and cancer. Oncogene, 29, 313–324.*

Derdak, Z., Mark, N.M., Beldi, G., Robson, S.C., Wands, J.R. & Baffy, G. (2008). *The mitochondrial uncoupling protein-2 promotes chemo resistance in cancer cells. Cancer Res., 68, 2813–2819.*

Dias, N. & Bailly, C. (2005). *Drugs targeting mitochondrial functions to control tumor cell growth. Biochem. Pharmacol., 70, 1–12.*

Diaz-Ruiz, R., Rigoulet, M. & Devin, A. (2011). *The Warburg and Crabtree effects: On the origin of cancer cell energy metabolism and of yeast glucose repression. Biochim. Biophys. Acta, 1807, 568–576.*

Díaz-Ruiz, R., Uribe-Carvajal, S., Devin, A. & Rigoulet, M. (2009). *Tumor cell energy metabolism and its common features with yeast metabolism. Biochim. Biophys. Acta,1796, 252–265.*

D'Souza, G.G. M., Wagle, M.A., Saxena, V. & Shah, A. (2011). *Approaches for targeting mitochondria in cancer therapy. Biochim. Biophys. Acta, 1807, 689–696.*

Dubois, M., Gilles, K.A., Hamilton, J.K., Rebers, P.A.& Smith, F. (1956). *Colorimetric method for determination of sugars and related substances. Anal. Chem., 28, 350–356.*

Eng, C., Kiuru, M., Fernandez, M.J. & Aaltonen, L.A. (2003). *A role for mitochondrial enzymes in inherited neoplasia and beyond. Nat. Rev. Cancer, 3, 193–202.*

Estabrook, R.W. (1967). *Mitochondrial respiratory control and the polarographic measurement of ADP: Oratios. Method. Enzymol., 10, 41–47.*

Fantin, V.R., St-Pierre, J. & Leder, P. (2006). *Attenuation of LDH-A expression uncovers a link between glycolysis, mitochondrial physiology, and tumor maintenance. Cancer Cell, 9, 425–434.*

Filomeni, G., Graziani, I., Rotilio, G. & Ciriolo, M.R. (2007). *Trans-Resveratrol induces apoptosis in human breast cancer cells MCF-7 by the activation of MAP kinases pathways. Genes Nutr., 2, 295–305.*

Fink, B.D., Reszka, K.J., Herlein, J.A., Mathahs, M.M. & Sivitz, W.I. (2005). *Respiratory uncoupling by UCP1 and UCP2 and superoxide generation in endothelial cell mitochondria. Am. J. Physiol. Endocrinol. Metab., 288, 71–79.*

Finkel, T. & Holbrook, N.J. (2000). *Oxidants, oxidative stress and the biology of ageing. Nature, 408, 239–247.*

Fliss, M.S., Usadel, H., Caballero, O.L., Wu, L., Buta, M.R., Eleff, S.M., Jen, J. & Sidransky, D. (2000). *Facile detection of mitochondrial DNA mutations in tumors and bodily fluids. Science, 287, 2017–2019.*

Floridi, A., Paggi, M.G., Marcante, M.L., Silvestrini, B., Caputo, A. & De Martino, C. (1981). *Lonidamine, a selective inhibitor of aerobic glycolysis of murine tumor cells. J. Natl. Cancer Inst., 66, 497–499.*

Frezza, C. & Gottlieb, E. (2009). *Mitochondria in cancer: Not just innocent bystanders. Semin. Cancer Biol., 19, 4–11.*

Fulda, S., Galluzzi, L. & Kroemer, G. Targeting mitochondria for cancer therapy. (2010). *Nat. Rev. Drug Discov., 9, 447–464.*

Furt, F. & Moreau, P. (2009). *Importance of lipid metabolism for intracellular and mitochondrial membrane fusion/fission processes. Int. J. Biochem. Cell Biol., 41, 1828–1836.*

Gallego, M.A., Ballot, C., Kluza, J., Hajji, N., Martoriati, A., Castera, L., Cuevas, C., Formstecher, P., Joseph, B., Kroemer, G., Bailly, C. & Marchetti, P. (2008). *Overcoming chemoresistance of non-small cell lung carcinoma through restoration of an AIF-dependent apoptotic pathway. Oncogene, 27, 1981–1992.*

Galli, S., Labato, M.I., Bal de Kier Joffe, E., Carreras, M.C. & Poderoso, J.J. (2003). *Decreased mitochondrial nitric oxide synthase activity and hydrogen peroxide relate persistent tumoral proliferation to embryonic behavior. Cancer Res., 63, 6370–6377.*

Galluzzi, L., Larochette, N., Zamzami, N. & Kroemer, G. (2006). *Mitochondria as therapeutic targets for cancer chemotherapy. Oncogene, 25, 4812–4830.*

Gatt, S. & Racker, E. (1959). *Regulatory mechanisms in carbohydrate metabolism: I. Crabtree effect in reconstituted systems. J. Biol. Chem., 234, 1015–1023.*

Gatzemeier, U., Cavalli, F., Haussinger, K., Kaukel, E., Koschel, G., Martinelli, G., Neuhauss, R. & von Pawel, J. (1991). *Phase III trial with and without lonidamine in non-small cell lung cancer. Semin. Oncol., 18, 42–48.*

Genova, M.L., Baracca, A., Biondi, A., Casalena, G., Faccioli, M., Falasca, A.I., Formiggini, G., Sgarbi, G., Solaini, G. & Lenaz, G. (2008). Is supercomplex organization of the respiratory chain required for optimal electron transfer activity? Biochim. Biophys. Acta, 1777, 740–746.

Gnaiger, E. (2009). Capacity of oxidative phosphorylation in human skeletal muscle.New perspectives of mitochondrial physiology. Int. J. Biochem. Cell Biol., 41, 1837–1845.

Gnaiger, E., Mendez, G. & Hand, S.C. (2000). High phosphorylation efficiency and depression of uncoupled respiration in mitochondria under hypoxia. Proc. Natl. Acad. Sci. U.S.A., 97, 11080–11085.

Gogvadze, V., Orrenius, S. & Zhivotovsky, B. (2008). Mitochondria in cancer cells: what is so special about them? Trends Cell Biol., 18, 165–173.

Gogvadze, V., Orrenius, S. & Zhivotovsky, B. (2009). Mitochondria as targets for cancer chemotherapy. Semin. Cancer Biol., 19, 57–66.

Goswami, P.C. (2009). Mutant mitochondria and cancer cell metastasis: Quest for amechanism. Cancer Biol. Ther., 8, 1386–1388.

Gottlieb, E. & Tomlinson, I.P. (2005). Mitochondrial tumour suppressors: a genetic and biochemical update. Nat. Rev. Cancer, 5, 857–866.

Gulbins, E., Dreschers, S. & Bock, J. (2003). Role of mitochondria in apoptosis. Exp. Physiol. 88, 85–90.

Guzy, R.D. & Schumacker, P.T. (2006). Oxygen sensing by mitochondria at complex III: the paradox of increased reactive oxygen species during hypoxia. Exp. Physiol., 91, 807–819.

Hackenbrock, C.R. (1968). Ultrastructural bases for metabolically linked mechanical activity in mitochondria: II. Electron transport-linked ultrastructural transformations in mitochondria. J. Cell Biol., 37, 345–369.

Hackenbrock, C.R., Rehn, T.G., Weinbach, E.C. & Lemasters, J.J. (1971). Oxidative phosphorylation and ultrastructural transformation in mitochondria in the intact ascites tumor cell. J. Cell Biol., 51, 123–137.

Hagen, T., Taylor, C.T., Lam, F. & Moncada, S. (2003). Redistribution of intracellular oxygen in hypoxia by nitric oxide: effect on HIF1alpha. Science, 302, 1975–1978.

Hail, N. (2005). Mitochondria: a novel target for the chemoprevention of cancer. Apoptosis, 10, 687–705.

Hammond, E.M. & Giaccia, A.J. (2005). The role of p53 in hypoxia-induced apoptosis. Biochem. Biophys. Res. Commun., 331, 718–725.

Hanahan, D. & Weinberg, R.A. (2000). The hallmarks of cancer. Cell, 100, 57–70.

Hardie, D.G. (2007). AMP-activated/SNF1 protein kinases: conserved guardians of cellular energy. Nat. Rev. Mol. Cell Biol., 8, 774–785.

Haworth, R.A. & Hunter, D.R. (1979). The Ca^{2+}-induced membrane transition in mitochondria. II. Nature of the Ca^{2+} trigger site. Arch. Biochem. Biophys., 195, 460–467.

Hervouet, E., Cízková, A., Demont, J., Vojtísková, A., Pecina, P., Franssen-van Hal, N.L., Keijer, J., Simonnet, H., Ivánek, R., Kmoch, S., Godinot, C. & Houstek, J. (2008). HIF and reactive oxygen species regulate oxidative phosphorylation in cancer. Carcinogenesis, 29, 1528–1537.

Hodgson, E. (2004). A Textbook of Modern Toxicology (3rd ed). New Jersey: John Wiley and Sons Inc.

Hong, C.Y., Lo, Y.C., Tan, F.C., Wei, Y.H. & Chen, C.F. (1994). Astragalus membranaceus and Polygonum multijlorum protect rat heart mitochondria against lipid peroxidation. Am. J. Chin. Med., 22, 63–70.

Horton, H.R., Moran, L.A., Ochs, R.S., Rawn, J.D. & Scrimgeour, K.G. (2002). Principles of Biochemistry (3rd ed). New Jersey: Science Press and Pearson Education North Asia Limited.

Hunter, D.R. & Haworth, R.A. (1979). The Ca^{2+}-inducedmembrane transition in mitochondria. I. The protective mechanisms. Arch. Biochem. Biophys., 195, 453–459.

Ibsen, K.H. (1961). The Crabtree effect: a review. Cancer Res., 21, 829–841.

Igney, F.H. & Krammer, P.H. (2002). Death and anti-death: tumour resistance to apoptosis. Nat. Rev. Cancer, 2, 277–288.

Indran, I. R.,Tufo, G., Pervaiz, S. & Brenner, C. (2011). Recent advances in apoptosis, mitochondria and drug resistance in cancer cells. Biochim. Biophys. Acta, 1807, 735–745.

Ishikawa, K., Takenaga, K. & Akimoto, M. (2008). ROS generating mitochondrial DNA mutations can regulate tumor cell metastasis. Science, 320, 661–664.

Ishitsuka, K., Hideshima, T., Hamasaki, M., Raje, N., Kumar, S., Hideshima, H., Shiraishi, N., Yasui, H., Roccaro, A.M. & Richardson, P. (2005). Honokiol overcomes conventional drug resistance in human multiple myeloma by induction of caspase-dependent and -independent apoptosis. Blood, 106, 1794–1800.

Iwama, K., Nakajo, S., Aiuchi, T. & Nakaya, K. (2001). Apoptosis induced by arsenic trioxide in leukemia U937 cells is dependent on activation of p38, inactivation of ERK and the Ca^{2+}-dependent production of superoxide. Int. J. Cancer, 92, 518–526.

Jacobson, M.D., Weil, M. & Raff, M.C. (1997). Programmed cell death in animal development. Cell, 88, 347–354.

Jang, M., Cai, L., Udeani, G.O., Slowing, K.V., Thomas, C.F., Beecher, C.W., Fong, H.H., Farnsworth, N.R., Kinghorn, A.D., Mehta, R.G., Moon, R.C. & Pezzuto, J.M. (1997). Cancer chemopreventive activity of resveratrol, a natural product derived from grapes. Science, 275, 218–220.

Johnson, L.V., Walsh, M.L., Bockus, B.J. & Chen, L.B. (1981). Monitoring of relative mitochondrial membrane potential in living cells by fluorescence microscopy. J. Cell Biol., 88, 526–535.

Juan, M.E., Wenzel, U., Daniel, H. & Planas, J.M., (2008). Resveratrol induces apoptosis through ROS-dependent mitochondria pathway in HT-29 human colorectal carcinoma cells. J. Agr. Food Chem., 56, 4813–4818.

Kann, O. & Kovács, R. (2007). Mitochondria and Neuronal Activity. Am. J. Physiol. Cell Physiol., 292, C641–C657.

Katabi, M.M., Chan, H.L., Karp, S.E. & Batist, G. (1999). Hexokinase type II: a novel tumorspecific promoter for gene-targeted therapy differentially expressed and regulated in human cancer cells. Hum. Gene Ther., 10, 155–164.

Khatri, S. & Plas, D.R. (2009). Targeting bioenergetics to enhance cancer chemotherapy: mitochondria SLP into apoptosis. Cancer. Biol. Ther., 8, 1659–1661.

Kirshner, J.R., He, S., Balasubramanyam, V., Kepros, J., Yang, C.-Y., Zhang, M., Du, Z., Barsoumand, J. & Bertin, J. (2008). Elesclomol induces cancer cell apoptosis through oxidative stress. Mol. Cancer Ther., 7, 2319–2327.

Klöhn, P.C., Soriano, M.E., Irwin, W., Penzo, D., Scorrano, L., Bitsch, A., Neumann, H.G. & Bernardi, P. (2003). Early resistance to cell death and to onset of the mitochondrial permeability transition during hepatocarcinogenesis with 2-acetylaminofluorene. Proc. Natl. Acad. Sci. U.S.A., 100, 10014–10019.

Kluza, J., Gallego, M.-A., Loyens, A., Beauvillain, J.-C., Sousa-Faro, J.-M.F., Cuevas, C., Marchetti, P. & Bailly, C. (2006). Cancer cell mitochondria are direct proapoptotic targets for the marine antitumor drug Lamellarin D. Cancer Res., 66, 3177–3187.

Ko, Y., Lin, Z., Flomenberg, N., Pestell, R., Howell, A., Sotgia, F., Lisanti, M. & Martinez-Outschoorn, U. (2011). Glutamine fuels a vicious cycle of autophagy in the tumor stroma and oxidative mitochondrial metabolism in epithelial cancer cells: Implications for preventing chemotherapy resistance. Cancer Biol. Ther., 12, 1085–1097.

Kovacevic, Z. & Morris, H.P. (1972). The role of glutamine in the oxidative metabolism of malignant cells. Cancer Res., 32, 326–333.

Koziel, K., Lebiedzinska, M., Szabadkai, G., Onopiuk, M., Brutkowski,W., Wierzbicka, K., Wilczynski, G., Pinton, P., Duszynski,J., Zablocki, K. &Wieckowski, M.R. (2009). Plasma membrane associated membranes (PAM) from Jurkat cells contain STIM1 protein is PAM involved in the capacitative calcium entry? Int. J. Biochem. Cell Biol., 41, 2440–2449.

Li, R., Chen, W. C., Wang, W.P. & Tian, W.Y. (2009). Extraction, characterization of Astragalus polysaccharides and its immune modulating activities in rats with gastric cancer. Carbohyd. Polym., 78, 738–742.

Li, X.T. (2012). *Investigation on the Mechanism of Qi-invigoration from a Perspective of Effects of Sijunzi Decoction on Mitochondrial Energy Metabolism. In: Hiroshi S. (Ed.) Alternative Medicine. Rijeka: InTech Publisher.*

Li, X.T. & Zhao, J. (2012). *An Approach to the Nature of Qi in TCM–Qi and Bioenergy. In: Kuang H. (Ed.) Recent Advances in Theories and Practice of Chinese Medicine. Rijeka: InTech Publisher.*

Li, X.T., Chen, R., Jin, L.M. & Chen, H.Y. (2009). *Regulation on energy metabolism and protection on mitochondria of Panax ginsengpolysaccharide. Am. J. Chin. Med., 37, 1139–1152.*

Li, X.T., Zhang, Y.K., Kuang, H.X., Jin, F.X., Liu, D.W., Gao, M.B., Liu, Z. & Xin, X.J. (2012). *Mitochondrial protection and anti-aging activity of Astragaluspolysaccharides and their potential mechanism. Int. J. Mol. Sci., 13, 1747–1761.*

Luo, Z., Zhong, L., Han, X., Wang, H., Zhong, J.& Xuan, Z. (2009). *Astragalus membranaceus prevents daunorubicin-induced apoptosis of cultured neonatal cardiomyocytes: Role of free radical effect of Astragalus membranaceus on daunorubicin cardiotoxicity. Phytother. Res., 23, 761–767.*

Mao, X.Q., Yu, F., Wang, N., Wu, Y., Zou, F., Wu, K., Liu, M. & Ouyang, J.P. (2009). *Hypoglycemic effect of polysaccharide enriched extract of Astragalus membranaceus in diet induced insulin resistant C57BL/6J mice and its potential mechanism. Phytomedicine, 16, 416–425.*

Mathupala, S. P., Ko, Y.H. & Pedersen, P.L. (2010). *The pivotal roles of mitochondria in cancer: Warburg and beyond and encouraging prospects for effective therapies. Biochim. Biophys. Acta, 1797, 1225–1230.*

Máximo, V. & Sobrinho-Simões, M. (2000a). *Hurthle cell tumours of the thyroid.A review with emphasis on mitochondrial abnormalities with clinical relevance. Virchows Arch., 437, 107–115.*

Máximo, V. & Sobrinho-Simões, M. (2000b). *Mitochondrial DNA 'common' deletion in Hurthle cell lesions of the thyroid. J. Pathol., 192, 561–562.*

Máximo, V., Lima, J., Soares, P. & Sobrinho-Simões, M. (2009). *Mitochondria and cancer. Virchows Arch., 454, 481–495.*

Mckee, T. & Mckee, J.R. (1999). *Biochemistry: An Introduction (2nd ed). New York: McGraw-Hill Companies Inc.*

Modica-Napolitano, J.S. & Aprille, J.R. (2001). *Delocalized lipophilic cations selectively target the mitochondria of carcinoma cells. Adv. Drug Deliv. Rev., 49, 63–70.*

Moll, U.M. & Schramm, L.M. *p53–an acrobat in tumorigenesis. (1998). Crit. Rev. Oral Biol. Med., 9, 23–37.*

Moreno-Sánchez, R., Rodríguez-Enríquez, S., Marín-Hernández, A. & Saavedra, E. (2007). *Energy metabolism in tumor cells. FEBS J., 274, 1393–1418.*

Muller-Hocker, J. (1992). *Random cytochrome-C-oxidase deficiency of oxyphil cell nodules in the parathyroid gland. A mitochondrial cytopathy related to cell ageing? Pathol. Res. Pract., 188, 701–706.*

Muller-Hocker, J. (2000). *Expression of bcl-2, Bax and Fas in oxyphil cells of Hashimoto thyroiditis. Virchows Arch., 436, 602–607.*

Muller-Hocker, J., Jacob, U. & Seibel, P. (1998). *Hashimoto thyroiditis is associated with defects of cytochrome-c oxidase in oxyphil Askanazy cells and with the common deletion (4, 977) of mitochondrial DNA. Ultrastruct. Pathol., 22, 91–100.*

Nakashima, R.A., Paggi, M.G. & Pedersen, P.L. (1984). *Contributions of glycolysis and oxidative phosphorylation to adenosine 5'-triphosphate production in AS-30D hepatoma cells. Cancer Res., 44, 5702–5706.*

Parker, N., Crichton, P.G., Vidal-Puig, A.J. & Brand, M.D. (2009). *Uncoupling protein-1 (UCP1) contributes to the basal proton conductance of brown adipose tissue mitochondria. J. Bioenerg. Biomembr., 41, 335–342.*

Pasdois, P., Devaud, C., Voisin, P., Bouchaud, V., Rigoulet, M. & Beauvoit, B. (2003). *Contribution of the phosphorylable complex I in the growth phase-dependent respiration of C6 glioma cells in vitro. J. Bioenerg. Biomembr., 35, 439–450.*

Pedersen, P.L. (1978). *Tumor mitochondria and the bioenergetics of cancer cells. Prog. Exp. Tumor Res., 22, 190–274.*

Pelicano, H., Carney, D. & Huang, P. (2004). *ROS stress in cancer cells and therapeutic implications. Drug Resist. Updat., 7, 97–110.*

Pelicano, H., Feng, L., Zhou, Y., Carew, J.S., Hileman, E.O., Plunkett, W., Keating, M.J. & Huang, P. (2003). *Inhibition of mitochondrial respiration: a novel strategy to enhance drug-induced apoptosis in human leukemia cells by a reactive oxygen species-mediated mechanism. J. Biol. Chem., 278, 37832–37839.*

Peskin, B. (2009). *Cancer and mitochondria defects: New 21st Century Research. Townsend letter–August/September.87–90.*

Peskin, B.S. & Carter, M.J. (2008). *Chronic cellular hypoxia as the prime cause of cancer: What is the de-oxygenating role of adulterated and improper ratios of polyunsaturated fatty acids when incorporated into cell membranes? Med. Hypotheses, 70, 298–304.*

Piccoli, C., Scrima, R., Boffoli, D. & Capitanio, N. (2006). *Control by cytochrome c oxidase of the cellular oxidative phosphorylation system depends on the mitochondrial energy state. Biochem. J., 396, 573–583.*

Pouyssegur, J., Dayan, F. & Mazure, N.M. (2006). *Hypoxia signalling in cancer and approaches to enforce tumour regression. Nature, 441, 437–443.*

Qu, Y., Wang, J., Sim, M.-S., Liu, B., Giuliano, A., Barsoum, J. & Cui, X. (2010). *Elesclomol, counteracted by Akt survival signaling, enhances the apoptotic effect of chemotherapy drugs in breast cancer cells. Breast Cancer Res. Tr., 121, 311–321.*

Rajagopalan, K.N. & DeBerardinis, R.J. (2011). *Role of glutamine in cancer: Therapeutic and imaging implications. J. Nucl. Med., 52, 1005–1008.*

Rodríguez-Enriquez, S., Juárez, O., Rodríguez-Zavala, J.S. & Moreno-Sánchez, R. (2001). *Multisite control of the Crabtree effect in ascites hepatoma cells. Eur. J. Biochem., 268, 2512–2519.*

Rodríguez-Enríquez, S., Pérez-Gallardo, J.C., Avilés-Salas, A., Marín-Hernández, A., Carreño-Fuentes, L., Maldonado-Lagunas, V. & Moreno-Sánchez, R. (2008). *Energy metabolism transition in multi-cellular human tumor spheroids. J. Cell. Physiol., 216, 189–197.*

Rodríguez-Enríquez, S., Vital-González, P.A., Flores-Rodríguez, F.L., Marín-Hernández, A., Ruiz-Azuara, L. & Moreno-Sánchez, R. (2006). *Control of cellular proliferation by modulation. Toxicol. Appl. Pharmacol., 215, 208–217.*

Ryan, M.T. & Hoogenraad, N.J. (2007). *Mitochondrial-nuclear communications. Annu. Rev. Biochem., 76, 701–722.*

Salt, I.P., Johnson, G, Ashcroft, S.J. & Hardie, D.G. (1998). *AMP-activated protein kinase is activated by low glucose in cell lines derived from pancreatic beta cells, and may regulate insulin release. Biochem. J., 335, 533–539.*

Samper, E., Morgado, L., Estrada, J.C., Bernad, A., Hubbard, A., Cadenas, S. & Melov, S. (2009). *Increase in mitochondrial biogenesis, oxidative stress, and glycolysis in murine lymphomas. Free Radic. Biol. Med., 46, 387–396.*

Savagner, F., Franc, B. & Guyetant, S. (2001). *Defective mitochondrial ATP synthesis in oxyphilic thyroid tumors. J. Clin. Endocrinol. Metab., 86, 4920–4925.*

Scatena, R., Bottoni, P., Pontoglio, A., Mastrototaro, L. & Giardina, B. (2008). *Glycolytic enzyme inhibitors in cancer treatment. Expert. Opin. Investig. Drugs, 17, 1533–1545.*

Schatz, G. (2007). *The magic garden.Annu. Rev. Biochem., 76, 673–678.*

Shao, B.M., Xu, W., Dai, H., Tu, P., Li, Z. & Gao, X.M. (2004). *A study on the immune receptors for polysaccharides from the roots of Astragalus membranaceus, a Chinese medicinal herb. Biochem. Biophys. Res. Commun., 320, 1103–1111.*

Shaw, R.J. & Cantley, L.C. (2006). *Ras, PI(3)K and mTOR signalling controls tumour cellgrowth. Nature, 441, 424–430.*

Shen, Z.X., Chen, G.Q., Ni, J.H., Li, X.S., Xiong, S.M., Qiu, Q.Y., Zhu, J., Tang, W., Sun, G.L. & Yang, K.Q. (1997). *Use of arsenic trioxide (As$_2$O$_3$) in the treatment of acute promyelocytic leukemia (APL): II. Clinical efficacy and pharmacokinetics in relapsed patients. Blood, 89, 3354–3360.*

Shetty, M., Loeb, J. N., Vikstrom, K. & Ismail-Beigi, F. (1993). *Rapid activation of GLUT-1 glucose transporter following inhibition of oxidative phosphorylation in clone 9 cells. J. Biol. Chem., 268, 17225–17232.*

Simonnet, H., Alazard, N., Pfeiffer, K., Gallou, C., Beroud, C. & Demont, J. (2002). *Low mitochondrial respiratory chain content correlates with tumor aggressiveness in renal cell carcinoma. Carcinogenesis, 23, 759–768.*

Simonnet, H., Demont, J., Pfeiffer, K., Guenaneche, L., Bouvier, R., Brandt, U., Schagger, H. & Godinot, C. (2003). *Mitochondrial complex I is deficient in renal oncocytomas. Carcinogenesis, 24, 1461–1466.*

Slater, E.C. (1977). *Mechanism of oxidative phosphorylation. Annu. Rev. Biochem., 46, 1015–1026.*

Slater, E.C. (2003). *Keilin, cytochrome, and the respiratory chain. J. Biol. Chem., 278, 16455–16461.*

Smolková, K., Bellance, N., Scandurra, F., Génot, E., Gnaiger, E., Plecitá-Hlavatá, L., Jezek, P. & Rossignol, R. (2010). *Mitochondrial bioenergetic adaptations of breast cancer cells to aglycemia and hypoxia. J. Bioenerg. Biomembr., 42, 55–67.*

Solaini, G. & Harris, D.A. (2005). *Biochemical dysfunction in heart mitochondria exposed to ischaemia and reperfusion. Biochem. J., 390, 377–394.*

Solaini, G., Baracca, A., Lenaz, G. & Sgarbi, G. (2010). *Hypoxia and mitochondrial oxidative metabolism. Biochim. Biophys. Acta, 1797, 1171–1177.*

Solaini, G., Sgarbi, G. & Baracca, A. (2011). *Oxidative phosphorylation in cancer cells. Biochim. Biophys. Acta, 1807, 534–542.*

Solaini, G., Sgarbi, G., Lenaz, G. & Baracca, A. (2007). *Evaluating mitochondrial membrane potential in cells. Biosci. Rep., 27, 11–21.*

Sonveaux, P., Végran, F., Schroeder, T., Wergin, M.C., Verrax, J., Rabbani, Z.N., De Saedeleer, C.J., Kennedy, K.M., Diepart, C., Jordan, B.F., Kelley, M.J., Gallez, B., Whal, M.L., Feron, O. & Dewhirst, M.W. (2008). *Targeting lactate-fueled respiration selectively kills hypoxic tumor cells in mice. J. Clin. Invest., 118, 3930–3942.*

Storz, P. (2005). *Reactive oxygen species in tumor progression. Front Biosci., 10, 1881–1896.*

Szewczyk, A. & Wojtczak, L. (2002). *Mitochondria as a pharmacological target. Pharmacol. Rev., 54, 101–127.*

Trachootham, D., Alexandre, J. & Huang, P. (2009). *Targeting cancer cells by ROS-mediated mechanisms: a radical therapeutic approach? Nat. Rev. Drug Discov., 8, 579–591.*

Um, S.H., D'Alessio, D. & Thomas, G. (2006). *Nutrient overload, insulin resistance, and ribosomal protein S6 kinase 1, S6K1. Cell Metab., 3, 393–402.*

Veech, R.L., Lawson, J.W., Cornell, N.W. & Krebs, H.A. (1979). *Cytosolic phosphorylation potential. J. Biol. Chem., 254, 6538–6547.*

Ventura-Clapier, R., Garnier, A. & Veksler, V. (2008). *Transcriptional control of mitochondrial biogenesis: the central role of PGC-1alpha. Cardiovasc. Res., 79, 208–217.*

Verdin, E., Hirschey M.D., Finley, L.W.S. & Haigis, M.C. (2010). *Sirtuin regulation of mitochondria: energy production, apoptosis, and signaling. Trends Biochem. Sci., 35, 669–675.*

Vetvicka, V., Volny, T., Saraswat-Ohri, S., Vashishta, A., Vancikova, Z. & Vetvickova, J., (2007). *Glucan and resveratrol complex – possible synergistic effects on immune system. Biomed. Pap. Med. Fac. Univ. Palacky Olomouc Czech. Repub., 151, 41–46.*

Wallace, D.C. (2005). *A mitochondrial paradigm of metabolic and degenerative diseases, aging, and cancer: a dawn for evolutionary medicine. Annu. Rev. Genet., 39, 359–407*

Wang, G.L. & Semenza, G. L. (1993). *General involvement of hypoxia-inducible factor 1 in transcriptional response to hypoxia. Proc. Natl. Acad. Sci. U.S.A., 90, 4304–4308.*

Wang, P., Zhang, Z., Ma, X., Huang, Y., Liu, X., Tu, P. & Tong, T. (2003). *HDTIC-1 and HDTIC-2, two compounds extracted from Astragali Radix, delay replicative senescence of human diploid fibroblasts. Mech. Ageing Dev. 124, 1025–1034.*

Wang, T.S., Kuo, C.F., Jan, K.Y. & Huang, H. (1996). *Arsenite induces apoptosis in Chinese hamster ovary cells by generation of reactive oxygen species. J. Cell Physiol., 169, 256–268.*

Wanga, F., Ogasawara, M.A. & Huang, P. (2010). Small mitochondria-targeting molecules as anti-cancer agents. Mol. Aspects Med., 31, 75–92.

Warburg, O. (1956). On the origin of cancer cells. Science, 123, 309–314.

Weinhouse, S. (1956). On respiratory impairment in cancer cells. Science, 124, 267–269.

Weinhouse, S. (1972). Glycolysis, respiration and anomalous gene expression in experimental hepatomas: G.H.A. Clawes memorial lecture. Cancer Res., 32, 2007–2016.

Weinhouse, S. (1976). The Warburg hypothesis fifty years later. Z. Krebsforsch. Klin. Onkol. Cancer Res. Clin. Oncol., 87, 115–126.

Wolvetang, E.J., Johnson, K.L., Krauer, K., Ralph, S.J. & Linnane, A.W. (1994). Mitochondrial respiratory chain inhibitors induce apoptosis. FEBS Lett., 339, 40–44.

Wu, M. (2007). Multiparameter metabolic analysis reveals a close link between attenuated mitochondrial bioenergetic function and enhanced glycolysis dependency in human tumor cells. Am. J. Physiol. Cell Physiol., 292, C125–C136.

Yin, X., Chen, L., Liu, Y., Yang, J., Ma, C., Yao, Z., Yang, L., Wei, L. & Li, M. (2010). Enhancement of the innate immune response of bladder epithelial cells by Astragalus polysaccharides through upregulation of TLR4 expression. Biochem. Biophys. Res. Commun., 397, 232–238.

Zhang, B.B., Zhou, G. & Li, C. (2009). AMPK: an emerging drug target for diabetes and themetabolic syndrome. Cell Metab., 9, 407–416.

Zheng, X.Y. (2005). Pharmacopoeia of the People's Republic of China(8th ed). Beijing: Chemical Industry Press.

Zhu, Z.Y., Liu, R.Q., Si, C.L., Zhou, F., Wang, Y.X., Ding, L.N., Jing, C., Liu, A.J. & Zhang, Y.M. (2011). Structural analysis and anti-tumor activity comparison of polysaccharides from Astragalus. Carbohyd. Polym., 85, 895–902.

Zini, R., Morin, C., Bertelli, A., Bertelli, A.A. & Tillement, J.P. (1999). Effects of resveratrol on the rat brain respiratory chain. Drugs Exp. Clin. Res., 25, 87–97.

Zoratti, M. & Szabo, I. (1995). The mitochondrial permeability transition. Biochim. Biophys. Acta, 1241, 139–176.

Nuclear Medicine Imaging in Cancer

Masha Maharaj
Department of Nuclear Medicine
University of Limpopo, Polokwane Campus, South Africa

Nisaar Korowlay
Division of Nuclear Medicine
Tygerberg Hospital, Stellenbosch University, South Africa

1   Introduction

The basic pathological unit in cancer is a colony of cells over which there is a loss of normal regulatory mechanisms. At a functional level this results in uncontrollable proliferation of an abnormal cell line driven by oncogenic signals, impaired differentiation, and invasion of other tissues leading to metastases. It has become increasingly obvious that the changes of a cancer observed on a molecular level bear increment value toward the outcome of therapy. In 2011, Hanahan and Weinberg (Hanahan & Weinberg 2011) described six biological hallmarks of cancer acquired during the multistep development of human tumours. The hallmarks constitute an organizing principle for rationalizing the complexities of neoplastic disease; sustaining proliferative signalling, evading growth suppressors, resisting programmed cell death (apoptosis), limitless replicative potential, sustained angiogenesis, tissue invasion and metastasis, changes in metabolism and tumour promoting inflammatory alterations and interactions (Multhoff & Radons, 2012; Marnett, 2012). The improved knowledge of tumour-specific and tumour-associated processes have motivated and resulted in the development of new tools for diagnosis (imaging) and targeted therapy in Nuclear Medicine (Jaffer & Weissleder, 2005; Beirsack *et al.*, 1992; Haberkorn *et al.*, 2011; Debergh *et al.*, 2012; Weisleder, 2006; Ray, 2011; Sullivan & Gatsonis, 2011; Valotassiou *et al.*, 2012).

The aim of this chapter is to assist the student and clinician in sufficient understanding of Nuclear Medicine pertinent to areas of imaging of cancer. The introduction briefly provides insight into the tracer and equipment in Nuclear Medicine. The radiopharmaceuticals have been discussed in parallel with the biological hallmarks of cancer; metabolic, proliferation, angiogenesis, hypoxia and apoptosis. Included in the chapter is summary of existing SPECT (single photon emission computer tomography) radiopharmaceuticals which have also made their mark in general imaging in cancer and cancer management. A brief introduction into Theranostics is provided at the end.

1.1   The Tracer Principle:

The tracer principle, founded by Nobel Hevesy G in 1912 (Leitha, 2009), suggested that radioactive elements had identical chemical properties to the nonradioactive form and therefore could be used to trace chemical behaviour in solutions or in the body. The basis of Nuclear Medicine involves the administration of small amounts of radiopharmaceuticals (radiolabelled tracer) that emit radiations such as gamma (γ)-rays, x-rays, beta (β)-particles, alpha (α)-particles or positrons. The administration of small amounts of the relevant tracer allows one to directly observe the physiological process under study, without disturbing that process under investigation. Imaging of the radiotracers allows for monitoring biological processes non-invasively. The administration of low dose radiopharmaceuticals exposes the patient to low levels of ionizing radiation which is consistent with ALARA (As Low As Reasonably Achievable). Avoiding harmful consequences of radiation of which carcinogenesis is a primary concern (Fahey, 2011).

1.2   Equipment

1.2.1   Single Photon Emission Computer Tomography (SPECT)

The Gamma camera, also called a Scintillation camera or Anger camera has been developed since 1944. It is a device used to use in Nuclear Medicine to image γ-radiation emitting radioisotopes (Table 1) to view and analyse images of the human body or the distribution of medically injected, inhaled, or ingested radionuclides emitting gamma rays, producing a two dimensional (2D) image, a technique known as scintigraphy. SPECT is a scintigraphic technique in which a computer-generated image of local radioactive tracer distribution in tissues is produced through the detection of single-photon emissions from radionuclides introduced into the body that is able to provide true three-dimensional (3D) information. This information is typically presented as cross-sectional slices through the patient, but can be freely reformatted or manipulated as required. SPECT camera may be combined with a computerised tomography (CT) unit to form a hybrid system and fusion imaging of the physiology and anatomy of the area/s being scanned. Combined SPECT/CT devices provide both the functional information from SPECT and the anatomic information from CT in a single examination. SPECT/CT acquisitions can include the whole body, a limited portion of the body, or an organ. The method of attenuation correction is the use of CT transmission data with SPECT/CT scanners (Mariani et al., 2008).

Nuclide	Half-life	Decay	Major emissions kilo electron volt (keV)
Technetium-99m (99mTc)	6 hours	Isomeric transition (I.T.)	140
Gallium-67 (67Ga)	78 hours	Electron Capture (E.C.)	93, 184, 296, 388
Indium-111 (111In)	67 hours	E.C.	172, 247
Iodine-123 (123I)	13 hours	E.C.	159
Iodine-125 (125I)	60 days	E.C.	27
Iodine- 131 (131I)	8 days	Beta emission(β-)	364
Thallium-201 (201Tl)	73 hours	E.C.	Hg daughter X-ray emission 69-81

Table 1: Selected radionuclides for SPECT imaging.

1.2.2. Positron Emission Tomography (PET)

PET has been in existence since the 1970s and has developed from a research technique to a current state-of-the-art clinical imaging tool. Through positron-emitting radionuclide labelling, PET allows in-vivo imaging of physiologically and pathologically important molecules containing basic organic chemical elements such as carbon, fluoride, oxygen and nitrogen. The molecular and/or metabolic information provides essential contribution to the diagnosis, evaluation and prognosis of disease. This has impacted on effective patient management.

PET radionuclides emit positrons (β^+) particles (positively charged electrons). The most commonly used radionuclide, fluorine-^{18} (^{18}F), has a median range of only 0.2 mm in tissue and a maximum range of 2.4 mm. At the end of its trajectory, the positron interacts with an electron in a nearby atom and both are annihilated resulting in the emission of two gamma (γ) photons, each with energy of 511 keV. These photons move away from the point of annihilation in opposite directions at almost 180° straight line.

PET is a volumetric technique optimized for detection of these annihilation photons. It allows precise tracking of the spatial and temporal distribution of positron emitting radiopharmaceuticals in patients and represents a unique functional tomographic imaging modality based on the biochemical handling of chemicals by tissues of the body (Zeigler, 2005; Schyler, 2004; Chen & Chen, 2011).

The two instrumental PET radionuclides currently in clinical use include ^{18}F and ^{68}Ga. ^{18}F is cyclotron produced with a physical half-life of 110 minutes. The development of the radiopharmaceutical ^{18}F-fluorodeoxyglucose (^{18}F-FDG), a glucose analogue taken up avidly by the majority of malignant tumours, has resulted in it being used routinely in the management of many cancer patients.

^{68}Ga has a physical half-life of 68 min. Its parent, Germanium- 68 (^{68}Ge) is accelerator produced on Ga_2O_3 targets with a half-life of 270.8 days and decays by electron capture. The major advantage of

^{68}Ga over ^{18}F is its production from an in-house generator, making ^{68}Ga supply independent of a nearby cyclotron. ^{68}Ge/^{68}Ga generator systems have been developed since the late 70's, however, their relevant clinical use and further use in development of PET radiopharmaceuticals has been launched recently (Khan *et al.*, 2009; Maecke *et al.*, 2005). Table 2 illustrates a summary of current regulatory status of PET tracers.

The last 15 years have seen an exponential growth of PET, and even more since the introduction of hybrid positron emission tomography/computed tomography (PET/CT). The term 'one-stop-shop' has been dubbed to indicate the proficiency of obtaining physiological and anatomical information in a single investigation. The advantages of combining PET and CT include its superior lesion localisation in accurate anatomical/functional registration; a better distinction between physiological uptake and pathological uptake; consolidation of functional and anatomical imaging; and a benefit in shorter total scan time enhancing patient comfort and minimizing issues with claustrophobia and movement.

Mechanism	Tracer	*PET (regulatory status)
Glucose metabolism	Glucose analogue	Food and Drug Administration (FDA) approved
Lipid and Fatty Acid metabolism	Choline Acetate	Investigational/ Institutional Clinical use
DNA metabolism	Thymidine analogues	Investigational/ Institutional Clinical use
Amino Acids and Protein metabolism	Dopamine Tumour specific Receptors Tumour targeting Antibodies Guanidine analogue Gene expression	Investigational/ Institutional Clinical use
Angiogenesis	Vacular endothelial growth factor and receptors Integrins Matrix metalloproteinases Other angiogenesis targets	Investigational/ Institutional Clinical use
Iodine metabolism	Iodine	Investigational/ Institutional Clinical use
Hypoxia	Nitromidazole derivatives	Investigational/ Institutional Clinical use
Apoptosis	Annexin-V	Investigational/ Institutional Clinical use

Table 2: Summary of PET tracers with current regulatory status (Hicks & Hofman, 2012).

2   Radiopharmaceuticals

Table 3 shows an overview of radiopharmaceuticals that will be discussed in this section.

2.1.   Metabolic

2.1.1.   Glucose metabolism

^{18}F-Fluorodeoxyglucose (^{18}F-FDG)

^{18}F -FDG provides information about the rate of glucose metabolism in the body. ^{18}F has a physical half-life of 110 minutes and suitable kinetics for imaging with optimal resolution (Gunn *et al.*, 2002). Malignant cells show increased glucose uptake in vitro and in vivo, and this process is thought to be mediated by glucose transporters. There are estimated 14 known glucose trans-porter (GLUT) protein subtypes,

Metabolic	Glucose metabolism	FDG
	Lipid and fat	Choline
		Acetate
	Proliferation (DNA metabolism)	Thymidine analogues
	Amino Acids and Protein metabolism	Radiolabelled amino Acids
		Radiolabelled peptides
		Somatostatin Receptor analogues
		Dopamine
		Tumour specific Receptors
		Monoclonal Antibodies
		Guanidine analogue (Metaiodobenzylguanidine)
		Gene expression
	Iodine metabolism	Iodine
Angiogenesis		Vacular endothelial growth factor and receptors Integrins Matrix metalloproteinases Other angiogenesis imaging targets
Hypoxia		Nitromidazole derivatives
Apoptosis		Annexin-V
General tumour imaging radiopharmaceuticals	Skeletal	Methylene Diphosphonate
		Flouride
	Mitochondrial activity	Methoxy-isobutyl-isonitrile
	Transferrin receptor mechanism	Gallium 67 citrate
	Na-K adenosine-tri-phosphatase (ATP) system	Thallium 201
	Lipophilic brain perfusion agent converted by glutathione	Hexamethyl propylamine oxime (HMPAO)
General use of Nuclear Medicine in management and monitoring in Cancer	Equilibrium-gated Radionuclide Angiocardiography	Red blood cells
	Sentinel Node Imaging	Colloid particles

Table 3: Overview of Radiopharmaceuticals discussed in Section 2

with Glut1 and Glut3 expressed to a greater degree in a variety of carcinomas. This up-regulation of Glut protein enhances tumour glucose metabolism (Kyoichi *et al.*, 2011). ^{18}F -FDG is transported into tumour cell and processed the same physiological way as glucose is processed. After phosphorylation to ^{18}F -FDG-6-phosphate by hexokinase, ^{18}F-FDG-6-phosphate cannot be metabolized further in the glycolytic pathway and becomes trapped in the cell because of its negative charge. In a normal cell this process is reversed by glucose-6-phosphatase. In most tumour cells there is overexpression of Hexokinase and down-regulation of glucose-6-phosphatase which results in the accumulation of ^{18}F-FDG-6-phosphate in the cell (Kyoichi *et al.*, 2001).

The assessment of uptake of FDG is subjective (visually) and objectively, using an FDG uptake index with Standard uptake values (SUV). The SUV method takes into account the injected dose of FDG as well as the patient's body mass and is calculated as: (counts within region of interest)/ (body weight x dose injected). Studies have demonstrated that SUVs may vary considerably depending on the clinical scenario; inflammation, size of lesion under 1 cm in size may be underestimated and benign lesions may express high SUV's. SUV is also subjective to other sources of variability which are not controlled such as glucose level, length of the uptake period, body weight, body composition, recovery coefficient and partial volume effect (PVE), image parameters and image protocols (Wiyaporn *et al.*, 2010). The pivotal role of the SUV would be in the follow-up of the patient in monitoring response to therapy (Joseph, 2004).

Gambhir *et al.*, 2001, from a collection of 419 articles from 1993 to 2000 estimated the average ^{18}F-FDG PET sensitivity and specificity across all indications in oncology at 84% (based on 18,402 patient studies) and 88% (based on 14,264 patient studies), respectively (Tinsu & Osama, 2008).

The European Association of Nuclear Medicine (EANM), British Nuclear Medicine Society (BNMS) and Society of Nuclear Medicine (SNM) guidelines have illustrated the current clinical indications of FDG-PET (SNM Procedure guidelines; BNMS Procedure guidelines; EANM Procedure guidelines). Assessment at primary presentation in the diagnosis of unknown primary malignancy, differentiation of benign and malignant lesions (such as a solitary lung nodule, especially in case of discrepant clinical and radiological estimates of the likelihood of cancer). Staging on presentation in non-small-cell lung cancer, T3 oesophageal cancer, Hodgkin's disease, non-Hodgkin's lymphoma, locally advanced cervical cancer, ENT tumours with risk factors and locally advanced breast cancer (Karaosmanoğlu & Blake, 2012). Evaluation of response to therapy in malignant lymphoma and GIST (Zanoni etal, 2011; Park *et al.*, 2011). Restaging in the event of potentially curable relapse for FDG avid tumours. Establishing and localizing disease sites as a cause for elevated serum markers (this includes colorectal, thyroid, ovarian, cervix, melanoma, breast and germ-cell tumours). Image guided biopsy and use in radiotherapy planning have made a colossal impact (Arens & Troost, 2011).

Variable physiological FDG Uptake is seen in normal structures brain, the nasal turbinates', pterygoid muscles, extraocular muscles, brown fat, vocal cord uptake, thyroid, parotid, submandibular glands, and lymphoid tissue of the adenoids, upper Waldeyers ring, brain, heart, kidneys and urinary tract. There is some degree of FDG accumulation in the muscular system, and is increased by exercise. Gastrointestinal tract uptake varies from patient to patient. Physiological thymic uptake may be present in children, in young adults and in patients with regenerating haemopoietic tissues.

False-positive findings include inflammation, infection, granulomatous processes and benign neoplasms. False negative results may arise from low FDG avidity tumours. These vary from well differentiated tumours such a prostate cancer and neuroendocrine tumours to metastatic lesions from FDG avid primaries such as sarcomas. Lack of uptake may arise from relatively low glucose metabolism, high mucin content, low proliferation rates and necrosis (Freeman& Blaufox, 2013). A modulatory factor for ^{18}F-FDG uptake has been associated with the overexpression of P-glycoprotein in tumours, the exact underlying mechanism and relationship to glucose metabolism remains unknown. Overexpression of P-glycoprotein is an in vivo marker of multidrug resistance (Satoru *et al.*, 2009). In vitro studies using cancer cell lines, the uptake of ^{18}F-FDG was markedly decreased by the inhibition of Glut1 or hypoxic inducible factor-1alpha (HIF-1α), whereas, Glut1 up-regulation by the induction of HIF-1α increased the ^{18}F-FDG uptake, indicating that cellular uptake of ^{18}F-FDG is mediated by Glut1 and that the expression of Glut1 protein was regulated by HIF-1α. (Kyoichi *et al.*, 2010). Although the mechanism is not fully understood, FDG negative soft tissue metastases of FDG avid primary sarcomas have been reported (Roberge *et al.*, 2012).

Interpretation of structures/lesions adjacent, within or in proximity to an anatomic structure with inherently high FDG uptake such as the brain or tonsils may make it difficult to distinguish pathologic from physiologic metabolic activity.

Interpretation may be limited by artefacts generated by CT-based attenuation correction. Metallic devices can demonstrate falsely elevated FDG uptake. Intravenous contrast material is present in venous structures during CT but not during the PET portion of the examination causing areas of linear artefact (mimicking intense FDG accumulation) on the attenuation-corrected PET. Respiration artefacts and motion artefacts are common. Truncation may cause artefacts due to differences in size of field of view (FOV) CT (50 cm) and PET (70 cm).

Preparation may vary in relation to the area being investigated as per centre protocol. Generally the patient should be kept warm to limit brown fat activity. They should be comfortable during uptake and scan. They should keep quiet at least 30 min prior to and after the injection. The protocol may require a head holder or frame. The patient should fast 6 hours prior to study. The random glucose level <7 mmol/l (or <120 mg/dl). All fertile females should have a pregnancy test prior to injection. It should be recorded when the last chemotherapy was done and usually at least 10 days is acceptable to perform the study. The study may be performed at least 3 months post radiation therapy and surgery. The patient must be able to lie still for 20-45 minutes. The average radiation dosimetry for 350MBq is 7mSv for PET and 3-5mSv for the low dose CT component. (Poeppel *et al.*, 2009)

2.1.2. Lipid and Fatty Acid Metabolism

Choline

All cells in the body absolutely require choline. Choline is needed for the synthesis of phospholipids in cell membranes, methyl metabolism, cholinergic neurotransmission, transmembrane signalling, and lipid-cholesterol transport and metabolism. The uptake mechanism of choline and fluorocholine in tumour cells is of great interest. The backbones of cell membranes are made of phospholipid bilayers, of which the major component is phosphatidylcholine. The cell membranes are duplicated at the same rate as the rate of cell duplication.

Choline is a precursor for the synthesis of the neurotransmitter, acetylcholine. In the cell, choline can be phosphorylated, acetylated or oxidized. On a basic molecular level, phosphorylcholine is converted into phosphatidylcholine (lecithin) which is then incorporated into membrane synthesis. The phosphorylation of choline is catalysed by the enzyme choline kinase which has been implicated in malignant transformation of cells associated with the induction of choline kinase activity resulting in increased levels of phosphorylcholine. There is an increased demand of choline and phosphorylcholine incorporated into tumour cells in order to match the rapid rate of cell turnover.

In 1997, [11]C Choline was introduced as a potential PET tracer to image brain and prostate cancer. The inconvenient short half-life of ^{11}C and the rapid oxidization of ^{11}C-choline in vivo encouraged the development of ^{18}F-labeled choline analogues (FCH) and ^{18}F-fluoroethylcholine (FECH). These radiotracers were found to be good substrates for the enzyme choline kinase, but not for the enzymes involved in the oxidation of choline. The uptake of radiolabeled choline and fluorocholine represents exactly the duplication rate of tumour cells, and radiolabeled compounds present as extremely useful tools in the molecular evaluation of cancer.

Studies in prostate cancer have shown using and comparing FCH and FDG, more lesions were identifiable with FCH, including lesions of the prostate, bone, and soft tissue. Oncological applications have included evaluating high grade gliomas, anaplastic astrocytomas and primary hepatocellular cancer (but have low affinity for metastatic lesions to liver from colorectal cancer). (Picchio & Castelluci, 2012; Jadvar, 2011).

Acetate

Acetate is taken up by cells and activated to acetyl-CoA in both the cytosol and mitochondria by acetyl-CoA synthetase. Acetyl-CoA is a common metabolic intermediate for synthesis of cholesterol and fatty acids, which are then incorporated into the membrane. In normal cells and in myocardium, Acetyl-CoA is oxidized in mitochondria to carbon dioxide and water. In tumour cells, acetate is converted into fatty acids by fatty acid synthetase (overexpressed enzyme in cancer cells).

Prostate cancer is the most prevalent tumour for which imaging by PET with ^{18}F-FDG has been found to be generally unsatisfactory (Jadvar, 2011). The 60%–70% sensitivity of ^{18}F-FDG PET for prostate cancer is not high enough to justify its routine clinical use for staging or restaging of this disease. The poor performance of ^{18}F-FDG PET is likely related to the low glucose metabolic rate that results from the relatively slow growth of most prostate cancers as well as to other factors, including significant excretion of ^{18}F-FDG into the adjacent urinary bladder, making detection of tumour uptake difficult. PET with ^{11}C-Acetate (^{11}C-ACE) has a high sensitivity for detection of prostate cancer and several other cancers that are poorly detected with ^{18}F-FDG. The short half-life of ^{11}C limits its general availability. ^{18}F-Fluoroacetate (^{18}F-FAC) is an analogue of acetate with a longer radioactive half-life. Results indicate that ^{18}F-FAC is retained longer in tumour tissue than in other organs, suggesting that it is a useful tracer for PET tumour imaging. The liver and kidney appear to be the major metabolic organs. It has not yet been determined as to the precise mechanism for the incorporation of ^{18}F-FAC into tumours. Several authors have indicated ^{18}F-FAC is a useful alternative to ^{11}C-ACE for the detection of prostate tumours. Future indications may include other neoplasms with relatively low glucose use.(Ponde *et al.*, 2007).

2.1.3.   Proliferation (DNA metabolism)

Thymidine Analogues

Increased cellular proliferation, increased mitotic rate, cell proliferation, and lack of differentiation were regarded as the main factors responsible for accelerated growth of malignant tissue. In the 1950s, ^{3}H-Thymidine was introduced to measure thymidine incorporation into DNA (thymidine labelling index) in tumour tissue. ^{11}C-thymidine was prepared but was not optimal for routine imaging studies due to the short half-life and the rapid catabolism of thymidine after injection. These limitations led to the development of analogues that are resistant to degradation and can be labelled with radionuclides more conducive to routine clinical use, such as [18]F (Kumar, 2008).

Thymidine analogues that have been studied the most are 39-deoxy-39-fluorothymidine (FLT) and 1-(29-deoxy-29-fluoro-1-b-D-arabinofuranosyl)-thymine (FMAU). Both are resistant to degradation and track the DNA synthesis pathway. FLT enters tumour cells both via a nucleoside transporter and partly via passive diffusion. Inside proliferating cells, FLT is accepted as a substrate by thymidine kinase 1 (TK-1), which phosphorylates it, thereby trapping it in cells. FLT-monophosphate is further phosphorylated to di- and triphosphate forms. FLT-triphosphate is not significantly incorporated into DNA, unlike other thymidine analogues. The majority of FLT persists as mono- and triphosphates in the cytosol (Shankar, 2007). Due to dephosphorylation of FLT-monophosphate by the enzyme deoxynucleotidase, some FLT is effluxed from cells, but at a slower rate, providing a significant period of relatively stable tracer retention for imaging (Bading & Shields, 2008).

The entrapment of the radiotracer within the cell and allows noninvasively measuring cellular proliferation in vivo in malignant tumours and organ tissues. It is incorporated by the normal proliferating marrow and is glucuronidated in the liver. FMAU can be incorporated into DNA after phosphorylation but shows less marrow uptake. It shows high uptake in the normal heart, kidneys, and liver, in part because of the role of mitochondrial thymidine kinase-2. Early clinical data for ^{18}F-FLT demonstrated that its uptake correlates well with in vitro measures of proliferation. Although [18]FFLT can be used to detect tumours, its tumour-to-normal tissue contrast is generally lower than that of ^{18}F-FDG in most cancers outside the brain. The most promising use for thymidine and its analogues is in monitoring tumour treatment response, as demonstrated in animal studies and pilot human trials. Further work is needed to determine the optimal tracer(s) and timing of imaging after treatment. Oncological applications thus far of Thymidine include primary lung cancer with recorded sensitivity of 72% and specificity of 89% (Yap *et al.*, 2006), brain malignancies mostly high grade gliomas iii/iv, lymphoma demonstrating high uptake in aggressive type cell, breast cancer for early assessment of response to chemotherapy within 2 weeks of therapy, colorectal cancer although it has not been found to be useful for liver metastasis, it was found useful in oesophageal cancer by van Westreenen, in head and neck cancer uptake correlates with the aggressiveness of the tumour, in melanoma and soft tissue sarcoma of the extremities (Plotnik *et al.*, 2010).

Treatment with chemotherapy and radiation has been shown to reduce FLT uptake in these cancer models.

FLT-PET should not be regarded as an overall staging tool for cancer. There is lower overall uptake of FLT in tumours and higher background activity in the liver and bone marrow. It is not expected to have the same outstanding sensitivity as FDG-PET for tumour detection. FLT-PET should be considered a powerful addition to staging by FDG-PET. Providing additional diagnostic specificity for proliferating tissues and important biological information that could have implications in treatment selection or monitoring (Salskov *et al.*, 2007).

2.1.4. Amino Acids and Protein Metabolism

Amino Acids (AAs) are precursors for many biomolecules, such as hormones or neurotransmitters, such as the DNA or RNA precursors adenine and cytosine, sphingosine (derived from serine), histamine (derived from histidine), thyroxine, adrenaline and melanine (all derived from tyrosine), and serotonin (derived from tryptophan). In addition to being metabolic precursors, amino acids can be crucial in metabolic cycles as they enter several metabolic cycles and undergo metabolism, transamination and decarboxylation. AAs may enter the cell by simple diffusion or are transported via more than 20 membrane transport systems. AAs may also originate within the cell being derived from intracellular protein recycling.

Proteins play crucial roles in virtually all biological processes. Nearly all chemical reactions in biological systems are catalysed by enzymes, and nearly all enzymes are proteins. Many small molecules are transported and stored through specific proteins. Proteins are the major component of muscle. They are important in mechanical support (collagen), in immune protection (antibodies), nerve impulse transmission (receptors) and in control of growth and differentiation (growth factors, DNA control proteins and others). A protein is built from a set of 20 amino acids. It is characterized by an amino- and a carboxyl-group and twenty side-chains, varying in size, shape, charge, hydrogen-bonding capacity and chemical reactivity. Polypeptide chains (proteins) are formed by linking amino acids through peptide bonds. The rate of protein synthesis depends on processes that are subject to complex regulations. Genes specify the unique amino acid sequence of proteins. Cells regulate which specific proteins are synthesized and also the total amount of protein synthesis. (Kanwar *et al.*, 2011; Mankoff *et al.*, 2008; Badgaiyan, 2011; Nil *et al.*, 2011).

Radiolabelled Amino Acids

Malignant transformation increases the use of amino acids for energy, protein synthesis, and cell division. Tumour cells often over-express transporter systems resulting in an overall increase in AA transport and /or an increase in protein synthesis rate by tumour cells. Carboxyl-^{11}C-L-leucine, ^{11}C-L-methionine, and ^{11}C-L-tyrosine were introduced as tumour-imaging agents for the estimation of protein synthesis approximately 30 years ago. ^{18}F-labeled tracers developed are based on tyrosine and phenylalanine AAs. The tumour uptake of the ^{18}F-labeled AAs is related to carrier-mediated active transport, and not to protein synthesis. ^{11}C-methionine is an amino-acid analogue. It has been found useful in low-grade glioblastoma, glioblastoma (mild uptake), and meningioma (high uptake). More recently, artificial amino acids such as L-3-^{123}I-iodo-alpha-methyl-tyrosine (IMT) or L-3-^{18}F-fluoro-alpha-methyl-tyrosine (FMT), O-2-^{18}F-fluoroethyl-L-tyrosine (FET), ^{18}F-fluoro-L-phenylalanine, ^{18}F-fluoro-L-proline and ^{11}C-methyl- alpha-aminoisobutyric acid have been studied.

Radiolabelled Peptides

Peptides have many key properties including fast clearance, rapid tissue penetration, and low antigenicity, and can be produced easily and inexpensively. However, there may be problems with in vivo catabolism, unwanted physiologic effects, and chelate attachment.

Somatostatin Receptor Analogues

The Somatostatin receptor (SSR) analogues have made their greatest impact in the management of neuro-endocrine malignancies. The hypothalamus, adrenals and the pancreas produce somatostatin, a cyclic tetradecapeptide (SST-14) and the congener SST-28. Somatostatin modulates neurotransmission in the central nervous system (as a neurotransmitter) and regulates the release of growth hormones and thyrotropin (as a neurohormone). It also has a regulatory role in the gastrointestinal tract, as well as in the exocrine and endocrine pancreas. The actions of SST are mediated through specific membrane receptors. These receptors are expressed in various organs and tissues such as the pituitary, the pancreas and cells of the immune system. To date five subtypes of human somatostatin receptors (SSTR1-5) have been cloned and characterized. The expression of high-affinity and -density SSTRs by certain class of neuroendocrine cancers made it attractive to use radionuclide-imaging techniques to detect, stage and diagnose these cancers and their distal metastases. SSTR are also expressed in renal cell carcinoma, small cell lung cancer, breast cancer, prostate cancer and malignant lymphoma.

[123]I-Tyr3-octreotide was the first radiopeptide SSTR tracer for which proof of principle was obtained. ^{111}In-DTPA-(D)Phe-1-octreotide is the commercially available radiopeptide SSTR tracer of choice for the detection and follow-up of neuroendocrine tumours (OctreoScan®, Tyco). It can be conveniently prepared using a kit. ^{111}In-DOTA-lanreotide is synthesized using the commercially available lanreotide (Somatuline ®) and 1,4,7,10-tetraazacyclo-dodecane-N,N′,N′′,N′′′-tetraacetic acid (DOTA) as starting materials. It is the most successful radiopeptide for tumour imaging. The use of OctreoScan as such analogue is being replaced with new peptides such as DOTATATE (DOTA-D-Phe^1-Tyr^3-Thr^8-octreotide) and DOTATOC (DOTA-Phe^1-Tyr^3-octreotide).

[99m]Tc-depreotide (NeoTect) is an SSTR receptor based radiopharmaceutical which, in contrast to octreotide based ligands, also binds to SSTR3 with high affinity. It is available from GE-Amersham in Europe and Schering in the USA. (NeoTect). It has a high sensitivity and specificity for lung cancer lesion detection.

[68]Ga is available from an in-house generator rendering ^{68}Ga radiopharmacy independent of an on-site cyclotron. [68]Ga has a half-life of 68 min and decays by 89% through positron emission. The parent, [68]Ge, is accelerator produced and decays with a half-life of 270.8 d by electron capture. Radiopeptides for ^{68}Ga labelling have been developed and tested preclinically for the targeting of somatostatin receptors, the melanocortin-1 receptor, and the bombesin receptor. The most valuable role of ^{68}Ga PET is in SSTR imaging. ^{68}Ga-DOTATOC and ^{68}Ga-DOTANOC ([68]Ga-[DOTA]-1-Nal[3]-octreotide) are the most prominent radiopharmaceuticals used currently. Clinical studies demonstrated higher sensitivity localizing neuroendocrine tumours with ^{68}Ga-DOTATOC compared to ^{111}In-Octreotide, ^{111}In-DTPA Octreotide and ^{18}F-FDG. The 2010 EANM 'Procedural guideline for PET/CT Tumour Imaging with ^{68}Ga-DOTA conjugated peptides: ^{68}Ga-DOTA-TOC, ^{68}Ga-DOTA-NOC, ^{68}Ga-DOTA-TATE,' stated the primary indication of ^{68}Ga-DOTA-conjugate peptides PET/CT is the imaging of NETs, which usually express high density of SST receptors. Less frequently it can be used in non-NET imaging, particularly if treatment with radio-labeled therapeutic SST analogues is considered. Currently available PET tracers are ^{68}Ga and ^{18}F somatostatin analogues and ^{64}Cu TETA-Octreotide. Oncological applications include identifying/localizing neuroendocrine tumours, evaluating disease extent, monitoring effects of therapy, selecting patients for therapy, prognostic indicator.(Laverman et al., 2012; Gnanasegaran et al., 2005; Baum et al., 2008; Baum et al., 2005; Rufini et al., 2006).

Radiolabelled peptide therapy is usually indicated for patients with widespread disease that is not amenable to focused radiation therapy or is refractory to chemotherapy. Radiolabelled peptides such as ^{111}In-pentetreotide, ^{90}Y-DOTA-Phe1-Tyr3-octreotide, ^{90}Y-DOTA-lanreotide, and ^{177}Lu-DOTA-octreotate are indicated for the treatment of patients with neuroendocrine malignancy. (Kam et al., 2012; Turaga &kvols, 2011).

Dopamine

Neuroendocrine tumours (NETs, APUDomas) can be small and situated almost throughout the body. This heterogeneous group of tumours take up amino acids, transform them into biogenic amines (dopamine and serotonin) by decarboxylation, and store the amines in vesicles; this is the so-called APUD (amino precursor uptake and decarboxylation) concept. L-Dihydroxyphenylalanine (L-DOPA) is a precursor of catecholamine's (dopamine, noradrenalin and adrenalin). Its conversion to dopamine is catalysed by the aromatic amino acid decarboxylase (AADC). Pancreatic islet cells take up L-DOPA where AADC converts it to dopamine. Ahlström et al. (1995) were the first to visualize pancreatic NETs with ^{11}C–L-dihydroxyphenylalanine (^{11}C-LDOPA) PET, and the same group in 1996 also demonstrated that the in vivo uptake was due to decarboxylation.

3,4-dihydroxy-6-^{18}F-fluoro-L-phenylalanine (^{18}F-FDOPA) was developed to examine the transport of dopamine precursor from the plasma (Seibyl et al., 2007). FDOPA in oncology has been proposed to evaluate melanomas, neuroendocrine tumours, medullary thyroid carcinoma, pheocromocytomas, gastro-intesitinal carcinoid tumours, brain tumours; mostly metastatic tumours and malignant gliomas superior in evaluating recurrent low-grade and high-grade gliomas. Tumor uptake of ^{18}F-FDOPA has been reported to be similar to that of 11C-methionine. ^{18}F-FDOPA accumulation is very high in the kidneys and urinary bladder which may be a problem in studying the tail of the pancreas (Fouge et al., 2011).

Jora, et al., did a comparative evaluation of ^{18}F-FDOPA, ^{13}N-AMMONIA, ^{18}F-FDG PET/CT and MRI in primary brain tumours and found ^{18}F-FDG uptake correlated with tumor grade (Jora et al., 2011). Although ^{18}F-FDOPA PET could not distinguish between tumor grades, it is more reliable than ^{18}F-FDG and ^{13}N-Ammonia PET for evaluating brain tumors. ^{18}F-FDOPA PET may prove to be superior to MRI in evaluating recurrence and residual tumor tissue. ^{13}N-Ammonia PET did not show any encouraging results (Oikonen, 2005).

Tumour Specific Receptors

Tumour receptors have been some of the earliest targets for cancer therapy, with notable successes in the treatment of endocrine-related cancers such as breast, prostate, and thyroid cancers. Advances in molecular cancer biology have revealed an ever-increasing number of tumour targets, many of which are receptors, such as the epidermal growth factor (EGF) receptor (EGFR). The ability to measure the expression of tumour receptors is essential for selecting patients for receptor-targeted therapy. Tumour receptor imaging emphasizes important emerging themes in molecular imaging: characterizing tumour biology, identifying therapeutic targets, and delineating the pharmacodynamics of targeted cancer therapy. The advantages of imaging include non-invasiveness, the ability to measure receptor expression for the entire disease burden and thereby to avoid the sampling error that can occur with heterogeneous receptor expression, and the potential for serial studies of the in vivo effects of a drug on the target. The estrogen receptor (ER) system is an illustrative example of a receptor system with relevance to cancer. (Mankoff *et al.*, 2008).

Flourine-^{18}-flouro-17-β-estradiol (FES)

Estradiol is the most potent form of estrogen in the body and binds to ERs. It is found in the cell nucleus of the female reproductive tract, breast, pituitary, hypothalamus, bone, liver, and also in various tissues in men. Estradiol is a naturally occurring agonist ligand for the ER. The molecular mechanism of estradiol action through the ER has been well studied. Estradiol is lipophilic, allowing access across cell membranes to the ER, a nuclear receptor. The ER has 2 receptor subtypes: ER-a and ER-b. ER-a serves mainly as an activator of downstream events related to breast and female sex organ function. The function of ER-b is less well understood; in some situations, ER-b may inhibit ER-a by forming a heterodimer with ER-a. Estradiol binding to ER-a in the nucleus results in dimerization of the receptor and allows interactions with specific DNA sequences known as the estrogen response elements, leading to the selective regulation of target gene transcription.

ER activation leads to different physiologic actions in different tissues. The ER Status: the growth of breast epithelial cells depends on estrogen acting through an ER and the induction of progesterone receptor. The ER status is an important prognostic factor in breast cancer. ER tumours have a slower rate of growth and a better response to hormonal therapy.

Despite the importance of tumour receptors in carcinogenesis and tumour growth, tumour receptors are not always effective targets for cancer treatment, because some cancers can sustain growth independently of receptor activation. In some situations, growth independence is accompanied by a loss of or a reduction in receptor expression, such as in ER negative (ER-) breast cancers. In such situations, the absence of receptor expression indicates a negligible chance of success of receptor-targeted therapy. In other situations, even though a receptor is still present, receptor pathway activation is not required for growth. In 30 to 40% of all breast cancers there is no estrogen receptors expression (ER-). Although 70% of breast cancers express the ER, only 50%–75% of ER-expressing primary breast cancers respond to endocrine therapy, and even fewer recurrent tumours respond. A non-invasive method to evaluate and quantify the presence of ER on the tumour and its metastases would better select patients for treatment, and predict the therapeutic response. The radiolabeled estrogen analogue identified is 16-^{18}F-fluoro-17-estradiol (FES) and has shown the most promise in quantifying the functional ER status of breast cancer, both in the primary tumour and in metastatic sites. ^{18}F-flourotamoxifen is still being investigated (Mankoff *et al.*, 2008).

Flourine ^{18}-Flouro- dihydrotestosterone

Androgen receptors play an important role in growth and proliferation of prostate cancer. The androgen status is a prognostic indicator. Dihydrotestosterone is the primary ligand for androgen receptors. Anti-androgen is one of the most effective treatments in the management of prostate cancer. Flourine-18-flouro-dihydrotestosterone (FDHT) is useful in monitoring treatment response. Androgen resistance of the lesion is shown by a negative FDHT scan and positive FDG scan. (Mankoff *et al.*, 2008).

Radioimmunoscintigraphy

Radioimmunodetection or radioimmunoscintigraphy uses tumour targeting antibodies or antibody fragments, labelled with a radionuclide suitable for external imaging, for the detection of specific cancers. Monoclonal antibodies have been developed against a variety of antigens associated with tumours and have been shown to target tumours with minimal side effects. Numerous radionuclides suitable for external imaging have been conjugated to antibodies, or antibody fragments, and the radioimmuno-conjugates have been shown to be stable in vivo. Several factors have accelerated the expansion of the role of antibodies in cancer imaging. It is the identification of cell surface biomarkers as imaging targets coupled with advances in antibody technology, which facilitate the generation of antibodies optimized for non-invasive imaging.

Radioimmunoscintigraphy has been shown to be of benefit in the detection of occult disease, in the management of patients with potentially resectable disease, and for the evaluation of lesion recurrence and therapeutic response. Radiolabelled antibody imaging in prostate cancer has been shown to be useful in risk stratification and in patient selection for loco-regional therapy. Antibody imaging can provide a sensitive, non-invasive means for molecular characterization of cell surface phenotype in vivo, which can in turn guide diagnosis, prognosis, therapy selection, and monitoring of treatment in cancer (Artiko *et al.*, 2011).

The clinical value of PET and immunoscintigraphy with ^{131}I or ^{111}In anti- CEA mAb for diagnosis of recurrent colorectal cancer has been confirmed by Ito *et al.*, who have concluded that PET/CT reflects more accurately the biological character of tumours, but cannot provide the specificity of immunoscintigraphy that enables us to distinguish patients for antibody-based therapy. The superior value of PET with FDG for detection of distant metastases (liver, bone, and lung) and lymph node involvement has been estimated in comparison to ^{99m}Tc-anti-CEA Fab for detection of recurrence of colorectal carcinoma. Immunoscintigraphy is superior for detection of local recurrent colorectal cancer, whereas PET is better for detection of distal metastases. Radioimmunoguided surgery (RIGS) enables intraoperative detection of small tumour deposits using special gamma probe systems, after intravenous administration of radiopharmaceuticals. Roveda *et al* have performed immunoscintigraphy with ^{131}I or ^{111}In anti-CEA and 19.9 mAb using a gamma probe, and have found it particularly useful for endoscopic study of the pelvis after anterior resection, which is difficult to achieve by other diagnostic procedures. Both immunoscintigraphy and RIGS enable a more accurate diagnosis according to Hladic *et al.* Florio *et al* have found positive intraoperative gamma probe detection, although negative for immunoscintigraphy. RIGS applied in primary colorectal cancer enables the detection of occult lymph node metastases. Imaging methods (CT, US, MRI) have an advantage for detection of liver metastases, whereas immunoscinitgraphy is more specific for the assessment of recurrence of abdominal tumours. Immunoscintigraphy may be applied in patients with suspected local recurrence and inconclusive results of routine diagnostic workup (Boermen &Oyen, 2011; Heine *et al.*, 2011).

Attention has also been given to PET specific tracers. [64]Cu anti-GD2 monoclonal antibody (mAb) target antigens overexpressed on neuroblastoma and melanoma. [124]I-, [64]Cu-, [86]Y-Labeled Antibodies are being studied with specific binding to tumour associated antigenic binding sites (such as CEA, PSMA, CD20 and CD22).

Radioimmunotherapy (RIT) is a treatment modality, which uses radiolabelled antibodies in the therapy of cancer. Monoclonal antibodies against a variety of tumour associated antigens have been developed and shown to target tumours with minimal side effects. Numerous radionuclides have been conjugated to antibodies and the radioimmunoconjugates have been shown to be stable in vivo. RIT for relapsed or refractory CD20-positive B-cell NHL means intravenous administration of ^{90}Y-labelled ibritumomab tiuxetan (Zevalin®) (Dillman, 2006). [90]Y(III)chloride is produced through decay of the radioactive precursor nuclide 90 Strontium (^{90}Sr). The decay of ^{90}Y is accompanied by the release of beta radiation with a maximum energy of 2.281 MeV (99.98%) into stable 90 Zirconium ([90]Zr), with a half-life of 64 h (2.7 d). Ibritumomab tiuxetan is a conjugated murine anti-CD20 antibody genetically engineered from Chinese hamster ovary (CHO) line using the MX-DTPA chelating agent. The ibritumomab tiuxetan antibody targets the CD20 antigen, which is expressed on the surface of normal (except for pre-B cells and secretory B cells) and malignant B lymphocytes.

Iodine (^{123}I/^{131}I) labelled Metaiodobenzylguanidine (MIBG)

MIBG is the combination of the benzyl group of bretylium and the guanidine group of guanethidine. It was developed in the early 1980s to visualise tumours of the adrenal medulla. MIBG structurally resembles norepinephrine. It enters neuroendocrine cells by an active uptake mechanism and is stored in the neurosecretory granules. [123]I/^{131}I-MIBG is used to image tumours of neuroendocrine origin, particularly those of the sympathoadrenal system (phaeochromocytomas, paragangliomas and neuroblastomas). Subsequent uptake in other neuroendocrine tumours (mostly carcinoids and medullary thyroid carcinoma) has also been reported. [123]I/^{131}I-MIBG has also been employed to study disorders of sympathetic innervation, such as that of the heart. MIBG can be labelled with either ^{131}I or [123]I. Theoretical considerations and clinical experience indicate that the ^{123}I-labelled agent is to be considered the radiopharmaceutical of choice, at least in children, as it has a more favourable dosimetry and provides better image quality. Nonetheless, ^{131}I-MIBG is widely employed for most routine applications mainly in adult patients because of its lower costs, its ready availability, longer half-life and the possibility of obtaining delayed images. It is an acceptable choice also in children especially when acquisitions are to be repeated over time. Paraganglioma, malignant paraganglioma, ganglioblastoma and neuroblastoma may all be detected with ^{123}I or ^{131}I-MIBG. Thyroid blockade with potassium iodide, lugol's iodine and perchlorate is indicated to limit the dosimetry of free iodine. The clinical indications for includes the localization of adrenal pheochromocytomas and extra-adrenal paragangliomas; the localization of metastatic adrenal medullary cancer secondary to pheochromocytoma; prior to ablation therapy of metastatic adrenal medullary cancer secondary to pheochromocytoma; the evaluation of patients with suspected neuroblastomas; the evaluation of patients with carcinoid and medullary thyroid cancer to determine if ^{131}I-MIBG therapy would be of benefit. (SNM Procedure guidelines; EANM Procedure guidelines)

Gene Expression

Differential expression between disease subgroups has been primarily seen in mitochondrial-, structural-, and transcription-related genes (Sanoudou *et al.*, 2004). 9-(4-18F-Fluoro-3-[hydroxymethyl]butyl)guanine (^{18}F-FHBG) is sensitive and specific for imaging the genes, herpes simplex 1 thymidine kinase (HSV1-tk) and its mutant HSV1-sr39tk. These genes have been demonstrated in the livers of hepatocellular cancer patients. Studies are being done on ^{68}Ga-labeled oligonucleotides target activated human K-ras oncogene.

Oncolytic adenoviruses can be engineered for better tumour selectivity, gene delivery and be armed for imaging and concentrating radionuclides into tumours for synergistic oncolysis (Gambhir *et al.*, 1999). Temporal and spatial changes in hNIS-expression during therapy were detected with SPECT, have demonstrated feasibility of evaluation of the combination therapy with hNIS-expressing adenoviruses and radioiodide (Fujiwara, 2011).

2.1.5. Iodine Metabolism

Iodine is an essential element which is used in the synthesis of thyroid hormone. Differentiated thyroid cancer (DTC) is among the most curable of cancers yet the presence of incidental thyroid micrometastases (diameter 1 cm or smaller) is 5% to 36% of autopsied adults. The management of DTC is one of the more debated topics in clinical medicine. Significant developments in monitoring and treatment during the past decade have changed many of the traditional approaches to the patient with DTC, some of which remain controversial. The most effective nonsurgical treatment and imaging for differentiated thyroid carcinoma is radioactive iodine (RAI). Radioiodine has 3 main indications in the postoperative management of patients with thyroid cancer: ablation of residual thyroid tissue with ^{131}I, imaging for possible recurrent disease with ^{123}I or ^{131}I, and treatment of residual or recurrent thyroid cancer with [131]I. The aim in therapy is to destroy any microscopic foci of disease remaining after the surgery and to destroy any remaining normal thyroid tissue to improve the value of serum Thyroglobulin (Tg) as a tumour marker. If all normal thyroid cells are eliminated by RAI, then any increase in serum Tg in the follow-up of these patients becomes more specific and indicates recurrence of thyroid cancer, and this also increases the specificity of ^{131}I scanning for detection of recurrent or metastatic disease by eliminating uptake by residual normal tissue (LiVolsi, 2011; McHenry & Phitayakorn, 2011). The use of [124]I in PET is currently investigational and limited to institutional clinical use.

According to the American Thyroid Association (ATA) revised guidelines (2009) (Cooper *et al.*, 2009), risk groups of patients may be classified into low-, intermediate- and high- risk. Low-risk patients have no local or distant metastases; all macroscopic tumour has been resected; there is no tumour invasion of locoregional tissues or structures; the tumour does not have aggressive histology (e.g., tall cell, insular, columnar cell carcinoma) or vascular invasion; and, if ^{131}I is given, there is no ^{131}I uptake outside the thyroid bed on the first post-treatment whole-body RAI scan (RxWBS). Intermediate-risk patients have microscopic invasion of tumour into the perithyroidal soft tissues at initial surgery; presence of cervical lymph node metastases or ^{131}I uptake outside the thyroid bed on the RxWBS done after thyroid remnant ablation; or tumour with aggressive histology or vascular invasion. High-risk patients have macroscopic tumour invasion, incomplete tumour resection, distant metastases, and may present with a thyroglobulinemia out of proportion to what is seen on the RxWBS.

The literature supports the use of [18]FDG-PET scanning for indications beyond simple disease localization in Tg-positive, RAI scan–negative patients. Current additional clinical uses of [18]FDG-PET scanning may include initial staging and follow-up of high-risk patients with poorly differentiated thyroid cancers unlikely to concentrate RAI in order to identify sites of disease that may be missed with RAI scanning and conventional imaging (Sandu etal, 2011). It has also been used for the initial staging and follow-up of invasive or metastatic Hurthle cell carcinoma.

2.2. Angiogenesis

Malignant tumours are characterised by the development of chaotic and leaky blood vessels a disturbed microcirculation, low oxygen tension, high interstitial pressure and ultimately insufficient delivery of chemotherapy. Many different features of vascularity permit the distinction between malignant and benign processes, some of which can be interrogated by imaging techniques. Structural and functional characteristics of malignant tumour vasculature include: spatial heterogeneity and chaotic structure; poorly formed, fragile vessels with high permeability to macromolecules; arteriovenous shunting, high vascular tortuosity and vasodilatation; intermittent or unstable blood flow due to transient rises in already raised interstitial pressure; extreme heterogeneity of vascular density with areas of low vascular density mixed with regions of high angiogenic activity. Studies have shown that monitoring tumour angiogenesis has prognostic value.

Angiogenesis is linked to an increased risk of local regional recurrence, distant metastases, and reduced survival in patients with cancers at various organs, including breast, lung, and ovary. A large number of local and circulating angiogenic factors are known to be involved in the angiogenic process, including vascular endothelial growth factor (VEGF), angiopoietins, and basic fibroblast growth factor (bFGF). These molecular processes are being currently studied by many investigators as potential targets for the development of angiogenesis imaging and for the development of novel radiotracers to evaluate both tumour angiogenesis and tumour response to various anti-angiogenesis drugs (Jeswani & Padhani, 2005; Missbach-Guentner *et al.*, 2011; Choe & Lee, 2077; Jansen *et al.*, 2010; Zhu *et al.*, 2010).

2.2.1. Vascular Endothelial Growth Factor and its Receptors (VEGF/VEGFRs)

VEGF is an important angiogenic factor induced by local hypoxia. VEGF induces various functions on endothelial cells by interacting with high affinity tyrosine kinase receptors. VEGF and VEGF receptors (VEGFR) are therefore considered potential targets for angiogenesis imaging. Both SPECT and PET imaging have been performed with radiolabeled anti-VEGF antibodies.

The more rational design is to use radiolabeled VEGF isoforms for SPECT or PET imaging of VEGFR expression. With SPECT imaging, recombinant human VEGF121 was labelled with ^{111}In and ^{99m}Tc through an "Adapter/Docking" strategy. VEGF121 has also been labelled with ^{64}Cu for PET imaging of tumour angiogenesis and VEGFR expression. Micro-PET imaging revealed the dynamic nature of VEGFR expression during tumour progression in that even for the same tumour model, VEGFR expression level can be dramatically different at different stages. The uptake of ^{64}Cu-DOTA-VEGF121 in the tumour peaked when the tumour size was about 100–250 mm^3.

Peptidic VEGFR antagonists can be labelled with short-lived isotopes such as ^{18}F. Labelling has also been reported with ^{188}Re for SPECT imaging of VEGFR in tumour-bearing nude mice. Planar imaging with SPECT demonstrated significant radioactivity accumulation in tumour 1 h after injection of the labelled peptide and disappearance of radioactivity 3 h later, facilitating repetitive imaging with the peptide for therapy response monitoring (Backer & Backer, 2012).

2.2.2   Integrins

Integrins are a family of receptors comprised of a family of heterodimeric glycoproteins, which are involved in the formation of new blood vessels in tumours. Integrins expressed on endothelial cells are related to cell survival and migration during angiogenesis, while integrins expressed on carcinoma cells modulate metastasis by facilitating invasion and movement across the vessels. The integrin member, which binds to arginine-glycine-aspartic acid (RGD)-containing components of the interstitial matrix such as vitronectin, fibronectin and thrombospondin, is expressed in a number of tumour types such as melanoma, late stage glioblastoma, ovarian, breast, and prostate cancer. Integrin ąvß3 promotes angiogenesis and endothelial cell survival and that antagonism of this integrin suppresses angiogenesis by inducing endothelial cell apoptosis in vitro and in vivo. Integrins are ideal pharmacological targets based on both the key role they played in angiogenesis, leukocytes function and tumour development and easy accessibility as cell surface receptors interacting with extracellular ligands.

^{18}F arginine-glycine-aspartic acid (RGD) peptide binds specifically to ąvß3 intergrins expressed at the surface of activated endothelial cells during angiogenesis. The (RGD) cell adhesion motif was discovered in fibronectin by Pierschbacher and Ruoslahti 20 years ago. This integrin is expressed on the luminal surface of neovasculature but is not found on the endothelial surface of mature capillaries. In addition it has been shown to be upregulated in tumour blood vessels that undergo continuous angiogenesis and has been implicated in metastasis. Synthetic RGD peptide antagonists were subsequently shown to inhibit growth of neovasculature and effect tumour regression in animal models, presumably by starving tumours of their blood supply. ^{18}F-Galacto-RGD has been developed for PET imaging of ąvß3 expression of a receptor involved in angiogenesis and metastases. Beer *et al* tested and established the feasibility of using this tracer in eleven patients with Head and neck squamous cell carcinoma (HNSCC). An important application of this new radiotracer would be in monitoring treatment response of anti-angiogenic therapy (Lewis, 2005).

A variety of radiometalated tracers have been developed as well, including peptides labelled with ^{111}In, ^{99m}Tc, ^{64}Cu, ^{90}Y, ^{188}Re, ^{89}Zr and ^{68}Ga. Most of them are based on the cyclic pentapeptide c(RGDfK) or c(RGDyK) and are conjugated via the ã-amino function of a lysine with different chelator systems, like diethylene triamine pentaacetic acid (DTPA), the tetrapeptide sequence H-Asp-Lys-Cys-Lys-OH, 1,4,7,10-tetraazacyclododecane-1,4,7,10-tetraacetic acid (DOTA) and 1,4,7-triazacyclononane-1,4,7-triacetic acid (NOTA). While all these compounds have shown high receptor affinity and selectivity and specific tumour accumulation, the pharmacokinetics of most of them still need to be improved (Shan, 2013; Zhanga *et al.*, 2011).

There are several issues and limitations regarding imaging of Integrins. Integrins are not only overexpressed on tumour endothelial cells but also on tumour cells. There is also heterogeneity of integrin expression between different tumours or even within the same tumour itself. In addition, tumour uptake and accumulation of imaging tracers is not only dependent on the receptor expression. Several other factors including vascular density and volume, vascular permeability and interstitial fluid pressure also affect the distribution (Haubner *et al.*, 1999).

2.2.3   Matrix metalloproteinases (MMPs)

MMPs are a family of zinc- and calcium-dependent endopeptidases which are responsible for the enzymatic degradation of connective tissue, and thus facilitate endothelial cell migration during angiogenesis. MMPs play an important role in new blood vessel formation. The MMP specific tracers have been labelled with several radionuclides such as ^{99m}Tc, ^{111}In and ^{64}Cu and are still currently under investigation. Significant improvements in tumour MMP targeting and in vivo pharmacokinetics are necessary before the use of MMP radiotracer imaging can be translated into clinical application.

2.2.4. Other Angiogenesis Imaging Targets

The angiogenic response is also modulated by the composition of the extracellular matrix (ECM) and intercellular adhesions, because endothelial cells must adhere to one another and to the ECM in order to construct new microvessels. Fibronectin and vitronectin recruited from plasma also play a key role in ECM remodelling during tumour growth and angiogenesis.

Fibronectin is a large glycoprotein and can be found physiologically in plasma and tissues. Extra-domain B of fibronectin (EDB), consisting of 91 amino acids, is not present in the fibronectin molecule under normal conditions, but expressed in the endometrium in the proliferative phase and some vessels of the ovaries. It is an angiogenesis marker in a variety of solid tumours.

A human antibody fragment scFv (L19) was identified and has been shown to efficiently localize on neovasculature in vivo. The L19 small immunoprotein (SIP) was labelled with ^{76}Br and ^{124}I for PET imaging.

Endoglin (CD105) is a cell membrane glycoprotein mainly expressed on endothelial cells and overexpressed on tumour vasculature. ^{111}In-labeled E-selectin antibody was used for imaging of inflamed human synovial vasculature. Other angiogenesis-related biomarkers, such as angiopoietins/Tie receptors, and CD276 are also potential targets for angiogenesis imaging.

2.3. Hypoxia

Increasing tumour size results in a reduced ability of the local vasculature to supply sufficient oxygen to rapidly dividing tumour cells. To identify and to quantify blood flow and tissue perfusion in tumours or to monitor response to chemotherapy later on, ^{15}O-labeled water was one of the first approved radiolabeled tracers in cancer patients (Wilson *et al.*, 1992; Tseng *et al.*, 2004). In these studies only functional changes due to alterations of volume distribution of radiolabeled water within the tumour tissue could be determined. Resulting hypoxia may inhibit new cell division or lead to cell death may also lead to activation of certain processes that will help cells survive and progress.

Well-oxygenated cells are more sensitive to the cytotoxic effects of ionizing radiation compared with poorly oxygenated cells. Hypoxia in tumour tissue is an important prognostic indicator of response to therapy. 2-Nitroimidazole (azomycin) was developed in the 1950s as an antibiotic targeted against anaerobic germs. It was only in 1979 that Chapman and coworkers proposed nitroimidazoles as markers of hypoxia and as a sensitizing factor for radiation therapy of hypoxic tumours. Hypoxic cell radiosensitizers (possessing a selective toxicity for the radioresistant hypoxic cells) tested in clinical trials included metronidazole, misonidazole, nimorazole, and tirapazamine.

Although SPECT is more commonly used than PET, and, in particular, ^{99m}Tc has a number of practical advantages that include ready availability at low cost, convenient half-life for hypoxia measurements and versatile chemistry as compared with ^{18}F, the superior spatial resolution and more accurate quantitation with PET makes the latter a better candidate for detection of tumoural hypoxia. Of all the PET tracers that are being evaluated as possible markers of tumour hypoxia, only three have been thoroughly evaluated in a clinical situation: ^{18}F-FMISO, ^{18}F-FDG and ^{64}Cu-ATSM (Mees *et al.*, 2009; Jordan &Sonveaux, 2012).

2.3.1. Iodine derivatives

^{123}I-IAZA and ^{125}I-IAZA (^{123}I/ ^{125}I-iodoazomycin arabinoside) have been used for studying tumour hypoxia. A study investigating the use of ^{123}I-IAZA in 51 human patients with newly diagnosed malignancies demonstrated hypoxia in small cell lung cancer and squamous cell carcinoma of head and neck but not in malignant gliomas. The study did, however, demonstrate the feasibility of ^{123}I-IAZA imaging in a clinical setting. Stypinski *et al.* reported the clinical pharmacokinetics of IAZA, the radiopharmacokinetics of ^{123}I-IAZA, total radioactivity kinetics and the radiation dosimetry estimates for six healthy volunteers and concluded that all supported its clinical use for imaging tissue hypoxia. Newer agents based on the azomycin-nucleoside structure such as iodoazomycin galactoside (IAZG), iodoazomycin pyranoside (IAZP), IAZGP and iodoazomycin xylopyranoside (IAZXP) have been developed and are being evaluated.

2.3.2. Technetium derivatives

BMS 181321 was the first ^{99m}Tc-labelled 2-nitroimidazole to be widely studied for imaging but was found not optimal for tumour hypoxia imaging because of in vitro and in vivo instabilities and high background levels in normal tissues. The nitro group of 2-nitroimidazole (NIM) enters the tumour cells and is bioreductively activated and fixed in the hypoxia cells. BRU59-21 is a second-generation analogue of BMS 181321 which shows greater stability in vitro and better characteristics. In a study by Zhang *et al.*, BRU59-21 and HL91 were compared directly in the same in vitro systems. Both tracers proved suitable for hypoxia imaging. Zhang *et al.* evaluated the efficacy of [^{99m}Tc]butylene amineoxime (^{99m}Tc-HL91) as a non-invasive marker of tumour hypoxia. Yutani *et al.* found that ^{99m}Tc-HL91 accumulated to significantly higher levels in hypoxic tumour areas and that ^{99m}Tc-HL91 uptake was strongly correlated with the expression of GLUT1 in the viable cancer cell area. Clinical studies concerning the clinical evaluation of ^{99m}Tc-HL91 are limited, however those done have demonstrated that ^{99m}Tc-HL91 is a safe radioligand and that metabolic binding in a large fraction but not all of local squamous cell carcinoma in Head and Neck tumour recurrences may be expected. In a study with 32 patients with non-small cell lung cancer, Li *et al.* showed that hypoxia imaging with ^{99m}Tc-HL91 before radiotherapy may predict tumour response and patient survival.

[99m]Tc-cyclam-2-nitroimidazole (^{99m}Tc-N4-NIM) has recently been developed for tumour hypoxia imaging. Planar imaging studies confirmed that the tumours could be visualized clearly with ^{99m}Tc-N4-NIM in animal models. Efficient synthesis of N4-NIM was achieved. ^{99m}Tc-N4-NIM may be useful in evaluating cancer therapy (Ali *et al.*, 2012).

2.3.3. [18]F derivatives

In 1984, ^{18}F-Fluoromisonidazole (FMISO) was introduced as a tracer for determining tumour hypoxia. It binds selectively to hypoxic cells. FMISO diffuses into cells, where it is reduced by enzymes. In necrotic cells, there is no reduction; therefore, no retention occurs. In normoxic cells, the FMISO is reoxidized and eventually diffuses out of the metabolic compartment. In hypoxic cells, further reduction of the FMISO results in cell retention. (Lee & Scott, 2007).

Its high lipophilicity, and slow clearance kinetics, necessitates imaging for longer periods of time post injection. It has been used to evaluate high grade gliomas, renal cell carcinoma low grade uptake, non-small cell lung carcinoma low uptake, and is widely used in head and neck tumours. Studies using FMISO have demonstrated variable, but significant levels of hypoxia in several tumour types. In addition,

FMISO PET imaging has been used as a prognostic indicator in several other studies. It has, however, failed to gain wider acceptance for routine clinical application because of a number of limitations such as: slow accumulation in hypoxic tumours; a low target to background ratio due to high non-specific binding resulting from its relatively high lipophilicity; and significant non-oxygen dependent metabolism leading to a considerable amount of radioactive metabolite products. ^{18}F-fluoroerythronitroimidazole (FETNIM), ^{18}F-fluoroetanidazole (FETA), and 1-(5-^{18}F-Fluoro-5-deoxy--D-arabinofuranosyl)-2-nitroimidazole (FAZA) have been developed with more favorable pharmacokinetics.

Several studies have tried to validate ^{18}F-FDG as an alternative marker for hypoxia imaging. The rationale behind this is that ^{18}F-FDG uptake during FDG PET imaging relies largely on the expression of proteins that are under control of HIF-1. As a result, the degree of ^{18}F-FDG uptake by tumours might indirectly reflect the level of hypoxia. This would obviate the need for more specific radiopharmaceuticals for hypoxia imaging. Reports trying to relate ^{18}F-FDG uptake with tumour hypoxia have given inconsistent results.

2.3.4. Other Pet tracers

^{64}Copper-diacetyl-bis-N4-methylthiosemicarbazone ([^{64}Cu]-CuATSM) is a neutral and lipophilic Copper-2-bis (thiosemicarbizone) that has shown rapid diffusion into cells and has been shown in vitro to be highly selective for hypoxic tissue (Kersemans *et al.*, 2011).

2.4. Apoptosis

'Programmed cell death' is central to homoeostasis, normal development and physiology in all multicellular organisms. Dysregulation can lead to the destruction of normal tissues in a variety of disorders; too much apoptosis may result from autoimmune and neurodegenerative diseases; too little apoptosis will result in the growth of tumours. The morphologic changes of apoptosis are preceded by an initiation phase triggered by an array of signals, including a lack of needed growth factors, antihormonal therapy, DNA damage, immune reactions, ischemic injury, ionizing radiation, and chemotherapy. The lag time between exposure to the trigger and the development of observable morphologic signs of apoptosis varies greatly, depending on cell type, type of trigger, intensity and duration of exposure, and the local environmental conditions of the cell. Effective therapy of tumours requires the iatrogenic induction of programmed cell death by radiation, chemotherapy, or both.

A non-invasive imaging method to serially detect and monitor this process in cancer patients undergoing conventional radiation and chemotherapy treatments as well as for the development and testing of new drugs would be desirable. Currently we can classify most apoptosis imaging agents being investigated into 4 categories on the basis of the cellular processes they detect: plasma membrane phospholipid asymmetry and phosphatidylserine (PS) exposure; caspase activation; mitochondrial membrane potential collapse. PS exposure has received the most attention as an imaging target in apoptosis for several reasons: The exposure is a near-universal event in apoptosis it occurs within a few hours of the apoptotic stimulus and it presents a very abundant target (millions of binding sites per cell) that is readily accessible on the extracellular face of the plasma membrane. PS exposure may also be increased in non-apoptic cells lines; in mitogen or anti-body stimulated B and T lymphocytes, granulocytes, mast cells. PS exposure is preceded by cell shrinkage and increased lipid mobility which are both inhibited by blockers of volume regulatory K+ and Cl- ion channels. Balsubramian *et al.*, found that PS exposure requires the sustained elevation of cytosolic calcium, an event that can be inhibited by Ca^{2+} channel blockers.

Annexin-V

Uncategorized Annexin-V is a protein which binds to PS lipid residues on inner cell membrane. Annexin V also known as annexin A5 has a molecular weight 36,000. It is an endogenous human protein that is widely distributed intracellularly. Very high concentrations in the placenta and lower concentrations in endothelial cells, kidneys, myocardium, skeletal muscle, skin, red cells, platelets, and monocytes. It is the most widely used phosphatidylserine-directed agent. Studies have been done in Head and neck, breast, non-small cell lung carcinoma, melanoma, bladder carcinoma and lymphoma (Schaper &Reutelingsperger, 2013). Its advantages include a very high affinity for apoptotic cells, ready production by recombinant DNA technology, lack of in vivo toxicity of the protein. ^{99m}Tc-HYNIC-Annexin V is available for imaging and has been used to determine the efficacy of chemotherapy in oncology patients stage 3-4 imaging within 24 hours of commencing chemotherapy. ^{18}F Annexin has since been developed and is one potential imaging agent to visualise programmed cell death. ^{124}I Annexin and ^{64}Cu labelled Streptokinase are still under investigation for cancer use (Blackenberg & Norfray, 2011).

3   General Tumour Imaging Radiopharmaceuticals

3.1. Skeletal Scintigraphy

The normal bone undergoes constant remodelling. There is a balance maintained between osteoclastic (resorptive) and osteoblastic activity. In the pathogenesis of bone metastases (Fili *et al.*, 2009), several factors are released by tumour cells that stimulate both osteoclast and osteoblast activity. Excessive new bone formation occurs around tumour cell deposits, resulting in low bone strength and potential vertebral collapse. Osteoclastic and osteoblastic activity releases growth factors that stimulate tumour cell growth, perpetuating the cycle of bone resorption and abnormal bone growth (Coxon *et al.*, 2004).

Bone metastases are the most common malignant bone tumour (Mundy, 2002). Skeletal involvement occurs in 30%-70% of all cancer patients, with breast cancer being the leading cause for bone metastases in women and prostate cancer in men, followed by lung cancer. Detection of bone metastases is essential for optimal tumour therapy. A malignant lesion may be detected on a bone scan as early as a year prior to being detected on anatomical imaging. It has been estimated that up to 75% reduction in bone density is required to visualize a metastasis on x-ray.

The purpose of imaging is to identify bone metastases as early as possible, to determine the full extent of disease, to evaluate the presence of complications that may accompany malignant bone involvement (including pathologic fractures and spinal cord compression), to monitor response to therapy, and, occasionally, to guide biopsy if histological confirmation is indicated.

3.1.1. Methylene Diphosphonate (MDP)

^{99m}Tc-MDP is the common agent used for bone imaging. It is an organic analogue of pyrophosphate and contains an organic P-C-P bond. The agent affixes to the bone surface by the process of chemisorption attaching to hydroxyapatite crystals in bone and calcium crystals in mitochondria. After administration, it is postulated that ^{99m}Tc-MDP dissociates into its technetium and MDP moieties which are then adsorbed onto the organic and inorganic (hydroxyapatite) phases, respectively. About 40-50% of the compound will be affixed to bone by 3 to 4 hours after injection. The labelling efficiency for ^{99m}Tc-MDP is typically 95%. Excretion is primarily renal. Clinicians have described early detection of renal pathology seen on a bone scan. By 6 hours, approximately 70% of the administered dose is eliminated. Bone scanning with ^{99m}Tc-MDP detects abnormalities of bone metabolism as early as 24 to 48 hours after the onset of pathology and is nearly always positive by 8 days. Thus, fractures and other manifestations of bone stress can be diagnosed very sensitively by bone scintigraphy. The oncological indications for bone scintigraphy with MDP are for primary tumours (e.g. Ewing's sarcoma, osteosarcoma); staging, evaluation of response to therapy and follow-up of primary bone tumours, secondary tumours (metastases); staging and follow-up of neoplastic diseases, and the distribution of osteoblastic activity prior to radiometabolic therapy (such as ^{89}Sr, ^{153}Sm-EDTMP and ^{186}Re-HEDP). (SNM Procedure guidelines; BNMS Procedure guidelines; EANM Procedure guidelines).

3.1.2. ^{18}F-Fluoride (^{18}F)

^{18}F-Fluoride was introduced as a bone-imaging agent by Blau *et al.* in 1962. The FDA approved the New Drug Application (NDA) for bone imaging to define areas of altered osteogenic activity in 1972. Fluoride ions are chemisorbed onto bone surface by exchanging with hydroxyl (OH) groups in hydroxyapatite ($Ca^{10}(PO_4)^6(OH)^2$) crystal of bone to form flouroapatite. Uptake is related to blood flow and bone remodelling or turnover. The use of ^{18}F in hybrid PET/CT imaging has significantly improved the specificity, because the CT component of the study allows morphologic characterization of the functional lesion and more accurate differentiation between benign lesions and metastases. ^{18}F bone scans may be used to identify skeletal metastases, including localization and determination of the extent of disease. (SNM Procedure guidelines)

3.2.   Methoxy-isobutyl-isonitrile (MIBI)

^{99m}Tc labelled MIBI was first described in 1984, by Jones *et al.*, as a myocardial perfusion tracer. In 1990, Delmon-Moingeon *et al.*, described MIBI as an in vivo tumour imaging agent and was fortuitously observed to show uptake in tumours of the lung, thyroid, brain, lymph node metastasis, bone and in breast cancer. MIBI has found a role in breast scintigraphy in the following indications: detection of breast cancer when mammography is doubtful, inadequate or indeterminate; as a complementary procedure in patients with doubtful microcalcifications or parenchymal distortions; scar tissue in the breast following surgery or biopsy in mammographically dense breast tissue; breasts with implants; identifying multicentric, multifocal or bilateral breast cancer in patients with a diagnosis of breast cancer (Bombardieri *et al.*, 2003).

The cellular uptake of MIBI is due to passive influx of the lypophilic cation and is driven by the plasma and mitochondrial membrane potentials generated in living cells. MIBI non-specifically localizes in mitochondria and the cytoplasm in response to elevated membrane potentials across the membrane bilayers of the cell and mitochondria. MIBI has been reported to localize non-specifically in a variety of malignant and non-malignant tumours. Enhanced uptake of ^{99m}Tc MIBI in malignant tumours is thought to reflect the increased numbers of mitochondria in cancer cells. Although the exact uptake mechanisms into the myocardial and tumour cells are not well understood, it is postulated to be related to blood flow, blood residence time, and the cellular uptake due to passive influx of the lipophilic cation, driven by the plasma and mitochondrial membrane potentials generated in living cells. Elevated potentials are directly related to metabolic state. A modulatory factor for MIBI uptake may be associated with the overexpression of P-glycoprotein in tumours, but it remains unknown about the exact underlying mechanism and relationship to MIBI. It has been observed that the lower MIBI uptake in certain histologically confirmed tumours such as bronchioloalveolar carcinoma was related to an overexpression of P-glycoprotein as an in vivo marker of multidrug resistance. MIBI is physiologically taken up by the salivary glands, thyroid, heart, liver, spleen, and skeletal muscle. There is physiological hepato-biliary and renal clearance. The advantages include a readily available kit, easy to prepare, cost effective for a large patient-base, reasonable radiation dosimetry with good quality images from the 140keV single gamma photon energy of ^{99m}Tc (Moretti *et al.*, 2005).

3.3. Gallium 67 Citrate (^{67}Ga)

^{67}Ga has been used for imaging a variety of solid tumours since 1969. ^{67}Ga is cyclotron produced. It has a physical half-life of 78 hours and a biological half-life of 2-3 weeks. After intravenous administration, ^{67}Ga is bound to transferrin in the blood, and distributed to liver, lacrimal glands, salivary glands, and soft tissue tumors. Within the cells of the liver and tumors, gallium is found in lysosomes, and rough endoplasmic reticulum. Within these organelles, ^{67}Ga is bound to a variety of macromolecules, including transferrin, ferritin, and a 45,000 molecular weight glycoprotein. ^{67}Ga imaging of neoplastic disease has shown the greatest utility in imaging lymphomas but it can also be used for other tumours. In addition, ^{67}Ga has been employed to detect chronic infections (such as sarcoidosis), to evaluate interstitial lung disease, and to examine patients with acquired immunodeficiency syndrome (AIDS). Clinical usefulness of ^{67}Ga has been suggested for the study of adults presenting with fever of unknown origin because of the possibility of locating pathological uptake (both malignant and benign). The main indication for ^{67}Ga scintigraphy is lymphoma (Hodgkin's disease, HD, and non-Hodgkin's lymphoma, NHL), for evaluation of response to treatment, assessing tumour viability in the presence of post-therapy residual disease detected by conventional radiological tools such as CT or MRI.

It is a prognostic indicator in the prediction of outcome; evaluation of disease extent. The accuracy of ^{67}Ga scan is not superior to that of CT or MRI in staging lymphomas at presentation; however, it may be useful prior to therapy as a reference for treatment monitoring. ^{67}Ga is more effective in restaging because of the frequent presence of anatomical distortions/alterations following treatment. ^{67}Ga uptake correlates with tumour cell type and proliferation rate. High ^{67}Ga avidity is shown by diffuse large cell lymphomas including diffuse histiocytic lymphoma and poorly differentiated lymphocytic lymphoma. Similar ^{67}Ga avidity is shown by high-grade and intermediate-grade lymphomas including Burkitt's lymphoma. ^{67}Ga avidity in low-grade lymphomas (e.g. well-differentiated lymphocytic lymphoma) seems to be low. For these reasons a gallium scan is necessary before therapy in untreated patients in order to evaluate whether lymphoma is gallium avid or not. If the ^{67}Ga scan is negative, it should not be repeated. Although the following non-lymphomatous tumours show ^{67}Ga avidity, the usefulness of ^{67}Ga scanning in these patients has not been clearly demonstrated. ^{67}Ga scanning can be employed to image lung cancer, head and neck tumours, hepatocellular carcinoma, germ cell tumours, neuroblastoma, sarcoma, multiple myeloma, and melanoma. ^{67}Ga is indicated for the examination of adults presenting with fever of unknown origin because of the possibility to locate pathological uptake (both malignant and benign) (SNM Procedure guidelines; EANM Procedure guidelines).

3.4. Thallium 201 (^{201}Tl)

^{201}Tl has been utilized in the study of a variety of tumours since 1976. ^{201}Tl is cyclotron produced. It has a physical half-life of 73 hours and a biological half-life of 11 days. It decays by electron capture and emits photons with an energy range of 68- 80keV. ^{201}Tl accumulates mainly within viable tumour tissue, less within connective tissue which contains inflammatory cells, and its accumulation is barely detectable in necrotic tissue. Cellular uptake of ^{201}Tl is not affected by steroids, chemotherapy, or radiation therapy.

Localization of ^{201}Tl within tumours is likely multifactoral and in part related to blood flow, tumour viability, the sodium-potassium adenosine-tri-phosphatase (ATP) system, the non-energy dependent co-transport system, the calcium ion channel system, vascular immaturity with leakage, and increased cell membrane permeability. Radiation therapy and chemotherapy do not appear to immediately inhibit ^{201}Tl uptake as they do ^{67}Ga accumulation. Imaging has been reported in Head and neck carcinomas, breast carcinoma, bone malignancies, lymphoma and soft tissue sarcomas. A baseline pretreatment determination of ^{201}Tl avidity in the tumour is crucial to its efficacy in therapeutic response assessment. The optimal time for ^{201}Tl tumour imaging is 20 to 60 minutes post injection. Delayed images at 3 hours are recommended when imaging lymphoma because of an improved lesion to background ratio on the later images. Spot views of the lesion should be 5 minute preset timed images using a high resolution collimator. The normal distribution of ^{201}Tl within the body is choroid plexus of the lateral ventricles, lacrimal glands, salivary glands, thyroid, myocardium, liver, spleen, splanchnic areas, kidneys, and testes. There is also uniform muscle uptake. Bone marrow activity should not be seen, and if noted indicates marrow hyperplasia. There is little uptake in healing surgical wounds. The kidneys are the critical organ. Unfortunately, ^{201}Tl does not demonstrate 100% specificity for tumours and false-positive uptake has been seen in histiocytosis X, benign bone tumours, stress fractures, and inflammation (Sugawara et $al.$, 2005).

3.5. ^{99m}Tc-labelled HMPAO

^{99m}Tc hexamethyl propylamine oxime (99mTc-HMPAO, Ceretec, Amersham Ltd., U.K.), also known as ^{99m}Tc-exametazime, is a lipid soluble macrocyclic amine. It is a brain perfusion imaging agent. Brain uptake of the radiotracer is rapid and reaches its maximum within 10 minutes post-injection time. The distribution of the radiotracer remains constant for many hours post-injection. Once it crosses the blood brain barrier, ^{99m}Tc-HMPAO is converted into a hydrophilic compound in the presence of intracellular glutathione and is trapped, with slow blood clearance. Both primary and metastatic brain tumour lesions present on SPECT brain perfusion imaging as localized defects that correspond to the mass lesions. This technique alone is of limited value in the primary diagnosis or evaluation of intracranial mass lesions. In conjunction with ^{201}Tl, however, SPECT brain perfusion imaging may be valuable in distinguishing between radiation necrosis and tumour recurrence in patients with malignant gliomas treated with high dose radiation. The study may also localize suspected recurrences for biopsy (Groshar et $al.$, 1993).

	Pathway	Tracers	Clinical/Investigated Applications
Metabolic	Glucose metabolism	FDG	Staging on presentation in non-small-cell lung cancer, T3 oesophageal cancer, Hodgkin's disease, non-Hodgkin's lymphoma, locally advanced cervical cancer, ENT tumours with risk factors and locally advanced breast cancer.
			Differentiation of benign and malignant lesions (such as a solitary lung nodule, especially in case of discrepant clinical and radiological estimates of the likelihood of cancer).
			Evaluation of response to therapy in malignant lymphoma and GIST.
			Restaging in the event of potentially curable relapse for FDG avid tumours.
			Diagnosis of unknown primary malignancy, Establishing and localizing disease sites as a cause for elevated serum markers (this includes colorectal, thy-

			roid, ovarian, cervix, melanoma, breast and germ-cell tumours). Image guided biopsy Radiotherapy planning.
	Lipid and fat	Choline	Evaluating prostate carcinoma, high grade gliomas, anaplastic astrocytomas and primary hepatocellular cancer
		Acetate	Evaluating Prostate carcinoma
	Proliferation (DNA metabolism)	Thymidine analogues	Primary lung carcinoma, high grade gliomas, lymphoma (aggressive cell type), breast cancer, (early assessment response to chemotherapy), colorectal carcinoma, head and neck carcinoma, melanoma, soft tissue sarcoma of extremities.
	Amino Acids and Protein metabolism	Radiolabelled amino Acids	Low grade glioblastoma, glioblastoma (mild uptake), meningioma (high uptake)
		Radiolabelled peptides	
		SSRI	Identify/localize Neuroendocrine malignancies, Evaluating disease extent, monitoring effects of therapy, selecting patients for therapy, and prognostic indicator.
		Dopamine	Evaluate melanomas, neuroendocrine tumours, medullary thyroid carcinoma, pheocromocytomas, gastrointesitinal carcinoid tumours, brain tumours; mostly metastatic tumours and malignant gliomas superior in evaluating recurrent low-grade and high-grade gliomas.
		Tumour specific Receptors	Mostly evaluating and monitoring treatment response in Breast and Prostate carcinomas
		Monoclonal Antibodies	Detection of occult disease, in the management of patients with potentially resectable disease, and for the evaluation of lesion recurrence and therapeutic response mostly Prostate and Colorectal carcinoma,
		Guanidine analogue (MIBG)	Tumours of neuroendocrine origin, particularly those of the sympathoadrenal system (phaeochromocytomas, paragangliomas and neuroblastomas).
		Gene expression	Hepatocellular carcinoma
	Iodine metabolism	Iodine	Differentiated Thyroid carcinoma
Angiogenesis		VEGF/VEGFRs Integrins MMPs	Melanoma, late stage glioblastoma, ovarian, breast, and prostate cancer
Hypoxia		Nitromidazole derivatives	Head and neck, high grade gliomas, and lung carcinoma
Apoptosis		Annexin-V	Head and neck, breast, non-small cell lung carcinoma, melanoma, bladder carcinoma and lymphoma
General tumour imaging radiopharmaceuticals	Skeletal	Methylene Diphosphonate	Evaluating primary tumours (e.g. Ewing's sarcoma, osteosarcoma); staging, evaluation of response to therapy and follow-up of primary bone tumours, secondary tumours (metastases); staging and follow-up of neoplastic diseases, and the distribution of osteoblastic activity prior to radiometabolic therapy.

		Flouride	Identify skeletal metastases, including localization and determination of the extent of disease
	Mitochondrial activity	MIBI	lung, thyroid, brain, lymph node metastasis, bone and in breast carcinoma
	Transferrin receptor mechanism	Gallium 67 citrate	Mostly lymphoma (Hodgkin's disease, HD, and non-Hodgkin's lymphoma, NHL), for evaluation of response to treatment, assessing tumour viability in the presence of post-therapy residual disease detected by conventional radiological tools such as CT or MRI
	Na-K adenosine-tri-phosphatase (ATP) system	Thallium 201	Head and neck, breast, bone, lymphoma and soft tissue sarcomas
	Lipophilic brain perfusion agent converted by glutathione	HMPAO	Used in conjunction with ^{201}Tl and other brain tumour agents to localize recurrences for biopsy.

Table 4: Summary list of tracers and clinical indications.

4   Theranostics

Theranostics is a combination of two words, therapy and diagnosis. The term theranostics epitomizes the inseparability of diagnosis and therapy, the pillars of medicine. Under ideal circumstances the diagnostician uses an agent that is highly specific for diagnosing the pathology. The therapist then utilizes a variation of the same agent so that the same disorder which the physician is dealing with and from which the patient is suffering is treated. The goal in management is maximum efficiency and minimum complications.

In Nuclear Medicine, this refers to the use of molecular targeting vectors (e.g. peptides). These vectors are labelled with diagnostic radionuclides [e.g. positron or gamma emitters], or with therapeutic radionuclides (e.g. beta or alpha emitters, Table 5) for diagnosis and therapy of a particular disease which is targeted specifically by the vector at its molecular level. Therefore molecular imaging and diagnosis of the disease can be effectively followed by personalized treatment utilizing the same molecular imaging vectors (Figure 1 and Figure 2 *adapted from General introduction to therapeutic nuclear medicine by C.A. Hoefnagel*). Table 5 represents a list of selected radionuclides currently being used for therapy and their characteristics which make them each unique for their purpose. The idea of tailored management and individualizing therapy has now been achieved and has opened a door for new and greater opportunities ahead (Lee & Li, 2011; Freeman & Blaufox, 2012; Baum & Kulkarni, 2012; Goldenberg *et al.*, 2012).

Acknowledgements

Dr Masha Maharaj: Thank You to the Lord Almighty who kept me focused on the work ahead and sustained me. I am truly grateful to my parents and my family for their support and encouragement in pursuit of excellence. A special thank you to my dear brother, Dr Shane Maharaj, who has through Christ Jesus conquered cancer and has inspired me in this field of Medicine. Thank you to my mentor and friend Prof Ajit Padhy. Finally, I thank the dedicated staff at Polokwane Provincial Hospital, Dr AG Frankl, Mr X Mqhayisa, Mrs F Rasool, Mr J Manamela and Mrs Kgakgudi for their support. Dr Nisaar Korowlay: I would like to thank my son Mohammed Baaqir for his love and support.

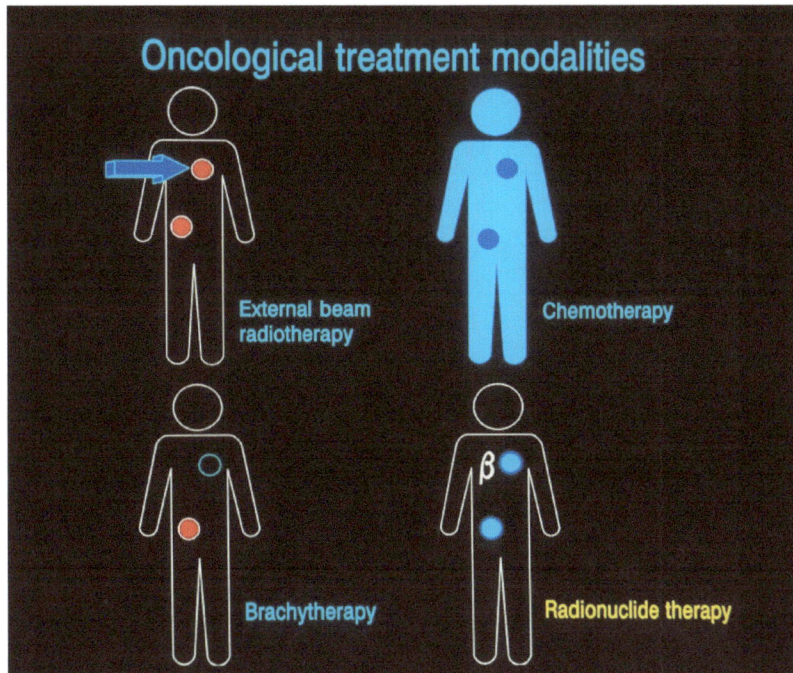

Figure 1: Oncological treatment modalities.

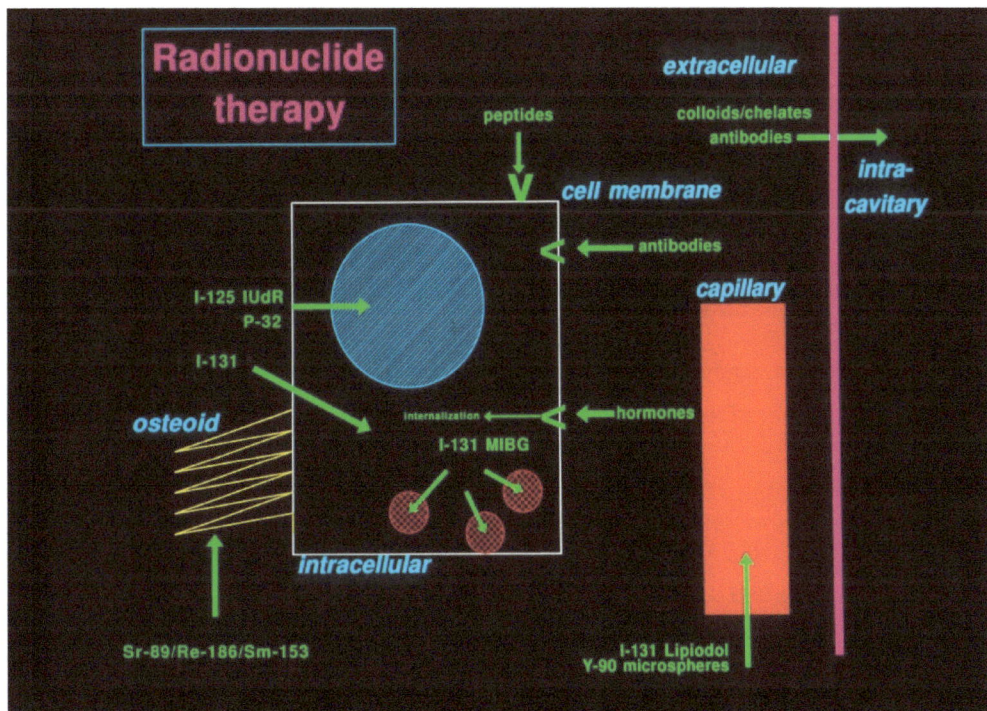

Figure 2: Multiple targeting vectors (Hoefnagel, 1998).

Radionuclide	Halflife	Emission	Maximum range in tissue
Bromiun-80m (80m Br)	4.42 h	Auger electrons	<10 nm
Iodine-125 (125I)	60 d	Auger electrons	10 nm
Astatine-211 (211At)	7.2 h	α	65 nm
Erbium-169 (169Er)	9.5 d	β-	1 mm
Lutetium-177 (177Lu)	6.71 d	β-/γ	2.1 mm
Copper-67 (67Cu)	2.58 d	β-/γ	2.2 mm
Iodine-131 (131I)	8.04 d	β-/γ	2.4 mm
Samarium-153 (153Sm)	1.95 d	β-/γ	3.0 mm
Gold-198 (198Au)	2.7 d	β-/γ	4.4 mm
Rhenium-186 (186Re)	3.77 d	β-/γ	5.0 mm
Dysprosium-165 (165Dy)	2.33 h	β-/γ	6.4 mm
Strontium-89 (89Sr)	50.5 d	β-	8.0 mm
Phosphorus-32 (32P)	14.3 d	β-	8.7mm
Yttrium-90 (90Y)	2.67 d	β-	12mm

Table 5 Selected radionuclides used for therapy and their characteristics

Conflict of interest

None.

References

Ali MS, Kong F, Rollo A, Mendez R. (2012). Development of 99mTc-N4-NIM for Molecular Imaging of Tumor Hy-poxia. Journal of Biomedicine and Biotechnology. Article ID 828139, 1-9

Arens J, Troost E. (2011). FDG-PET/CT in radiation treatment planning of head and neck squamous cell carcinoma. Q J Nuc Med Mol Imaging. 55: 521-528

Artiko V, Marković A, Šobić-Šaranović D, Petrović M. (2011). Monoclonal immunoscintigraphy for detection of metastasis and recurrence of colorectal cancer. World J Gastroenterol. 17(19): 2424-2430

Backer MV, Backer JM. (2012). Imaging Key Biomarkers of Tumor Angiogenesis. Theranostics. 2(5):502-515

Badgaiyan R. (2011). Neurotransmitter Imaging: Basic Concepts and Future Perspectives. Current Medical Imaging Reviews. 7, 98-103

Bading J, Shields A. (2008). Imaging of Cell Proliferation: Status and Prospects. J Nucl Med. 49:64S–80S

Baum R, Kulkarni HR. (2012). THERANOSTICS: From Molecular Imaging Using Ga-68 Labelled Tracers and PET/CT to Personalized Radionuclide Therapy – The Bad Berka Experience. Theranostics. 2(5):437-447

Baum RP, Niesen A, Leonhardi J, et al. (2005). Receptor PET/CT imaging of neuroendocrine tumours using the Ga-68 labelled, high affinity somatostatin analogue DOTA-1-Nal3-octreotide (DOTA-NOC): clinical results in 327 patients. Eur J Nucl Med Mol Imaging. 32:S54 (abstr)

Baum RP, Prasad V, Hommann M, Horsch D. (2008). Receptor PET/CTimaging of neuroendocrine tumours. Recent Results. Cancer Res 170:225–42.

Beirsack H, Briele B, Hotze A, Oehr P. (1992). The role of Nuclear Medicine in Oncology. Annals of Nuclear Medicine. Vol 6 (3): 131-136

Blankenberg F, Norfray F. (2011). Multimodality Molecular Imaging of Apoptosis in Oncology. AJR. 197:308–317

Boerman O, Oyen J. (2011). Immuno-PET of Cancer: A Revival of Antibody Imaging. J Nucl Med. Vol. 52 • No. 8: 1171-1172

Bombardieri E, Aktolun C, Baum RP, Bishof-Delaloye A, Buscombe J, et al. (2003). Breast scintigraphy procedure guidelines for tumour imaging. EANM Guidelines.

Chen K, Chen X. (2011). Positron Emission Tomography Imaging of Cancer Biology: Current Status and Future Prospects. Semin Oncol. 38(1): 70–86

Choe Y, Lee KH. (2007). Targeted In Vivo Imaging of Angiogenesis: Present Status and Perspectives. Current Pharmaceutical Design. 13, 17-31

Cooper DS, Doherty GM, Haugen BR, Kloos RT, Lee Sl. et al. (2009). Revised American Thyroid Association Management Guidelines for Patients with Thyroid Nodules and Differentiated Thyroid Cancer. THYROID. Volume 19, Number 11

Coxon JP, Oades GM, Colston KW, Kirby RS. (2004). Advances in the use of bisphosphonates in the prostate cancer setting. Prostate Cancer Prostatic Dis. 7(2):99-104.

Debergh I, Vanhove C, Ceelen W. (2012). Innovation in Cancer Imaging. Eur Surg Res. 48:121–130

Dillman RO. (2006). Radioimmunotherapy of B-cell lymphoma with radiolabelled anti-CD20 monoclonal antibodies. Clin Exp Med. 6:1–12

Fahey H, Treves T, Adelstein J. (2011). Minimizing and Communicating Radiation Risk in Pediatric Nuclear Medicine. J Nucl Med. 52:1240–1251

Fili S, Karalaki M, Schaller B. (2009). Mechanism of bone metastasis: the role of osteoprotegerin and of the host-tissue microenvironment-related survival factors. Cancer Lett. 283(1):10-9

Fouge C, Suchorska B, Bartenstein P, Kreth F. (2011). Molecular imaging of gliomas with PET: Opportunities and limitations. Neuro-Oncology. 13(8):806–819

Freeman L, & Blaufox D. (2012). Theranostics. J.Semnuclmed. Vol 42(3): 145-146

Freeman L, Blaufox D. (2012). PET/CT in Radiation Oncology. J.Semnuclmed. Vol 42(5): 281-282

Freeman LM, Blaufox D. (2013). Letter from the Editors: Low-Sensitivity FDG-PET Studies. J. Semnuclmed. Vol 42 (5): 219-220

Fujiwara T. (2011). A Novel Molecular Therapy Using Bioengineered Adenovirus for Human Gastrointestinal Cancer. Acta med Okayama. Vol 65. 3. 151-162

Gambhir SS, Barrio JR, Phelps ME, Lyer M. (1999). Imaging adenoviral-directed reporter gene expression in living animals with positron emission tomography. Proc. Natl. Acad. Sci. Vol. 96, pp. 2333–2338

Gambhir SS, Czernin J, Schwimmer J, Silverman D, Coleman R, et al. (2001). A Tabulated Summary of the FDG PET Literature. J Nucl Med 42:1S–93S

Gnanasegaran G, Kapse N, Buscombe J. (2005). Recent Trends in Radionuclide Imaging and Targeted Radionuclide Therapy of Neuroendocrine Tumours. IJNM. 20(3): 55-66

Goldenberg M, Chang CH, Rossi E, McBride W. (2012). Pretargeted Molecular Imaging and Radioimmunotherapy. Theranostics. 2(5):523-540

Groshar D, McEwan A, Parliament M, Urtasun R, Golberg L, et al. (1993). Imaging Tumor Hypoxia and Tumor Perfusion. J Nucl Med. 34:885-888

Gunn R, Gunn S, Turkheimer F, AstonJ, Cunningham V. (2002). Positron Emission Tomography Compartmental Models: A Basis Pursuit Strategy for Kinetic Modelling. J Cereb Blood Flow Metab. Dec;22(12):1425-39

Haberkorn U, Markert A, Eisenhut M, Mier W, Altmann A. (2011). Development of molecular techniques for imaging and treatment of tumours. Q J Nuc Med Mol Imaging. 55: 655-670

Hanahan D, Weinberg RA. (2011). Hallmarks of cancer: the next generation. Cell. 144(5):646-74

Haubner R, Wester H, Reuning U, Senekowitsch-Schmidtke R. (1999). Radiolabeled $\alpha V \beta 3$Integrin Antagonists: A New Class of Tracers for Tumor Targeting. J Nucl Med. 40:1061-1071

Heine M, Nollau P, Masslo C, & Nielsen P. (2011). Investigations on the Usefulness of CEACAMs as Potential Imaging Targets for Molecular Imaging Purposes. PLoS ONE. Vol 6 (12): e28030

Hicks, R, Hofman, M. (2012). Is there still a role for SPECT-CT in oncology in the PET-CT era? Nature Reviews Clinical Oncology. 9, 712-720

Hoefnagel C. (1998). Radionuclide cancer therapy. Annals of Nuclear Medicine. Vol 12, No. 2, 91-70

Jadvar H. (2011). Prostate Cancer: PET with 18F-FDG, 18F- or 11C-Acetate, and 18F- or 11C-Choline. J Nucl Med. 52:81–89

Jaffer F & Weissleder R. (2005). Molecular Imaging in the Clinical Arena. JAMA. 293(7):855-862

Jansen J, Koutcher J, Shukla-Dave A. (2010). Non-invasive imaging of angiogenesis in head and neck squamous cell carcinoma. Angiogenesis. 13(2): 149–160

Jeswani_T, Padhani.AR. (2005). Imaging tumour angiogenesis. Cancer Imaging. 5, 131–138

Jora C, Mattakarottuc J, Aniruddha PG, & Mudalsha R. (2011). Comparative evaluation of 18F-FDOPA, 13N-AMMONIA, 18F-FDG PET/CT and MRI in primary brain tumours - A pilot study. Indian J Nucl Med. Apr-Jun; 26(2): 78–81

Jordan B, Sonveaux P. (2012). Targeting tumour perfusion and oxygenation to improve the outcome of anticancer therapy. Frontiers in Pharmacology: Pharmacology of Anti-Cancer Drugs. Vol 3; Article 94: 1-15

Joseph AT. (2004). Understanding the Standardized Uptake Value, Its Methods, and Implications for Usage. J Nucl Med. vol. 45 no. 9 1431-1434

Kam B, Teunissen JM, Krenning EP, De Herder W. (2012). Lutetium-labelled peptides for therapy of neuroendocrine tumours. Eur J Nucl Med Mol Imaging. Vol 39 (Suppl 1):S103–S112

Kanwar JR, Roy K, Kanwar RK. (2011). Chimeric aptamers in cancer cell-targeted drug delivery. Critical Reviews in Biochemistry and Molecular Biology. 46(6): 459–477

Karaosmanoğlu A, Blake M. (2012). Applications of PET-CT in patients with esophageal cancer. Diagn Interv Radiol. 18:171–182

Kersemans V, Cornelissen B, Hueting R, Tredwell M, Hussien K, et al. (2011). Hypoxia Imaging Using PET and SPECT: The Effects of Anesthetic and Carrier Gas on [64Cu]-ATSM, [99mTc]-HL91 and [18F]-FMISO Tumor Hypoxia Accumulation. PLoS ONE. 6(11): e25911

Khan MU, Khan S, El-Refaie S, Win Z, Rubello D, Al-Nahhas A. (2009). Clinical indications for Gallium-68 positron emission tomography imaging. EJSO 35 561-567

Kumar R. (2008). Oncological PET tracers beyond [18F] FDG and the novel quatitative approaches in PET imaging. Q J Nuc Med Mol Imaging. 52: 50-65

Kyoichi K, Masahiro E, Masato A, Kazuo N, Yasuhisa O, et al. (2010). Biologic Correlation of 2-[18F]-Fluoro-2-Deoxy-D-Glucose uptake on Positron Emission Tomography in Thymic Epithelial Tumors. J Clin Oncol. 28:3746-3753

Kyoichi K, Noboru O, Noriaki S, Tamotsu I, Shimizu K, et al. (2011).A systemic review of PET and biology in lung cancer. Am J Transl Res. 3(4):383-391

Kyoichi K, Takehiro O, Yasuhisa O, Toshiaki T, Haruyasu M, et al. (2011). Correlation Between 18F-FDG Uptake on PET and Molecular Biology in Metastatic Pulmonary Tumors. J Nucl Med 52:705–711

Larson S. (1978). Mechanisms of localization of gallium-67 in tumors. Seminars in Nuclear Medicine. Vol.8. Issue 3, 193–203

Laverman P, Sosabowski J, Boerman O, Oyen W. (2012). Radiolabelled peptides for oncological diagnosis. Eur J Nucl Med Mol Imaging. 39 (Suppl 1):S78–S92

Lee D, Li KP. (2011). Molecular Theranostics: A Primer for the Imaging Professional. AJR. . 197:318–324

Lee SZ, Scott A. (2007). Hypoxia Positron Emission Tomography Imaging With 18F-Fluoromisonidazole. Semin Nucl Med 37:451-461

Leitha T. (2009). Nuclear medicine: proof of principle for targeted drugs in diagnosis and therapy. Curr Pharm Des. 15(2):173-87

Lewis MR. (2005). Radiolabeled RGD Peptides Move Beyond Cancer: PET Imaging of Delayed-Type Hypersensitivity Reaction. J NucI Med. Vol. 46 (1): 2-4

LiVolsi V. (2011). Papillary thyroid carcinoma: an update. Modern Pathology. Vol 24, S1–S9

Maecke HR., Hofmann M; Haberkorn U. (2005). 68Ga-Labeled Peptides in Tumor Imaging. J Nucl Med. 46:172S–178S

Mankoff D, Link JM, Linden HM, Sundararajan L. (2008). Tumor Receptor Imaging. J Nucl Med. 49:149S–163S

Mariani, G, Flotats, A, Israel, O, Kim, E.E, Kuwert, T. (2008). Clinical Applications of SPECT/CT: New Hybrid Nuclear Medicine Imaging System. IAEA Doc.

Marnett LJ. (2012). Inflammation and Cancer: Chemical Approaches to Mechanisms, Imaging, and Treatment. J. Org. Chem. 77, 5224−5238

McHenry CR, Phitayakorn R. (2011). Follicular Adenoma and Carcinoma of the Thyroid Gland. The Oncologist 16:585–593

Mees G, Dierckx R, Vangestel C, Van de Wiele C. (2009). Molecular imaging of hypoxia with radiolabelled agents. Eur J Nucl Med Mol Imaging. Vol 36:1674–1686

Missbach-Guentner J, Hunia J, Alves F. (2011). Tumor blood vessel visualization. Int. J. Dev. Biol. 55: 535-546

Moretti J, Hauet N, Caglar M, Rebillard O, Burak Z. (2005). To use MIBI or not to use MIBI? That is the question when assessing tumour cells. Eur J Nucl Med Mol Imaging. 32:836–842

Multhoff &, Radons J. (2012). Radiation, inflammation, and immune responses in cancer. Frontiers in Oncology: Molecular and Cellular Oncology. Vol 2 (58): 1-18

Mundy GR.(2002). Metastasis to bone: causes, consequences and therapeutic opportunities. Nature reviews: Cancer. Vol 2: 284-293

Ni1 X, Castanares M, Mukherjee A, Lupold S. (2011). Nucleic acid aptamers: clinical applications and promising new horizons. Curr Med Chem. 18(27): 4206–4214

Oikonen V. (2005). NET and [18F]FDOPA PET: Literature review. Turku PET Centre Modelling report. TPCMOD0018

Park JW, Cho CH, Jeong DS, Chae HD. (2011). Role of 18F-fluoro-2-deoxyglucose Positron Emission Tomography in Gastric GIST: Predicting Malignant Potential Pre-operatively. J Gastric Cancer. 11(3):173-179

Picchio M, and Castellucci P. (2012). Clinical Indications of 11C-Choline PET/CT in Prostate Cancer Patients with Biochemical Relapse. Theranostics. 2(3): 313-317

Plotnik D, Emerick L, Krohn K, Unadkat J, L Swartz. (2010). Different Modes of Transport for 3H-Thymidine, 3H-FLT, and 3H-FMAU in Proliferating and Nonproliferating Human Tumor Cells. J Nucl Med. 51:1464–1471

Poeppel TD, Krause BJ, Heusner TA, Boy C, Bockisch A, et al. (2009). PET/CT for the staging and follow-up of patients with malignancies. Eur J Radiol. 70(3):382-392

Ponde DE, Dence CS, Oyama N, Kim J. (2007). 18F-Fluoroacetate: A Potential Acetate Analog for Prostate Tumor Imaging - In Vivo Evaluation of 18F-Fluoroacetate Versus 11C-Acetate J Nucl Med. 48:420–428

Procedure guidelines: British Nuclear Medicine Society (BNMS). http://www.bnms.org.uk

Procedure guidelines: European association of Nuclear Medicine (EANM). http://www.eanm.org

Procedure Guidelines. Society of Nuclear Medicine (SNM). http://interactive.snm.org/index

Ray P. (2011). Multimodality molecular imaging of disease progression in living subjects. J. Biosci. 36(3): 499–504

Roberge D, Vakilian S, Alabed YZ, Turcotte RE, Freeman CR, et al. (2012). FDG PET/CT in Initial Staging of Adult Soft-Tissue Sarcoma. Sarcoma, vol. Article ID 960194, 1-7

Rufini V, Calcagni ML, Baum RP. (2006). Imaging of Neuroendocrine Tumors. Semin Nucl Med. 36:228-247

Salskov A, Tammisetti VS, Grierson J, Vesselle H. (2007). FLT: Measuring Tumor Cell Proliferation In Vivo With Positron Emission Tomography and 3=-Deoxy-3=-[18F]Fluorothymidine. Semin Nucl Med. 37:429-439

Sandu N, Pöpperl G, Toubert E, Arasho B, Spiriev T, et al. (2011). Molecular imaging of potential bone metastasis from differentiated thyroid cancer: a case report. Journal of Medical Case Reports. Vol 5:522

Sanoudou D, Frieden LA, Haslett JN, Kho AT, Greenberg SA, et al. (2004). Molecular classification of nemaline myopathies: "nontyping" specimens exhibit unique patterns of gene expression. Neurobiol Dis. Apr;15(3):590-600

Satoru S, Etsuro H, Tatsuya H, Akio N, Yuji N, et al. (2009). P-glycoprotein expression affects 18F-fluorodeoxyglucose accumulation in hepatocellular carcinoma in vivo and in vitro. Int J Oncol. 34(5):1303-12

Schaper F and Reutelingsperger C. (2013). 99mTc-HYNIC-Annexin A5 in Oncology: Evaluating Efficacy of Anti-Cancer Therapies. Cancers 5, 550-568

Schlyer D. (2004). PET tracers and radiochemistry. Ann Acad Med Singapore. 33: 146-154

Seibyl J, Chen W, Silverman DHS. (2007). 3,4-Dihydroxy-6-[18F]-Fluoro-L-Phenylalanine Positron Emission Tomography in Patients With Central Motor Disorders and in Evaluation of Brain and Other Tumors. Semin Nucl Med. 37:440-450

Shan L. (2013). 111In-Labeled multifunctional single-attachment-point reagent-c [RGDfK]: [111In-MSAP-RGD]. MICAD. PMID: 22934321. [Pubmed]

Shankar V. (2007). 18F-Labeled Positron Emission Tomographic Radiopharmaceuticals in Oncology: An Overview of Radiochemistry and Mechanisms of Tumor Localization. Semin Nucl Med. 37:400-419

Sugawara Y, Kikuchi T, Kajihara M, Semba T, Ochi T, et al. (2005). Thallium-201 scintigraphy in bone and soft-tissue tumors: a comparison of dynamic, early and delayed scans. Annals of Nuclear Medicine Vol. 19, No. 6, 461–468,

Sullivan DC, Gatsonis C. (2011). Response to Treatment Series: Part 1 and Introduction, Measuring Tumor Response— Challenges in the Era of Molecular Medicine. AJR. 197:15–17

Tinsu P and Osama M. (2008). PET/CT in radiation oncology. Med. Phys. 35, 4955

Turaga K, Kvols LK. (2011). Recent Progress in the Understanding, Diagnosis, and Treatment of Gastroenteropancreatic Neuroendocrine Tumors. CA Cancer J Clin. 61:113–132

Valotassiou V, Leondi A, Angelidis G, & Psimadas D. (2012). SPECT and PET Imaging of Meningiomas. The Scientific World Journal. Article ID 412580, 1-11

Weissleder R. (2006). Molecular Imaging in Cancer. Science. Vol 312: 1168-1171

Wiyaporn K, Tocharoenchai C, Pusuwan P, Ekjeen T, Leaungwutiwong S, et al. (2010). Factors Affecting Standardized Uptake Value (SUV) of Positron Emission Tomography (PET) Imaging with 18F-FDG. J Med Assoc Thai. 93 (1): 108-14

Zanoni L, Cerci J, Fonti S. (2011). The use of PET/CT to evaluate response to therapy in Lymphoma. Q J Nucl Med Mol Imaging. 55: 633-647

Zhanga Y, Hongb H, Cai W. (2011). PET Tracers Based on Zirconium-89. Curr Radiopharm. 4(2): 131–139

Zhu L, Niu G, Fang X, Chen X. (2010). Preclinical Molecular Imaging of Tumor Angiogenesis. Q J Nucl Med Mol Imaging. 54(3): 291–308

Ziegler, SI. (2005). Positron Emission Tomography: Principles, Technology, and Recent Developments. Nuclear Physics A 752 679c–687c

Preliminary Studies on Chest X-ray by Digital Tomosynthesis Imaging

Tsutomu Gomi
School of Allied Health Sciences
Kitasato University, Japan

1   Introduction

In tomography, an X-ray tube and X-ray film receptor are positioned on either sides of an object. The relative motion of the tube and film is predetermined on the basis of the location of the in-focus plane (Ziedses des Plantes, 1932). Only a single image plane is generated by a scan; therefore, multislice computed tomography (CT) scans are necessary to provide a sufficient number of planes to cover the selected structure in the object. Tomosynthesis acquires only a single set of discrete X-ray projections, which can be used to reconstruct any plane of the object retrospectively (Grant, 1972). The application of this technique to angiography and the imaging of the chest, hand joints, lungs, teeth, urinary organs (Well *et al.*, 2011), and breasts (Stiel *et al.*, 1993; Duryea *et al.*, 2003; Sone *et al.*, 1995; Niklason *et al.*, 1997; Dobbins *et al.*, 2003; Johnsson *et al.*, 2012; Savalkvist *et al.*, 2012; Quaia *et al.*, 2012; Yamada *et al.*, 2011) has been investigated.

Existing tomosynthesis algorithms can be classified into two categories: back-projection and filtered backprojection (FBP) algorithms. The projected images can be shifted and added (SAA) to coincide either the circles or the triangles (i.e., focus) with the smeared out complementary object. The basis for FBP is the backprojection of the data acquired from projections obtained over all angles. When this procedure is performed for each pixel in a projection and for all possible angles of the projected data, then a simple back-projected image of the object is created (Figure 1). The back-projection algorithm is referred to as "SAA," in which the projected images captured at different angles are electronically SAA to generate an image plane focused at a certain depth below the surface. The projection shift is adjusted such that the visibility of features in the selected plane is enhanced, whereas that in other planes is blurred. By using a digital detector, image planes at all depths can be retrospectively reconstructed from one set of projections. The SAA algorithm is valid only if the X-ray focal spot moves parallel to the detector.

FBP algorithms are widely used in CT, in which many projections acquired at greater than 360° are used to reconstruct cross-sectional images. The number of projections typically ranges between a few hundreds to approximately thousands. In two-dimensional (2D) CT imaging, the projection of an object corresponds to sampling the object along the direction perpendicular to the X-ray beam in Fourier space (Kak *et al.*, 1988). For many projections, information about the object is properly sampled, and the object can be restored by combining the information from all projections. In three-dimensional (3D) cone-beam imaging, information about the object in Fourier space is related to the radon transform of that object. The relationship between the radon transform and cone-beam projections has been studied satisfactorily, and solutions to cone-beam reconstruction have been provided (Smith, 1985). The FBP algorithm generally provides a high degree of precision for 3D-reconstructed images when an accurate algorithm is employed (Feldkamp *et al.*, 1984). Therefore, this method is adopted for the image reconstruction in 3D tomography and multidetector cone-beam CT.

Tomosynthesis is a limited-angle method of image reconstruction. In this technique, the projection dataset of an object acquired at regular intervals during a single acquisition pass is used to reconstruct planar sections *post priori*. Tomosynthetic slices that are planes parallel to the detector plane exhibit high resolution. Tomosynthesis enhances the existing advantages of conventional tomography, i.e., low radiation dose, short examination time, as well as easy and low-cost availability of longitudinal tomographs, which do not include the partial-volume effect. This technique is developed by improving the older technique of geometric tomography, which is not preferred for chest imaging because of positioning difficulties, high radiation dose, and residual blur caused by out-of-plane structures. Tomosynthesis overcomes these difficulties by enabling the reconstruction of numerous image slices from a single low-dose image data. Tomosynthesis images are invariably affected by blurring because of objects present outside the plane of interest and superimposition on the focused image of the fulcrum plane by a limited acquisition angle. This results in poor object detectability in the in-focus plane. In this section, we report phantom studies that involve a comparison between tomosynthesis with CT and that with radiography to detect artificial pulmonary nodules. In addition, we cite a few clinical cases.

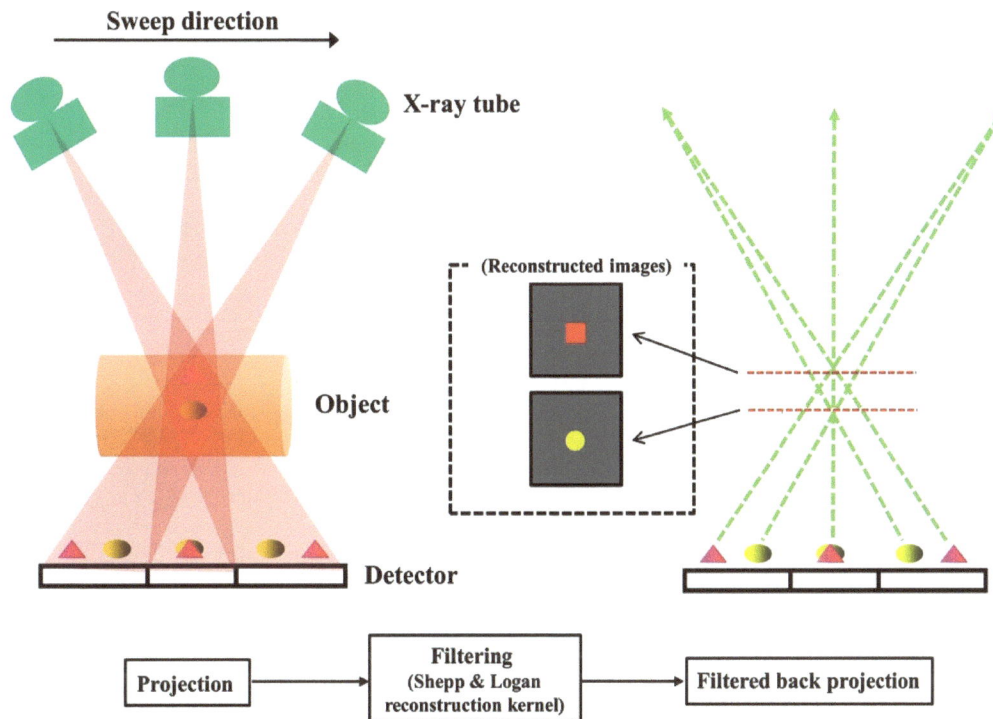

Figure 1: The basis for filtered back projection is the back projection of the data acquired from projections obtained over all angles. To create a simple back-projected image of an object, this procedure is performed for each pixel in a projection and for all the possible angles of the projected data.

2   Device

2.1   Tomosynthesis and Radiography System

The tomosynthesisand radiography system (Sonial Vision Safire II, Shimadzu Co., Kyoto, Japan) comprises an X-ray tube with a 0.4mm focal spot and a $432 \times 432\text{mm}^2$ amorphous selenium digital flat-panel detector with a detector element size of 150×150 μm^2. The tomosynthesis projection images were sampled during a single tomographic pass (74 projections) with a matrix size of 1280×1280 by 12 bits. Tomosynthesis-reconstruction processing was used to reconstruct the tomograms of a desired height. The tomosynthesis images (357.46×357.46 mm^2, 0.28mm/pixel) were reconstructed using FBP. In addition, an antiscatter grid was used (focused type, grid ratio 12:1).

2.2   CT system

CT scan was performed on a multislice CT scanner (64slice Somatom Definition scanner; Siemens Medical Systems, Forchheim, Germany) with a 120kVp, 110mA, a detector configuration of 64 × 0.6 mm and 0.5s gantry rotation time at a beam pitch of 0.8. The clinical task was to assess the lung. A slice thickness of 5 mm is routinely used in clinical practice. In this study, we applied the slice thickness used during screenings; therefore, the axial reconstructed images were obtained with a 5mm slice thickness at 5mm reconstruction intervals. Both standard and sharp reconstruction kernelswere used (B35f, standard kernel; B60f, sharp kernel).

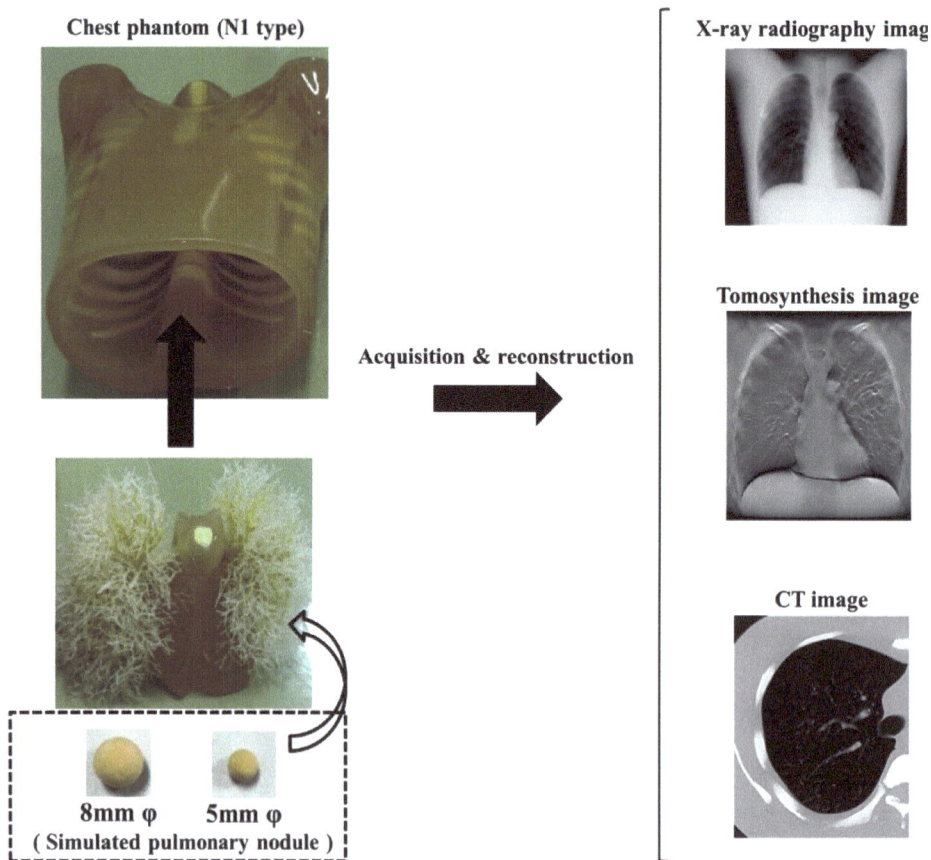

Figure 2: Illustration of the chest phantom N1 (Kyoto Kagaku Co., Tokyo, Japan) and artificial pulmonary nodules.

3   Specifications of Phantom and Artificial Pulmonary Nodules

The Chest Phantom N1 (Kyoto Kagaku Co., Tokyo, Japan) is constructed from synthetic materials (i.e., polyurethane, epoxy resin, and calcium carbonate) in a configuration that resembles soft tissue and vessels. The artificial pulmonary nodules resemble the ground glass in terms of their opacity (5 and 8 mm in diameter, urethane foam) with a homogenous composition (Figure 2). These are arranged in each lung region, and the nodules that were adjacent to the edges of the lungs or mixed with the blood vessels were observed. The target contrast (ΔCT) of the artificial pulmonary nodules (ΔCT = 200HU) was determined on the basis of the lung parenchyma with an artificial background.

4 Evaluation of Artificially Detected Pulmonary Nodule

4.1 Comparison between Tomosynthesis and CT

Detecting and characterizing pulmonary nodules is one of the most challenging tasks in thoracic imaging; even experienced chest radiologists may overlook up to 30% of such lesions on conventional chest radiographs (Stitik et al., 1978). Nodules are frequently visible retrospectively only while reviewing the previous images of patients with a known history of nodules (Muhm et al., 1983), and identifying them prospectively is difficult. Because of its high sensitivity, normal-dose helical CT is currently considered as the standard method to diagnose lung cancer. Early reports indicate that low-dose helical CT can detect lung cancer in its initial stage, thereby decreasing morbidity (Yankelevitz et al., 2000). In addition, CT solves the problem of impaired visibility due to overlapping anatomical structures, which leads to lower detection rates.

X-ray CT has progressed over the last three decades, and now, it is a powerful tool for medical diagnosis. CT has become an essential noninvasive-imaging technique especially since the advent of spiral CT in the 1990s, which has led to shorter scan times and improved 3D spatial resolution. Although CT provides high resolution in the tomographic plane, it has a limited axial resolution. Therefore, the partial-volume effect (PVE) may complicate the evaluation of structures that are not oriented in the direction of the CT tomographic plane.

CT, particularly high-resolution CT (HRCT), has considerably improved the evaluatation of pulmonary lesions; moreover, it has replaced conventional tomography to a great extent (Siegelman et al., 1986; Zwirewich et al., 1991; Murata et al., 1986; Webb, 1991). HRCT reveals a detailed configuration of localized and diffuse parenchymal abnormalities and facilitates the recognition of their anatomical distribution. However, because of PVE, this modality continues to encounter difficulties when used in pulmonary imaging, for example, while displaying or recognizing lesions in addition to related bronchovascular structures in longitudinal sections and while displaying small calcifications.

Tomosynthesis, which enhances the existing advantages of conventional tomography, also provides the additional benefits of digital imaging (Miller et al., 1971; Grant, 1972; Baily et al., 1973; Krunger et al., 1983; Sone et al., 1991, 1995). The effective dose of a chest examination by tomosynthesis is approximately twice of that by a conventional examination [International Commission on Radiological Protection Publication 60; two-view radiography, 0.056 mSv; tomosynthesis, 0.124 mSv; average chest CT, 7 mSv (Sabol et al., 2009)].In addition, tomosynthesis provides some of the tomographic benefits of CT at a reduced radiation dose and cost by an approach that can be easily implemented in conjunction with chest radiography.

In this study, we performed two experiments to measure the detection capabilities of a tomosynthesis imaging system for use as an effective screening method and compared the results with those of CT imaging (Gomi et al., 2012).

4.1.1 Conditions for Data Acquisition

We evaluated two items to compare the performance of tomosynthesis with CT.Tomosynthesis was performed with a linear tomographic movement and a total acquisition time of 6.4 s. Each projection image was acquired at 120 kVp, 200 mA, and with a 5ms exposure time for X-rays. The tomosynthesis reconstruction images were obtained with a 5mm slice thickness at 5mm reconstruction intervals.

4.1.2 Detectability Index

Detectability index (DI) provides a figure-of-merit (FOM) that incorporates the basic system performance and imaging and offers an objective function for system optimization and design:

$$d'^2 = \iint \frac{MTF^2_{2D}(u,v)}{NPS_{2D}(u,v)} W^2_{Task}(u,v) \, du \, dv \tag{1}$$

where d' is DI, u and v are spatial frequencies, $MTF(u, v)$ denotes the modulation transfer function [International Commission on Radiation Units and Measurement (ICRU) report 54, 1996],and $NPS(u, v)$ denotes the noise power spectrum (ICRU report 54, 1996). MTF was obtained by the 2D Fourier transformation of the line-spread function (tomosynthesis, copper wire images; CT, tungsten microsphere images). NPS was obtained using the fast Fourier transform of a 2D noise pattern of an exposure image. The measured NPS in terms of the pixel value was converted to that in terms of relative X-ray intensity by using the system-response characteristic curve. The trend correction used a quadratic polynomial approximation. Two-dimensional integration was performed over the Nyquist region. The term $W_{Task}(u, v)$ denotes the task function, a frequency-domain representation of the imaging task (ICRU report 54, 1996). The task function was derived from the Fourier transform of the difference between the two hypotheses:

$$W_{Task}(u,v) = \left| F\left[h_1(x,y) - h_2(x,y) \right] \right| \tag{2}$$

where F denotes the Fourier transform, and $h_1(x, y)$ and $h_2(x, y)$ denote the functions that describe the signal in the spatial domain for the two hypotheses. DI for a background and a spherical image were considered. Therefore, $h_1(x, y) = 0$ and $h_2(x, y)$ corresponded to the 2D image profile of a sphere derived from the attenuated signal passing through a 5-mm-diameter sphere. Attenuation data were used to model a solid lesion ($\Delta CT = 370$, materials: polyurethane and hydroxyapatite). In this form, DI could also be interpreted as a weighted sum of the task function with the noise-equivalent quanta. The resulting DI was used in various applications as an FOM for system optimization (Richard et al., 2005). Then, DI was evaluated to compare the effectiveness of chest-tomosynthesis imaging (acquisition angles, 8°, 20°, 30,° and 40°; 2D images) with that of CT imaging (2D images) for detecting artificial pulmonary nodules.

4.1.3 Observer Study

Five thoracic radiologists, two with 20 and three with 12 years of experience in chest radiology, evaluated the images for the presence of artificial pulmonary nodules by using the free-response receiver-operating characteristic (FROC) paradigm. The images were evaluated with ViewDEX 2.0 software (Södra Älvsborgs Sjukhus, Sahlgrenska University and University of Gothenburg, Gothenburg, Sweden) (Sodra, 2009), which is designed for displaying images. We examined the 50 samples of artificial pulmonary nodules (5 and 8 mm in diameter) using both tomosynthesis (acquisition angle, 40°; 2D images) and CT (standard kernel, 2D images) imaging. The artificial pulmonary nodules were placed at various locations in the chest phantom, after which CT and tomosynthesis images were acquired. The radiologists were presented with both CT and tomosynthesis images at different times and were not allowed to change the window width, levels, or use the pan or zoom functions. We standardized the gradation specifications of each image to avoid differences in indications. The observers were informed that nodule to non-nodule cases were in the ratio 38:25 and that there could be multiple nodules per case (one nodule/image, 12 cases; two nodules/image, 13 cases; no nodules/image, 25 cases; and total 50 samples of each modality). Before each session, five educational cases that were not included in the study were shown. Each observer was instructed to detect any artificial pulmonary nodules on the tomosynthesis and CT images and describe the presence of each nodule on a scale of 1 – 4, where 4 represented the highest degree of confidence (definitely a nodule), and 1 represented the lowest degree of confidence (probably not a nodule). Observers were requested to search for nodules in the entire field of the chest phantom; therefore, they had to repeat the search using 100 individual images in which the nodules of different sizes were placed at different locations in the phantom. The given marks, along with ratings and locations, were extracted from the logfile produced by the ViewDEX 2.0 software and were compared with the actual locations. Thus, each mark was classified as a lesion or a non-lesion localization. The time frame between image interpretations was 1 – 2 weeks. Because of the substantial difference between the appearances of the tomosynthesis and CT images, this procedure was considered appropriate to avoid recall bias.

The FROC data were analyzed with the jackknife FROC (JAFROC) method (Ruschin *et al.*, 2007), which was implemented in the JAFROC software version 2.3a (Chakraborty DP, University of Pittsburgh, Pittsburgh, USA) (Chakraborty, 2006, 2008). This software computes an FOM, which is defined as the probability of a lesion-localization rating exceeding all non-lesion-localization ratings in a normal case. Thus, only the highest non-lesion-localization ratings in normal cases were included in the analysis. The computation of FOM is identical to the calculation of the Wilcoxon-test statistic for the two samples (Ruschin *et al.*, 2007). JAFROC version 2.3a calculates the mean FOM of each modality and determines the difference between the means with 95% confidence intervals (CI). In general, the importance of a nodule in the statistical analysis can be considered by assigning a weighting factor to each nodule. However, the importance of artificial nodules was not analyzed in this study; therefore, the weighting factors were identical for all nodules in the same sample.

4.1.4   Results of Comparison between Tomosynthesis and CT

Contrast was found to be greater when tomosynthesis imaging increased the acquisition angle of images from the same location (Figure 3). In tomosynthesis imaging, contrast was higher in images with large nodules; a similar tendency was exhibited by CT imaging (Figure 4).

For each increased acquisition angle, the tomosynthesis image was similar to the CT image (Figure 3 and 4). We compared CT and tomosynthesis in terms of DI and found that they were identical (Figure 5 upper).

Figure 5 (lower) shows the FROC curves according to the readings given by the five observers. The detectability difference between tomosynthesis and CT was not statistically significant. The observer-averaged JAFROC FOM was 0.617 (95% CI, 0.49, and 0.72) for tomosynthesis and 0.5765 (95% CI, 0.46, and 0.68) for CT; this difference was not statistically significant (difference, 0.0363; 95% CI, −0.18, 0.26; F-statistic = 0.101; $p = 0.75$). JAFROC analysis possessed sufficient sensitivity to judge the ability of tomosynthesis and CT for detecting artificial pulmonary nodules. In Figure 5 (lower), the FROC curves for the three observers show that at the lower threshold of the non-lesion localization fraction (NLF < 0.2), CT clearly outperforms tomosynthesis, whereas at the upper threshold of NLF (> 0.2), tomosynthesis clearly outperforms CT. In the observer experiment, the detectability rates of tomosynthesis and CT were approximately equivalent.

Chest images obtained by tomosynthesis and CT in a clinical case were compared. Tomosynthesis and CT appear to have a similar accuracy in detecting pulmonary nodules, but tomosynthesis has a greater clinical potential (Figure 6).

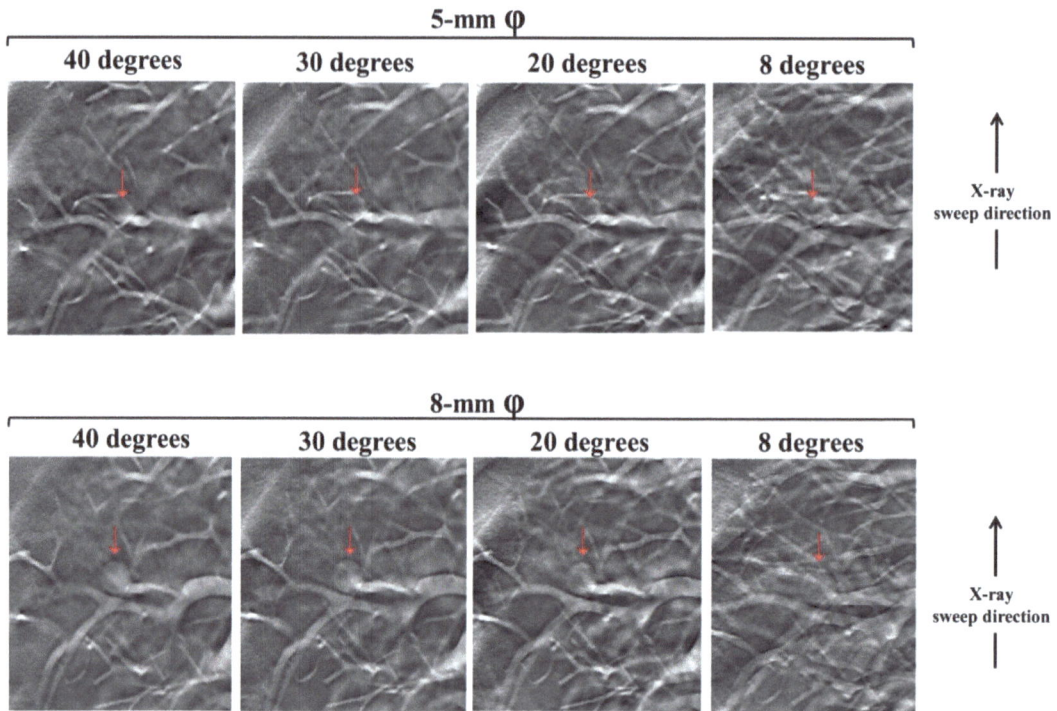

Figure 3: Tomosynthesis image with the different acquisition angles of the same slice, demonstrating the content of the artificial pulmonary nodules.

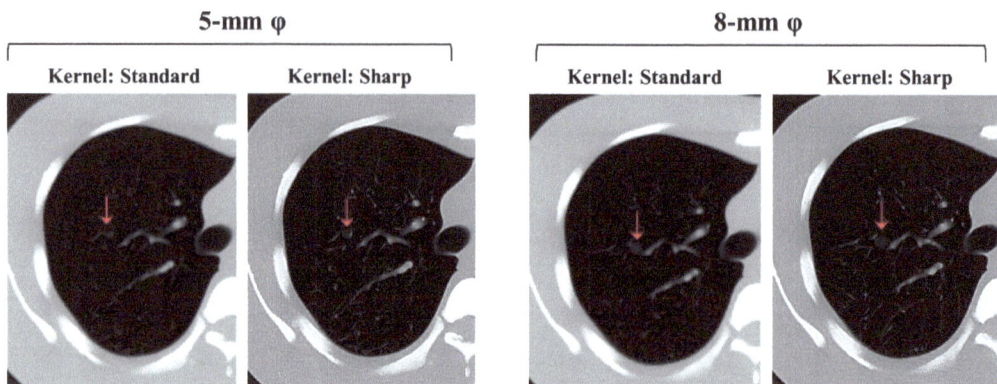

Figure 4: Computed tomography (CT) image from the different reconstruction kernels of the same slice, demonstrating the content of artificial pulmonary nodules.

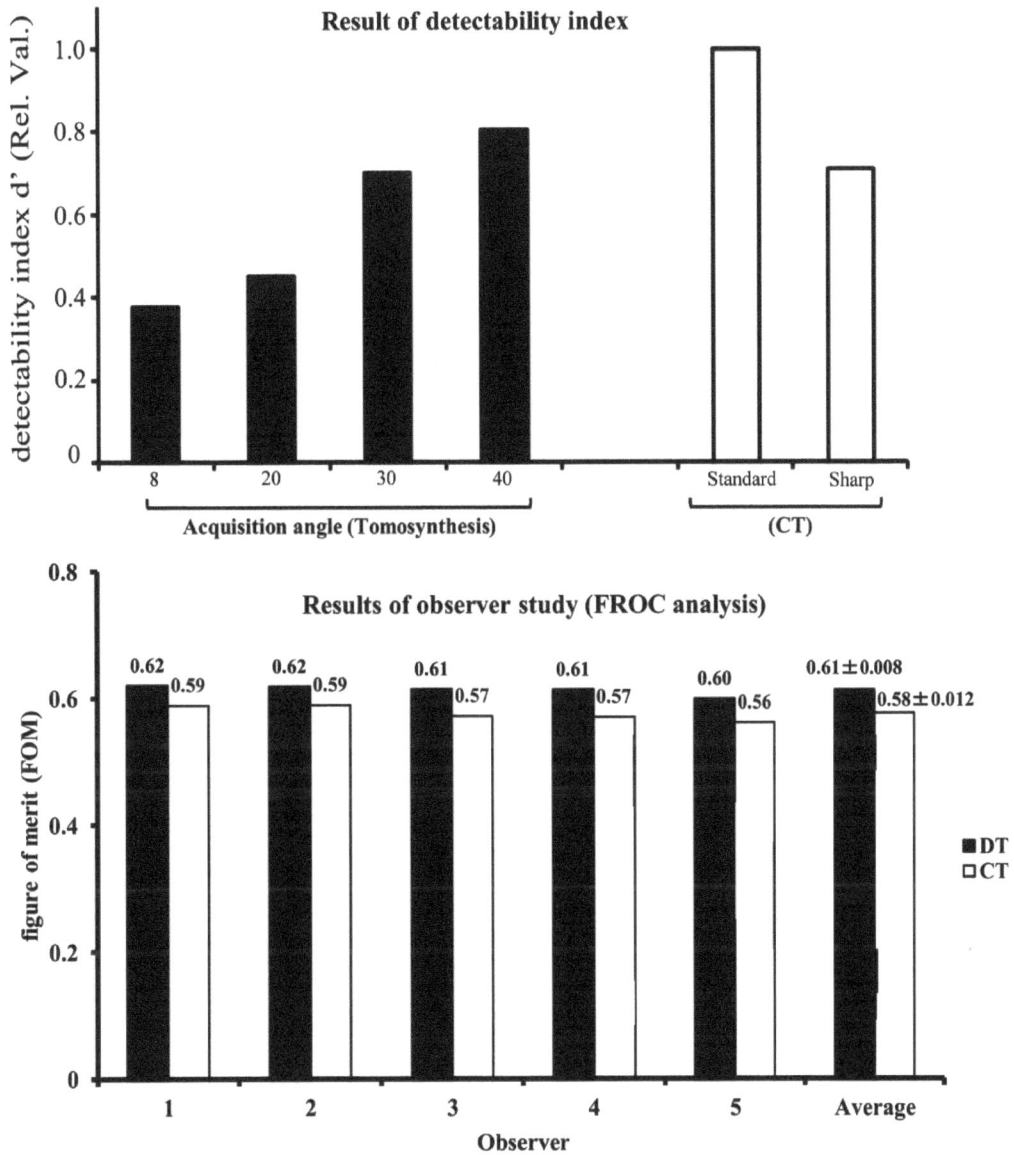

Figure 5: (upper) Tomosynthesis and CT images showing the detectability index (DI). At the 40° acquisition angle, the high-detectability phantom case demonstrated clear detectability by tomosynthesis imaging, which produced increased DI values for identical planes.(lower) Jackknife free-response receiver operating characteristics for tomosynthesis and CT for observers. Uncertainty bars represent 95% confidence intervals. (DT, tomosynthesis; CT, computed tomography)

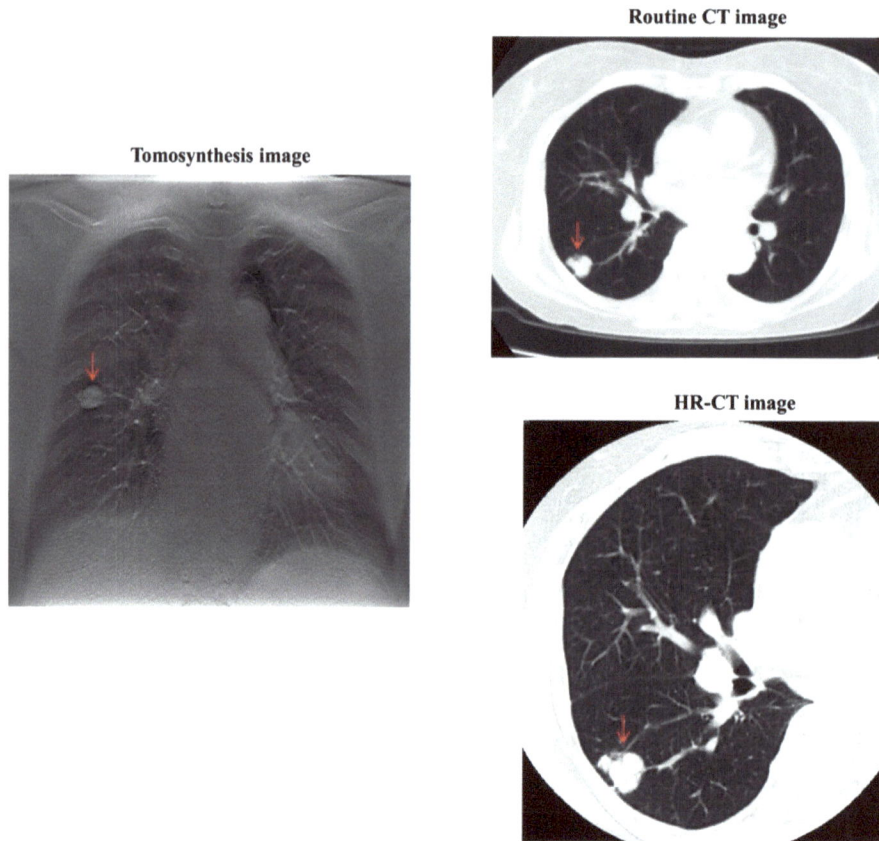

Figure 6: Lung cancer in a 64-year-old female

4.2   Comparison between Tomosynthesis and Radiography

Currently, lung cancer is the primary cause of cancer death, and its occurrence continues to increase worldwide. Because of its high sensitivity, normal-dose helical CT is currently considered as the gold standard for lung-cancer detection. Previous studies have cited that low-dose helical CT can detect early-stage lung cancer, thereby decreasing morbidity (Yankelevitz *et al.*, 2000). CT is advantageous because it is insusceptible to the problem of reduced accuracy due to the overlapping anatomy. However, it has disadvantages such as high radiation dose and cost compared to those of chest radiography. In contrast, the advantages of chest radiography include short examination time, low cost, and easy access; however, low sensitivity and specificity are its prominent disadvantages. In chest radiography, the 3D view of the chest is projected onto a 2D image; therefore, for many analyses, the capability to detect pathological findings is limited by the overlapping anatomy rather than quantum noise. Chest radiography has been shown to have a relatively low sensitivity for detecting pulmonary nodules. This poor sensitivity precludes its use as a screening method despite its low cost, low dose, and the widespread availability of radiographic devices.

Two radiographic findings indicate a benign lesion while differentiating between benign and malignant pulmonary masses: the presence of calcifications in the mass and mass stability (Godwin, 1983; Littleton, 1983; Siegelman *et al.*, 1980, 1986; Zerhouni *et al.*, 1988). A benign pattern of calcifications has been considered necessary to eliminate malignancy (Littleton, 1983; Fraser *et al.*, 1986; McLendon *et al.*, 1985; O'Keefe *et al.*, 1957; Siegelman *et al.*, 1983). For evaluating diffusely disseminated pulmonary nodules, the identification of calcifications in the nodules has been helpful in restricting differential diagnosis (Burgener *et al.*, 1991). Conventional radiography and tomography have been used to detect calcifications, but they have been replaced by CT to a great extent (Siegelman *et al.*, 1980, 1986). However, CT has several inherent problems, including motion artifacts and variation in the reconstruction algorithms used by different scanners. Despite recent developments in CT techniques, difficulties persist, such as slice-level shifting in thin-section CT images acquired during different breaths as well as the ability to clarify the characteristics and distribution of calcifications relative to the soft tissue components of the mass.

With respect to the images of nodules with similar sizes, the contrast was greater when tomosynthesis imaging was used for processing as compared with that when radiography was used. From the three most recent reports, first, the detectability of pulmonary nodules is considerably higher with chest tomosynthesis than that with chest radiography. Sensitivity was increased, especially for nodules smaller than 9 mm (Vikgren *et al.*, 2008). Second, tomosynthesis is an advantageous new technique for detecting pulmonary nodules (Zachrisson *et al.*, 2009). Third, tomosynthesis showed considerably improved sensitivity in the detection of known small lung nodules in all three size groups [< 5, 5 – 10, and > 10 mm] when compared with chest radiography (Dobbins *et al.*, 2008). According to these reports, in terms of detectability, tomosynthesis is better than radiography.

Dual-energy-subtraction (DES) imaging has been proposed and investigated by many researchers to reduce the impact of anatomical "noise" during disease detection by chest radiography. DES involves forming the two radiographic projections of the patient with the X-ray beams of different energies. By exploiting the difference between the energy dependence of attenuation for the bone and soft tissue, the contrast of the bone can be reduced, thereby producing a soft-tissue-only image, whose contrast can be reduced to produce the image of a bone (Brody *et al.*, 1981). Recent computed radiography (CR) systems have been hampered by poor subtraction effectiveness, workflow inconveniences, and detective-quantum-efficiency limitations of the CR technology. However, DES radiography is useful in detecting calcifications (Littleton *et al.*, 1983; Zerhouni *et al.*, 1988; Hickey *et al.*, 1987; Ishigaki *et al.*, 1986, 1988; Nishitani *et al.*, 1986). Projected images acquired by DES techniques exhibit the disadvantage of overlapping anatomical features (e.g., calcifications superimposed over the ribs or spine).

We developed a DES tomosynthesis system to address the problem associated with projection-type DES images (Gomi *et al.*, 2011). In this study, we reported the results of previous studies that compared the accuracy of chest DES tomosynthesis with those of DES radiography for detecting artificial pulmonary nodules with and without calcifications.

4.2.1   Conditions for Data Acquisition

We compared the performances of DES tomosynthesis and DES radiography. In both DES-tomosynthesis and DES-radiography imaging, pulsed X-ray exposures were used involving rapid switching between low (60 kVp) and high (120 kVp) exposures. Tomography was performed with a linear tomographic movement of the system, scan time of 6.4 seconds, and swing angle of 40°. Thirty-seven low- and high-voltage projected images were sampled during a single tomographic pass. Each projected image was acquired at 200 mA and 20 – 25 ms exposure time for low-voltage X-rays, and at 200 mA and 25 ms or less for high-voltage X-rays. DES radiography images were processed from low- and high-voltage projected images by two double-exposure acquisitions. Bone or soft tissue images were produced by weighted subtraction for each different absorption coefficient (Figure 7).

Calcification was composed of hydroxyapatite (powder type). The amount of calcification for the nodules of 5mm and 8mm diameters were 100 mg/mL and 200 mg/mL, respectively. The different concentrations of hydroxyapatite were painted onto the surface of glass disks having the same size. Calcifications were associated adequately closely with the nodules so that they appeared in the same reconstructed slice.

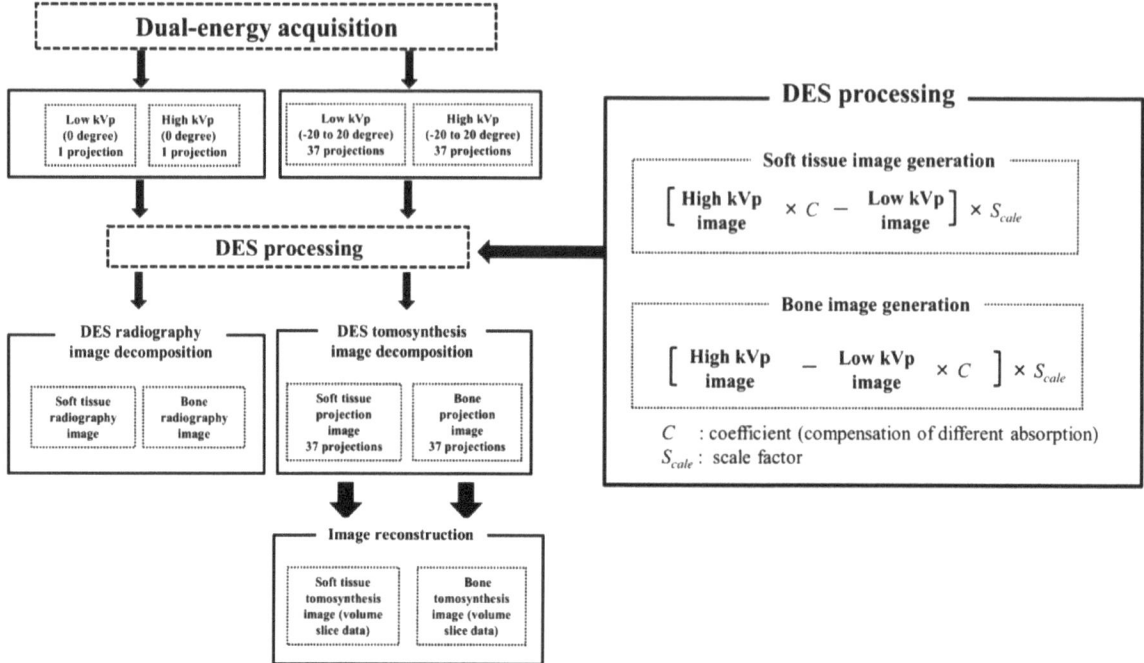

Figure 7: Illustration of the imaging sequence and processing by dual-energy-subtraction (DES) tomosynthesis imaging and DES radiography.

4.2.2   Contrast-to-noise ratio

To compare the effectiveness of chest DES tomosynthesis with that of DES chest radiography for detecting artificial pulmonary nodules, these nodules were arranged in the lung region (middle-lobe position). Our analysis considered the contrast-to-noise ratio (CNR) of different sizes and the calcification degrees of the artificial pulmonary nodules. In the phantom study, CNR was calculated for DES tomosynthesis and DES radiography techniques. CNR is defined in equation (3).

$$CNR = \frac{N_1 - N_0}{\sigma_0} \tag{3}$$

where N_1 is the mean pixel value in the line within the region of artificial pulmonary nodules with and without calcification, N_0 is the mean pixel value in the line in a background area, and σ_0 is the standard deviation of pixel values in the base line. Throughout these results, σ_0 includes structure noise that can obscure the object, besides photon statistics and electronic noise.

4.2.3   Observer Study

Five thoracic radiologists examined the images for detecting artificial pulmonary nodules by using the receiver-operating-characteristic (ROC) paradigm. We examined 30 samples with and 30 samples without the different degrees of each artificial pulmonary nodule with and without calcifications by both DES tomosynthesis and DES radiography. The artificial pulmonary nodules were randomly arranged in the lung region. Each case occurred only once in each group. The locations of the nodules were determined by a random number generator, which was also used to determine the reading order. The readers presented the important slice and both the DES-radiography and DES-tomosynthesis images at different times. The observers were not allowed to change window width and window level or use the pan and zoom functions. Before each session, the two image sets of the 10 educational cases were shown. Each observer was instructed to detect artificial pulmonary nodules using DES-tomosynthesis images and DES-radiography images and to separately describe the presence of an artificial pulmonary nodule on a continuous scale from 1 to 100. For artificial pulmonary nodules without calcifications, the score 100 indicated the highest degree of confidence (probably a nodule), and the score 0 indicated the lowest degree of confidence (probably not a nodule). For artificial pulmonary nodules with calcifications, the score 100 indicated the highest degree of confidence (probably a calcification), and the score 0 indicated the lowest degree of confidence (probably not a calcification). The time frame between reading the images was 1–2 weeks. Because of the considerable difference between the appearances of tomosynthesis images and radiographs, this procedure was considered appropriate to avoid recall bias.

The ROC-analysis software used was DBM MRMC Version 2.2 (Derbaum, 2009). The detectability of the artificial pulmonary nodules was described by the area under the ROC curves (Hanley et al., 1982, 1983). For statistical analysis, the average area under the curve (AUC) and standard deviation were obtained by individually fitting the ROC curves to the confidence ratings of each observer and averaging the estimated areas across observers. AUC values were used to test the significance of the differences via the paired F-test.

4.2.4   Results of the Comparison between Tomosynthesis and Radiography

CNR was evaluated for DES-tomosynthesis and DES-radiography processing, as shown in Figure 8. Both the methods of DES processing for the high-contrast detectability phantom having clear contrast detectability increased the contrast in the same-level images. In these images, contrast was greater with DES-tomosynthesis processing than that with DES-radiography processing. The CNR and quality of the DES-tomosynthesis images were significantly superior to those obtained by DES radiography. For DES tomosynthesis, CNR for the 5-mm-diameter nodules was 31% (without calcification) and 96% (with calcification); these values increased with size to a CNR of 59% for the 8-mm-diameter nodules (without calcification) and 49% (with calcification).

On the basis of the results of ROC-performance analysis (Figure 9), the detection ability of our DES tomosynthesis was considerably better than that of DES radiography (8-mm-diameter nodules without calcification at $p < 0.03$ and with calcification at $p < 0.003$). ROC analysis was simple in DES tomosynthesis because it easily detects calcification and large (8mmdiameter) artificial pulmonary nodules. Calcification may be buried all over the rippled pattern. We can expect to improve calcification detection if the effect of the rippled pattern is excluded.

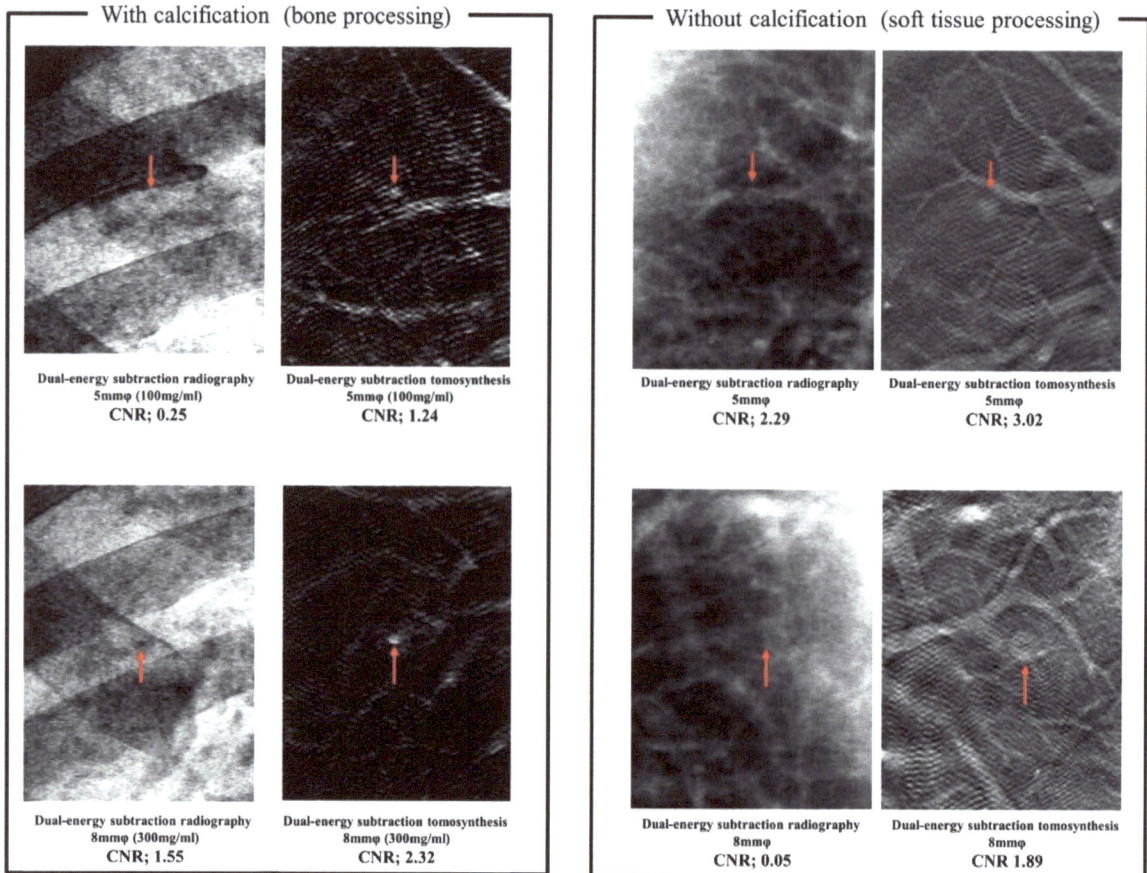

Figure 8: DES tomosynthesis image and DES radiograph of the same slice, which demonstrates the content of artificial pulmonary nodules with and without calcifications. The case of the high-contrast-detectability phantom having a clear contrast detectability increased the contrast-to-noise ratio values for identical planes by DES tomosynthesis imaging.

Chest images obtained by DES tomosynthesis (with and without DES processing) and DES radiography (with and without DES processing) in a clinical case were compared. The high-contrast-detectability case having clear contrast detectability with and without DES tomosynthesis imaging produced identical planes (Figure 10 and 11).

5   Potential Artifact

5.1   Blur

Ideally, structures in a given plane of interest should be clearly displayed in the corresponding tomosynthesis-reconstruction plane, those located outside that plane should not be visible. Essentially, the limited angular range of the tomosynthesis-image-acquisition geometry dictates that spatial resolution is restricted to the dimension perpendicular to the detector plane. Therefore, out-of-plane structures cannot be completely removed from the reconstruction plane. Out-of-plane structures are present in every recon

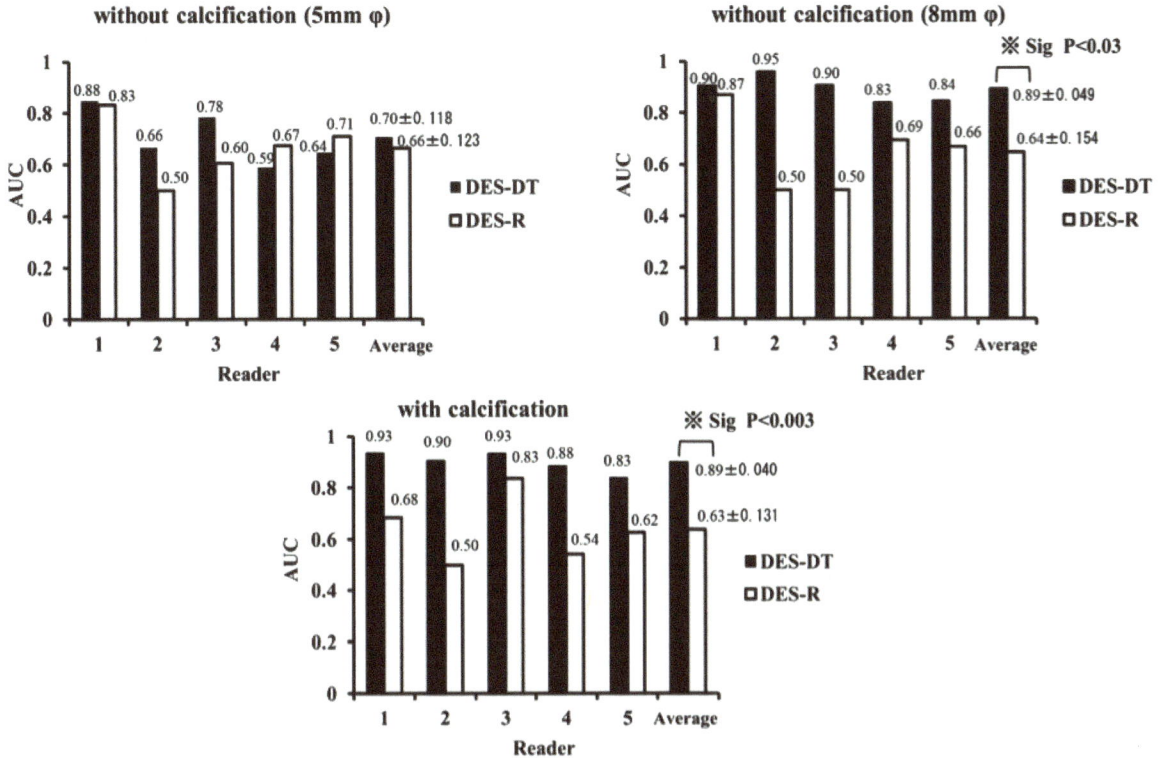

Figure 9: Comparison of the area under the curve to detect the accuracy of DES tomosynthesis imaging and DES radiography by the observers. (DES–DT,DES tomosynthesis,DES radiography)

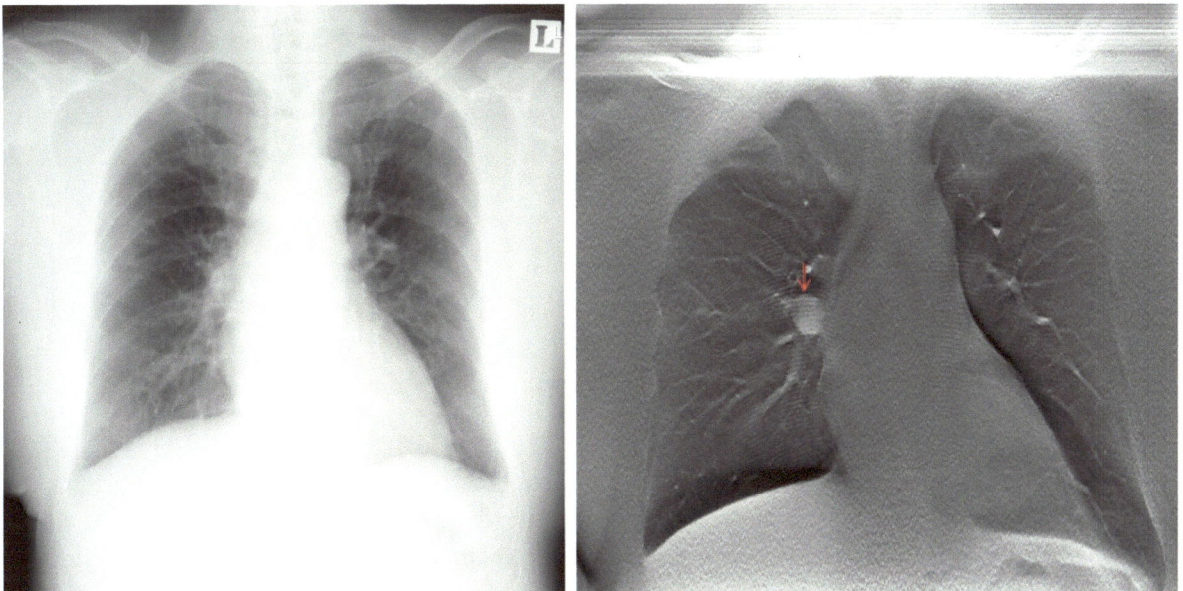

Figure 10: Lung cancer in a 74-year-old male (tomosynthesis at 120 kVp, 200 mA, and 5ms exposure time; radiography at 120 kVp, 200 mA, and 20ms exposure time). **Left:** X-ray radiography image. **Right:** Tomosynthesis image.

**DES tomosynthesis image
(bone processing)**

**DES tomosynthesis image
(tissue processing)**

**DES radiography image
(bone processing)**

**DES radiography image
(tissue processing)**

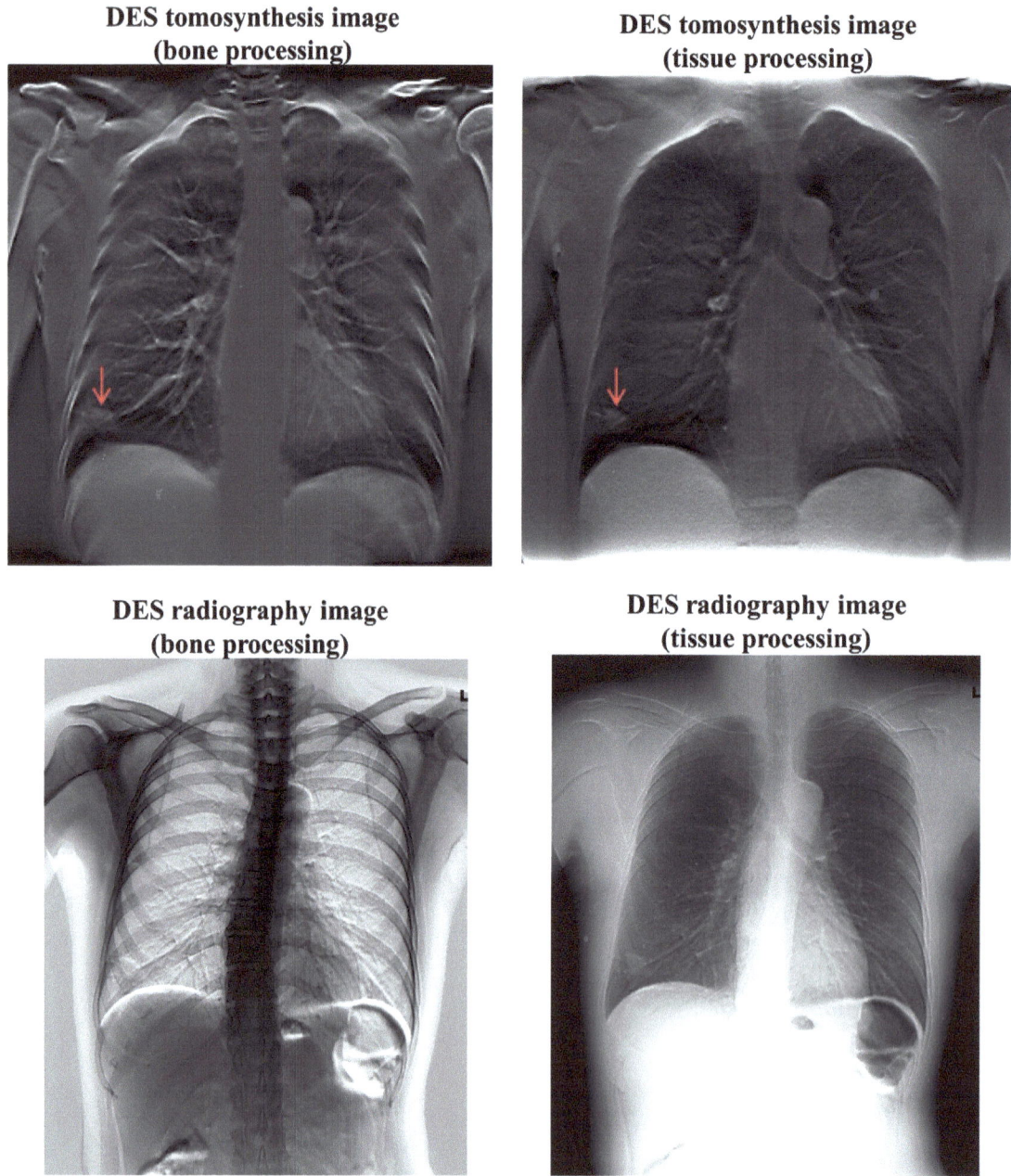

Figure 11: Lung cancer in a 74-year-old female.

struction plane, but most of the structures are invisible because various low-amplitude structures from projections overlap each other in the reconstruction plane; therefore, these structures are blurred. Out-of-plane structures with high-attenuation features cannot be blurred. They appear as the multiple replicates of the particular feature in every reconstruction plane except for the one in which the actual high-attenuation feature is located. At one projection angle, these shadowing features are distributed along the line formed by the X-ray source and actual feature (Figure 12).

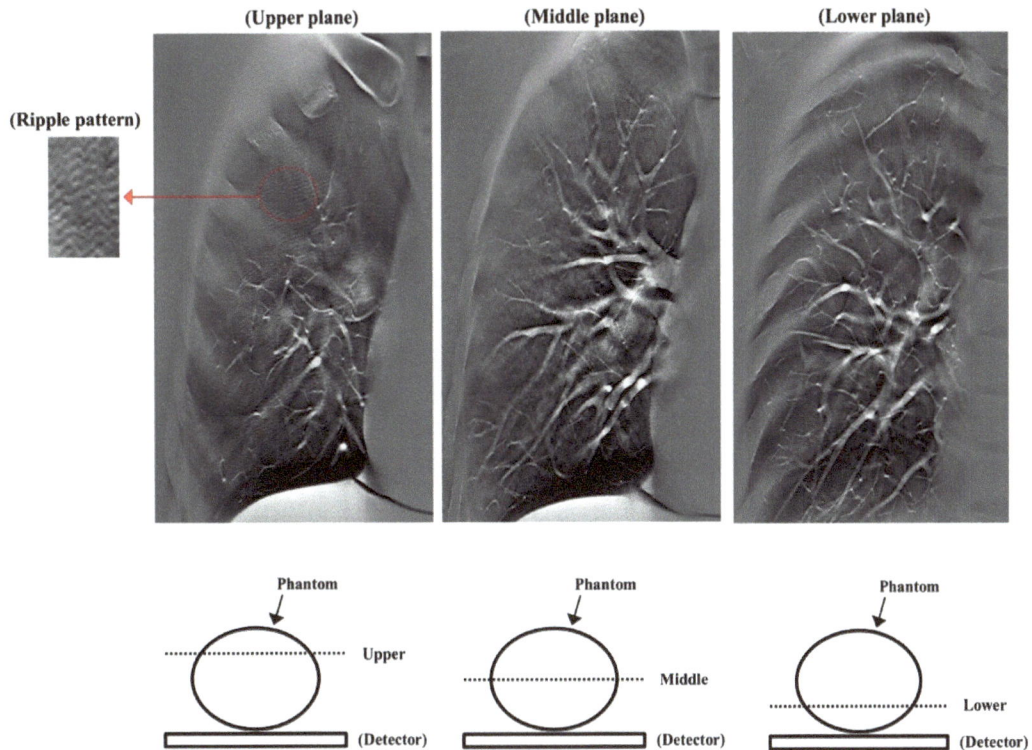

Figure 12: Out-of-plane structures are present in every reconstruction plane, but most of them are invisible because various structures from projections overlap each other in the reconstruction plane; therefore, these structures are blurred.

5.2   Ripple

Quantum noise plays an important role in the degradation of the contrast resolution of radiographs. It increases inversely with the X-ray exposure and constitutes the dominant noise source at low radiation-exposure levels. Because of quantum noise, the technical factors used to reduce the radiation dose in our system are limited to the levels usually employed in conventional tomography. However, synthesized tomograms can be obtained with technical factors same as those used for radiography when quantum noise can be endured. Any calcifications are visible in the presence of the overwhelmingly rippled artifact on DES tomosynthesis images (Figure 12). This artifact is a consequence of the inherent misalignment between the low and high kVp images because the X-ray tube moves continuously. These features may be amenable to filtration, but such filtration may eliminate the desired clinical features.

6   Discussions

Tomosynthesis systems have a few limitations. For example, patients undergoing this procedure have to stand still and hold their breath firmly. In addition, tomosynthesis has a limited depth resolution, which may explain the difficulty in detecting pathologies in the subpleural region and the occurrence of artifacts in medical devices (Johnsson *et al.*, 2010).

Our observer study also had a few potential limitations. Because of the learning effect, the frequency with which artificial pulmonary nodules were detected by the observers increased with each reading session. This was expected considering that the phantom model remained the same while the artificial pulmonary nodules changed in each configuration. However, this factor was corrected in the observer-study design and statistical-analysis model.

The observers were forewarned that the objective of the test was to detect artificial pulmonary nodules and that half of the cases was normal. The study did not assess other thoracic abnormalities encountered in clinical practice, in which diagnostic decisions are more complex than the mere detection of pulmonary nodules. A more stringent criterion should be investigated, especially one that would considerably lower the number of false positive ratings and increase the sensitivity estimates. Because of the artificial nature of our study, its results should be compared with those observed in an actual clinical setting. Therefore, the performance of the observers was probably optimized when compared with a physician's performance in routine clinical practice. However, this effect should not have led to bias of the results of this study in favor of or against either of the systems used.

7   Conclusion

In conclusion, the advantages of tomosynthesis over CT are its decreased radiation dose and the practical accessibility of such an examination. Therefore, tomosynthesis may be a useful alternative to CT as a screening method to detect pulmonary nodules. The results of our phantom study were probably corrected in the observer-study design and statistical-analysis model to facilitate use in an actual clinical setting. Therefore, the tomosynthesis system may become available for clinical use in the near future.

Initial data from our study suggest that DES tomosynthesis will substantially enhance sensitivity and specificity in pulmonary-nodule detection. Despite its potential, DES tomosynthesis is a new technique. Therefore, there is no guidance for its integration into the clinical practice of chest radiography. The most reliable signs for discriminating between benign and malignant masses are the growth rate of the mass and the presence or absence of calcifications within the mass. Because calcifications are commonly observed in benign masses and no other radiographic characteristic is specific to characterizing masses, it is important to detect and characterize calcification within lesions.

References

Ziedses des, Plantes BG. (1932).Eine neue methode zur differenzierung in der roentgenographie (planigraphie).Acta radiologica, 13, 182-192.

Grant DG. Tomosynthesis. (1972).A three-dimensional radiographic imaging technique.IEEE transactions on bio-medical engineering, 19, 20-28.

Well IT, Raju VM, Rowberry BK, Johns S, Freeman SJ, Wells IP. (2011). Digital tomosynthesis –a new lease of life for the intravenous urogram?. The British Journal of Radiology, 84, 64-68.

Stiel G, Stiel LG, Klotz E. Nienaber CA.(1993).Digital flashing tomosynthesis: A promising technique for angiographic screening.IEEE transactions on medical imaging,12, 314-321.

Duryea J, Dobbins JT, Lynch JA. (2003).Digital tomosynthesis of hand joints for arthritis assessment. Medical Physics, 30, 325-33.

Sone S, Kasuga T, Sakai F, Kawai T, Oguchi K, Hirano H, Li F, Kubo K, Honda T, Haniuda M.(1995).Image processing in the digital tomosynthesis for pulmonary imaging.European Radiology, 5, 96-101.

Niklason LT, Christian BT, Niklason LE, Landberg CE, Slanetz PJ, Giardino AA, Moore R, Albagli D, DeJule MC, Fitzgerald PF, Fobare DF, Giambattista BW, Kwasnick RF, Liu J, Lubowski SJ, Possin GE, Richotte JF, Wei CY, Wirth RF.(1997).Digital tomosynthesis in breast imaging.Radiology, 205, 399-406.

Dobbins JT III, Godfrey DJ. (2003).Digital x-ray tomosynthesis: curent state of the art and clinical potential.Physics in medicine and biology,48, R65-106.

Johnsson AA, Fagman E, Vikgren J, Fisichella VA, Boijsen M, Flinck A, Kheddache S, Svalkvist A, Bath M. (2012). Pulmonary nodule size evaluation with chest tomosynthesis. Radiology, 265, 273-282.

Svalkvist A, Johnsson AA, Vikgren J, Hakansson M, Ullman G, Boijsen M, Fisichella V, Flinck A, Molnar D, Mansson LG, Bath M. (2012). Evaluation of an improved method of simulating lung nodules in chest tomosynthesis. Acta Radiologica, 53, 874-884.

Quaia E, Baratella E, Cernic C, Lorusso A, Casagrande F, Cioffi V, Cova MA. (2012). Analysis of the impact of digital tomosynthesis on the radiological investigation of patients with suspected pulmonary lesions on chest radiography. European Radiology, 22, 1912-1922.

Yamada Y, Jinzaki M, Hasegawa I, Shiomi E, Sugiura H, Abe T, Sato Y, Kuribayashi S, Ogawa K. (2011). Fast scanning tomosynthesis for the detection of pulmonary nodules: diagnostic performance compared with chest radiography, using multidetector-row computed tomography as the reference. Investigative Radiology, 46, 471-477.

Kak A, Slaney M. (1988).Principles of computerized tomographic imaging.IEEE, ISBN 0-89874-494-X, New York

Smith DB. (1985).Image reconstruction from cone-beam projections: necessary and sufficient conditions and reconstruction methods. IEEE transactions on medical imaging,Ml-4, 14-25.

Feldkamp LA, Davis LC, Kress JW. (1984).Practical cone-beam algorithm. Journal of the Optical Society of America, A1, 612-619.

Stitik FP, Tockman MS. (1978).Radiographic screening in the early detection of lung cancer. Radiologic Clinics of North America16, 347-366.

Muhm JR, Miller WE, Fontana RS, Sanderson DR, Uhlenhopp MA.(1983).Lung cancer detected during a screening program using four-month chest radiographs. Radiology 148, 609-615.

Yankelevitz DF, Reeves AP, Kostis WJ, Zhao B, Henschke CI.(2000).Small pulmonary nodules: volumetrically determined growth rates based on CT evaluation. Radiology 217, 251-56.

Siegelman SS, Khouri NF, Leo FP, Fichman EK, Braverman RM. Zerhouni EA.(1986).Solitary pulmonary nodules: CT assessment. Radiology 160, 307-312.

Zwirewich CV, Vedal S, Miller RR, Muller NL.(1991).Solitary pulmonary nodules: High resolution CT and radiologic-pathologic correlation. Radiology 179, 469-476.

Murata K, Itoh H, Todo G, Kanaoka M, Noma S, Itoh T, Furuta M, Asamoto H, Torizuka K.(1986).Centrilobular lesions of the lung: Demonstration by high-resolution CT and pathologic correlation. Radiology 161, 641-645.

Webb WR. (1991).High resolution lung computed tomography. Normal anatomic and pathologic findings. Radiologic Clinics of North America 29, 1051-1063.

Miller ER, McCurry EM, Hruska B. (1971).An infinite number of laminagrams from a finite number of radiographs. Radiology 98, 249-255.

Grant DG. Tomosynthesis: A three-dimensional radiographic imaging technique. (1972).IEEE Transactionon Biomedical Engineering 19, 20-28.

Baily NA, Lasser EC, Crepeau RL. (1973).Electrofluoro-plangigraphy. Radiology 107, 669-671.

Kruger RA, Nelson JA, Ghosh-Roy, Miller FJ, Anderson RE, Liu PY.(1983).Dynamic tomographic digital subtraction angiography using temporal filtration. Radiology 147, 863-867.

Sone S, Kasuga T, Sakai F, Aoki J, Izuno I, Tanizaki Y, Shigeta H, Shibata K.(1991).Development of a high-resolution digital tomosynthesis system and its clinical application. Radiographics 11, 807-822.

Sabol JM. (2009).A Monte Carlo estimation of effective dose in chest tomosynthesis. Medical Physics 36, 5480-5487.

Gomi T, Nakajima M, Fujiwara H, Takeda T, Saito K, Umeda T, Sakaguchi K. (2012). Comparison between chest digital tomosynthesis and CT to detect artificial pulmonary nodules for screening: a phantom study. The British Journal of Radiology85, e622-e629.

Dobbins JT III, Godfrey DJ. (2003).Digital x-ray tomosynthesis: current state of the art and clinical potential. Physics in Medicine and Biology 48, R65-R106.

Internal commission on radiation units and measurements (ICRU), 'Medical imaging-The assessment of image quality,' ICRU Report No.54 (Bethesda, MD, 1996).

RichardS, Siewerdsen JH, Jaffray DA, Moseley DJ, Bakhtiar B. (2005).Generalized DQE analysis of radiographic and dual-energy imaging using flat-panel detectors. Medical Physics 32, 1397-1413.

Södra Älvsborgs Sjukhus. ViewDEX 2.0. http://www.vgregion.se/sas/viewdex/. Published 2009; Accessed 5 October 2009.

Ruschin M, Timberg P, Båth M, Hemdal B, Svahn T, Saunders RS, Samei E, Andersson I, Mattsson S, Chakrabort DP, Tingber A.(2007).Dose dependence of mass and microcalcification detection in digital mammography: free response human observer studies. Medical Physics 34, 400-407.

Chakraborty DP. (2006).Analysis of location specific observer performance data: validated extensions of the jackknife free-response (JAFROC) method. Academic Radiology 13, 1187-1193.

Chakraborty DP. JAFROC software 2.3a. http://www.devchakraborty.com/. Published 2008; Accessed 17 April 2008. Godwin JD (1983). The solitary pulmonary nodule. Radiologic Clinics of North America 21, 709-21.

Littleton JT (1983). Pluridirectional tomography in diagnosis and management of early bronchogenic carcinoma. In: sectional imaging methods. A comparison, edited by Little JT & Durizch ML. University Park Press, 155.

Siegelman SS, Zerhouni EA, Loe FP, Khouri NF, Stitik FP. (1980). CT of the solitary pulmonary nodule. American Journal of Roentgenology135, 1-13.

Zerhouni EA, Caskey C, Khouri NF (1988). The pulmonary nodules. SeminarsinUltrasound, CT, andMRI9, 67-78.

Fraser RG, Hickey NM, Niklason LT, Sabbagh EA, Luna RF, Alexander CB, Robinson CA, Katzenstein AL, Barnes GT. (1986). Calcification in pulmonary nodules. detection with dual-energy digital radiography. Radiology 160, 595-601.

McLendon RE, Roggli VL, Foster WL Jr, Becsey D (1985). Carcinoma of the lung with osseous stromal metaplasia. Arcjhivesof Pathology& Laboratory Medicine109, 1051-3.

O'Keefe ME Jr, Good CA, McNonald JR (1957). Calcification in solitary nodules of the lung. American Journal of Roentgenology77, 1023-33.

Siegelman SS, Zerhouni EA (1983). Computed tomography of the solitary pulmonary nodule. In: Sectional imaging methods. A comparison, Edited by Littleton JT and Durizch ML. Baltimore: University Park Press, 155.

Burgener FA, Kormano M (1991). Differential diagnosis in conventional radiology. Berlin : Thieme Verlag.

Vikgren J, Zachrisson S, Svalkvist A, Johnsson AA, Boijsen M, Flink A, Kheddache S, Båth M. (2008). Comparison of chest tomosynthesis and chest radiography for detection of pulmonary nodules: human observer study of clinical cases.

Radiology 217, 251-256.

Zachrisson S, Vikgren J, Svalkvist A, Johnsson AA, Boijsen M, Flinck A, Månsson LG, Kheddache S, Båth M. (2009). Effect of clinical experience of chest tomosynthesis on detection of pulmonary nodules. Acta Radiologica 50, 884-891.

Dobbins JT III, Mcadams HP, Song JW, Li CM, Godfrey DJ, Delong DM, Paik SH, Martinez-Jimenez S. (2008). Digital tomosynthesis of the chest for lung nodule detection: interim sensitivity results from an ongoing NIH-sponsored trial. Medical Physics 35, 2554-2557.

Brody WR, Butt G, Hall A, Macovski A. (1981). A method for selective tissue and bone visualization using dual-energy scanned projection radiography. Medical Physics 8, 353-357.

Hickey NM, Niklason LT, Sabbagh E, Fraser RG, Barnes GT. (1987). Dual-energy digital radiographic quantification of calcium in simulated pulmonary nodules. American Journal of Roentgenology 148, 19-24.

Ishigaki T, Sakuma S, Horikawa Y, Ikeda M, Yamaguchi H. (1986). One-shot dual-energy subtraction imaging. Radiogy 161, 271-3.

Ishigaki T, Sakuma S, Ikeda M (1988). One-shot dual-energy subtraction chest imaging with computed radiography. Radiology 168, 67-72.

Nishitani H, Umezu Y, Ogawa K, Yuzuriha H, Tanaka H, Matsuura K. (1986). Dual-energy projection radiography using condenser X-ray generator and digital radiography apparatus. Radiology 161, 533-5.

Gomi T, Nakajima M, Fujiwara H, Umeda T. (2011). Comparison of chest dual-energy subtraction digital tomosynthesis imaging and dual-energy subtraction radiography to detect simulated oulmonary nodules with and without calcifications. Academic Radiology 18, 191-196.

Derbaum K. DBM MRMC software 2.2. URL: http://perception.radiology.uiowa.edu (published June 24, 2008; accessed January 7, 2009).

Hanley JA, McNeil BJ. (1982). The meaning and use of the area under receiver operating characteristic (ROC) curves. Radiology 143, 29-36.

Hanley JA, McNeil BJ. (1983). A method of comparing the areas under receiver operating characteristic curves derived from the same cases. Radiology 148, 839-843.

Johnsson AA, Vikgren J, Svalkvist A, Zachrisson S, Flinck A, Boijsen M, Kheddache S, Månsson LG, Båth M. (2011). Overview of two years of clinical experience of chest tomosynthesis at Sahlgrenska University Hospital. Ratiation Protection Dosimetry, 139, 124-129.

Multiscale Fractal Descriptors to Quantify Behaviours of Healthy and Diseased Tissues in Mammographic Images

Leandro Alves Neves
Department of Computer Science and Statistics
São Paulo State University, São José do Rio Preto, Brazil

Marcelo Zanchetta do Nascimento
Faculty of Computer Science
Federal University of Uberlândia, Brazil

Moacir Fernandes de Godoy
Transdisciplinary Center for Study of Chaos and Complexity
São José do Rio Preto Medical School, Brazil

1   Introduction

Mammography is considered a relevant imaging method and it has been effective aid for radiologists, mainly in the early detection of occult breast cancers. This method contributes to reduce the mortality rate by as much as 41% according to one South Australian study (Verma *et al.*, 2010). However, the overlapping of structures and physical effects present in the process of image acquisition can influence the accuracy and reliability of diagnosis (do Nascimento *et al.*, 2008). As a result, radiologists fail to detect 10% – 30% of malignant lesions on mammograms during the exam (Gupta *et al.*, 2006). Radiologists employed double reading of the same screening mammogram to improve the accuracy of mammography system (Wei *et al.*, 2011). Obviously, this procedure is too expensive, complex, and time consuming, particularly in screening programs where a high number of mammographic images have to be read (Mencattini *et al.*, 2010).

An alternative is the development of computer-aided diagnosis (CAD) as second reader. This system has been applied to mammographic images to assist radiologists on lesion analysis such as microcalcification and mass. The sensitivity of the CAD system for masses is considerably lower than the corresponding performance for microcalcifications (Astley & Gilbert, 2004). Masses are more difficult to detect than microcalcifications because their features can be obscured or similar to normal breast parenchyma. Masses often occurred in the dense areas of the breast tissue and have smoother boundaries than microcalcifications.

In the literature there are studies with CAD proposals to support the diagnosis of breast cancer. Algorithms for image processing together with artificial intelligence techniques are used in order to detect and classify breast cancer. The analysed features can describe the behaviour of structures identified in healthy or diseased, (Duncan & Ayache, 2000; Cheng *et al.*, 2003; Kallergi, 2004; Hukkinen & Pamilo, 2005; Gennaro & di Maggio, 2006; Dantas *et al.*, 2012). These models are used for identification of lesions in the breast by extraction of the area of interest in mammograms. Typically, two classes of features are extracted from mammograms with these algorithms, namely morphological and non-morphological features. Morphological features are used to quantify information related to the morphology of a lesion, such as size or shape. Texture analysis is an important class that represents gray level properties of images used to describe non-morphological features. Texture can be very useful for experiments of medical image classification and identification. In mammographic image processing, these features are used to distinguish density patterns that indicate different levels of risk to developed malignant lesions (Qian *et al.*, 2001). However, regions of interest (ROIs) selected with a square or rectangular window can include background regions with different behaviours of healthy or diseased patterns. The background regions are commonly identified as partial pixels (PP), which have different features of diseased or healthy tissue (Mencattini *et al.*, 2008b).

Methodologies have been proposed for texture analysis of medical images. Many of these proposals evaluate the local behaviour of the texture via statistical (Gupta *et al.*, 2006), structural (Ayres & Rangayvan, 2005) and spectral (Ramos *et al.*, 2012; Gorgel *et al.*, 2009) properties of the image. A study shows that these methods fail to distinguish many natural textures and examples of these indistinct textures include mammographic images (Kaplan, 1999). To represent these natural textures, we can use models employing methods that behave similarly to natural phenomena. For such, the fractal techniques are potential alternatives as natural descriptors of textures (Backes *et al.*, 2012). The fractal and lacunarity techniques are alternatives to analyse images with self-similar content (M. Ivanovici, 2011), such as texture (Backes *et al.*, 2012), mainly when observed on different scales. This association is known as the multiscale fractal signature (Coelho & Costa, 1995; Chaudhuri & Sarkar, 1995; Plotnick *et al.*, 1996). The application of these descriptors is an efficient approach for quantifying and qualifying of information in different areas of knowledge (Emerson *et al.*, 1999; Du & Yeo, 2002; Plotze *et al.*, 2005; Goldberger *et al.*, 1990; Baish & Jain, 2000; Mancardi *et al.*, 2008; Neves *et al.*, 2011).

The applicability of fractal descriptors for medical diagnostics leaves no doubt of their potential to quantify different phenomena. Pulmonary alveolar structure and capillary network are examples that demonstrate the fractal properties present in parts of living organisms (Mandelbrot, 1995). There is evidence that fractal properties are present in the human body. Then, it is possible to quantify the structures and establish correlations between fractal properties in healthy and diseased cells (Goldberger *et al*., 1990; Baish & Jain, 2000; Mancardi *et al*., 2008).

In mammography, an approach that can still be explored is the characterisation of the normal and diseased breast structures based on texture. In this work is presented a study to discriminate the behaviours of normal and diseased breast structures, considering measures of lacunarity and fractal dimension with the corresponding texture signatures (Stojic *et al*., 2006; Pruess, 2007; H Li, 2007; Chaudhuri & Sarkar, 1995; Dua *et al*., 2010). Furthermore, the quantification of the adjacent structures for the malignant nodules are presented, considering the multilevel segmentation method based on maximum entropy. In our experiments, the texture signatures were calculated and the fractal behaviours were defined for the breast structures. The quantification presented here provides important information about these structures and may contribute with the developments of CAD systems. For experimental evaluation, a data set of mammography images of Digital Database for Screening Mammography (DDSM) was used.

The study is structured as follows: In Section 2.1, we present the groups of mammography cases selected from a public database, the Digital Database for Screening Mammography (DDSM). In sections 2.2 and 2.3 are described, respectively, the procedures used to determine the regions of interest (ROIs) and regions defined as partial pixels (PP). The details of the proposed segmentation method applied on ROIs are presented in Section 2.4. Next, in Sections 2.5, we describe the quantification of ROIs using the fractal dimension and lacunarity. The method used to show the distinctions between the groups investigated was described in Section 2.6. Finally, Section 3 discusses the results of applying the proposed method for evaluation of normal and diseased breast structures.

2   Materials and Methods

An overview of the research methodology of model for quantifying mammographic image made up of an segmentation method based on maximum entropy and multiscale fractal techniques is shown in Figure 1.

2.1   Data Set

The database used in this work was taken from the Digital Database for Screening Mammography (DDSM) (Heath et al, 1998). The DDSM project is a joint effort of researchers from the Massachusetts General Hospital (D. Kopans, R Moore), the University of South Florida (K. Bowyer), and the Sandia National Laboratories - EUA (P. Kegelmeyer). The DDSM database has been widely used as a benchmark for numerous articles on the mammographic area, for being free of charge and having a vast and diverse quantity of cases. It is constituted of mammographic images and its corresponding technical and clinical information, including exam dates, age of patients, digitalization equipment (as well as resolution, number of rows, pixels per row and bits per pixel of the acquired images), lesion types, according to Breast Imaging Reporting and Data System (BIRADS), and existent pathologies.

The data set consisted of 164 mammographic images in mediolateral oblique (MLO) and craniocaudal (CC) views taken from the DDSM, half containing a mass, rated as abnormal images, and half with no lesions distributed in two group: malignant nodule (MN), with 54 cases (29 CC and 29 MLO) and the group

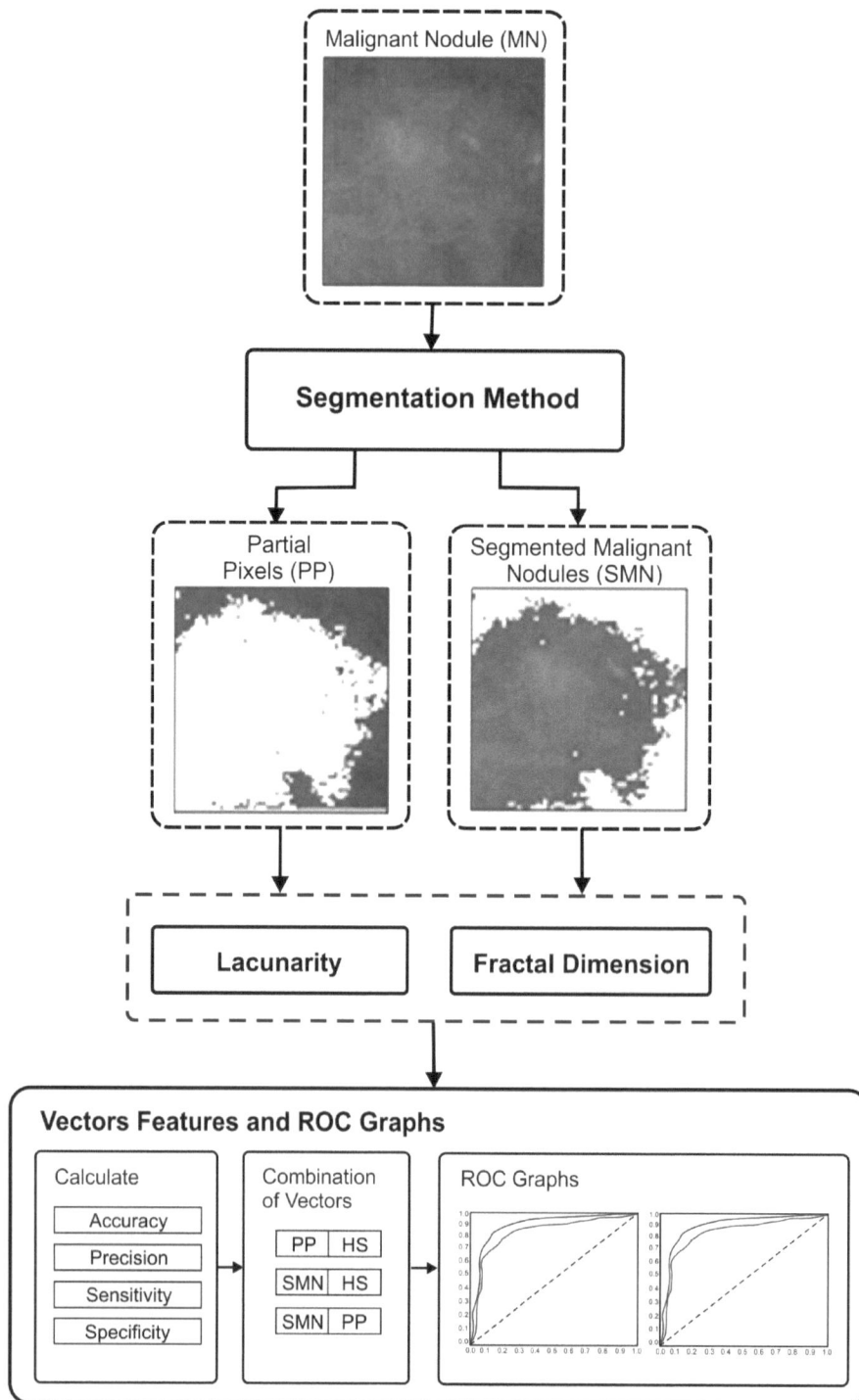

Figure 1: Flow chart of the proposed system in this work.

healthy structure (HS), with the other images (54 CC and 54 MLO). The normal images have been used for estimating the false-positive ratio, and positive examples were extracted from malignant cases. We selected digitised images with a Lumisys laser film scanner at 50 μm pixel size. Each image has a resolution of 256 gray level tones. In these experiments only the images obtained by the Lumisys scanner were selected because questions related to standardisation of resolution.

2.2   Selection of ROIs

In order to quantify the groups malignant nodule (NM) and healthy structure (HS) were obtained the ROIs of mammographic images. ROIs of the group HS were extracted from mammograms without the presence of lesions. The lesions of the group NM were taken from the code-chain of the file .ics, which is available at the DDSM project. We used this information to extract ROIs, which are square regions (sub-images) from original mammograms. In our approach, the ROIs were defined using a window of size 64 $\times$ 64 pixels, whose centers correspond to the centers of the presented lesions. Some lesions selected by a radiologist in the images of the CC and MLO views are shown in Figure 2. The study of lesions using ROIs is a process commonly adopted in the majority of works of literature (Mencattini *et al.*, 2008a).

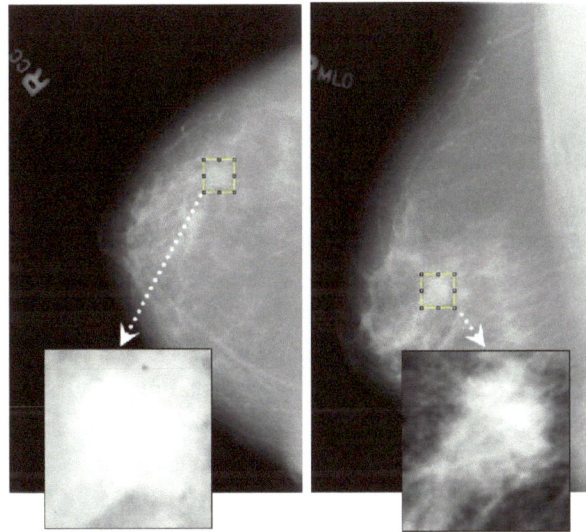

Figure 2: Mammographic image and regions of interest.

2.3   Definition of Partial Pixels (PP)

The stage of definition of the ROIs in which extracts square sub-images with mass region can include background region, i.e., adjacent tissues. This region defined as partial pixels (PP) influences the measurements and distinctions of the patterns. In this study, the regions PP were quantified separately to demonstrate their differences in relation to other groups evaluated (Mencattini *et al.*, 2008a). Segmentation algorithm was applied in ROIs of the group NM to define the group PP. This step resulted in the group consisting only with the segmented malignant nodule (SMN) and the group with the adjacent tissues, which was defined as PP. The measurements based in multiscale fractal techniques were performed for each group mentioned.

2.4   Automatic Multilevel Thresholding Method

The characterisation of healthy and diseased tissues based on texture with fractal depends on the appropriate segmentation stage of the ROIs. This stage allows the separation of an object into parts based on a uniformity criterion (Dougherty & Henebry, 2001). In order to obtain high-quality segmentation, image processing systems primarily use thresholding, which consists of determining an intensity value at which an object is best distinguished from the background region. In the literature, there are different automatic thresholding methods based on different criteria (Borys *et al.*, 2008; Gonzalez & Woods, 2008; Brink, 1996; Kapur *et al.*, 1985; Abutableb, 1989; Otsu, 1979). In many cases, however, a single threshold is not sufficient in furnishing adequate segmentation for the entire image. In such situations, variable and multilevel thresholding methods are used (Sahoo *et al.*, 1988). Aboud Neta (Neta *et al.*, 2008) proposes one such method, but its sensitivity leads to high rates of non-significant threshold values, which can compromise the assessment of the image.

The automatic multilevel thresholding method determines the threshold value based on the identification of maximum entropy, which compare the entropy values in different regions of the histogram of the image evaluated (Neves *et al.*, 2011). This method is an improvement over the proposed approach by Aboud Neta (Neta *et al.*, 2008), allowing better control over the threshold values identified. For such, properties were added to the method mentioned, such as the division of the histogram into classes, analysis of the slope percentage and maximum entropy to define the threshold values.

2.4.1   Quantification of Histogram

In this step the histogram of gray levels was calculated for all the images of the group MN. The histogram was divided into classes for each image. A class is one or more gray levels values that make up the histogram. For this division, it is necessary to predefine the class size. If the class size informed is 1, the process evaluates each level of intensity of the histogram. For values greater than 1, the increment considered in the iteration process of the method is the predefined value. To exemplify the proposed approach consider a class made up of 10 intensity levels and a histogram with 256 gray levels. The first class encompasses levels 0 to 9, the second encompasses 10 to 19, and so forth, totalling 25 classes with 10 levels of gray and one class with 6 gray levels (Figure 3).

2.4.2   Valleys Analysis

This stage consists of the identification of classes with relevant valley regions (sharper peaks) to the specification of the threshold values. The method automatically identifies these classes by means of sign transition, examining the following features: the average of the points contained in the first half of the analysed class is compared with the average of the points in the second half of the same class. If the value of the first half is smaller, the values of the histogram are increasing toward a peak and the sign attributed to the class is positive. Otherwise, a negative sign is attributed to the class, indicating movement toward a valley. The sign of the next class is determined. If there is a transition from a negative to a positive sign, the valley is relevant to the specification of a threshold value (Figure 4).

The determination of threshold values based on valley analysis may be influenced by homogeneous regions in the histogram (with no valleys or with non-significant valleys). To solve this problem, the proposed method determines that a class is relevant if it has a slope percentage greater than a predefined value. This value can be adjusted to the type of image being studied. A slope percentage is the percentage difference between the averages of the points in the first and second halves of the analysed class. Two or more classes are grouped together when the slope percentage is lower than the predefined value. This resource allows controlling the sensitivity of the multilevel thresholding method. A threshold value is established when the slope percentage of the class is greater than the predefined value.

In the study of mammographic images, the values used for the input parameters for segmentation were classes of size 10 and slope with 35%. These values were established empirically to segment the ROIs considering the features present in the tissues of the groups SMN and PP.

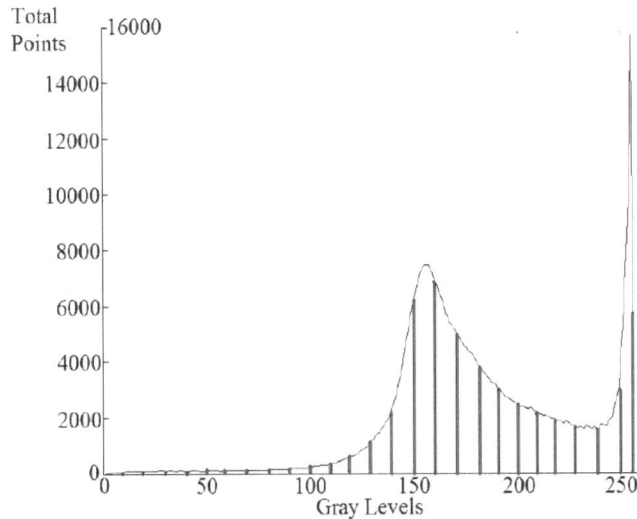

Figure 3: Example to demonstrate the proposed approach considering a histogram that was divided into 26 classes: 25 containing 10 levels and one containing 6 levels; vertical lines delimit classes.

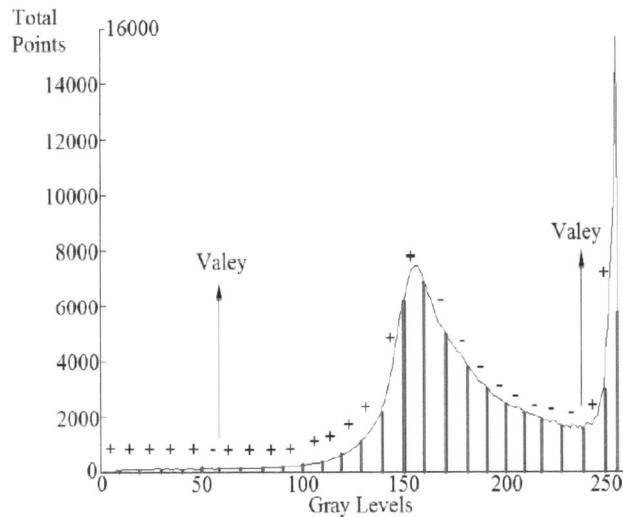

Figure 4: Example of histogram divided into 26 classes with indication of two relevant valleys to the determination of threshold values - one at gray levels 50-59 and another at gray levels 230-239.

2.4.3   Threshold Identification Using Maximum Entropy

For each relevant class identified, we calculated a threshold value based on entropy considering a probability of an intensity correctly segmenting a given group of objects. For such, the image was taken as the result of a random process in which probability p corresponds to the probability of a pixel in the image taking on an intensity value i ($i=1,..,n$) (Gonzalez & Woods, 2008), as shown in equations 1 and 2. The intensity or gray level of the class with the greatest entropy was identified as a threshold value (Sahoo *et al.*, 1988).

$$H = -\sum_{i=1}^{n} p_i log\,(p_i),\tag{1}$$

$$p_i = \frac{n_i}{N},\tag{2}$$

in which H is the entropy of the image; n is the total number of outputs (number of gray levels in the image); p_i is the probability of gray level i being found in the image; n_i is the number of pixels with intensity i; and N is the total number of pixels in the image.

The results obtained by segmentation stage defined two new groups: the group only in the region of the segmented malignant nodule (SMN) and adjacent tissues, partial pixels (PP). Quantification was performed for each image contained in SMN, PP and HS based on the fractal descriptors.

2.5   Quantification of ROIs

The texture in an image is characterised by the repetition of a model over a region: the model may be repeated exactly or with slight variations (Dougherty & Henebry, 2001). The texture analysis allows distinguishing regions with the same reflectance features, which is a process used for the recognition, analysis, description and classification of digital images. There are different approaches to the study of texture described in the literature (Dougherty & Henebry, 2001). This work present the quantification of texture features of ROIs using more natural methods, such as the fractal dimension and lacunarity.

2.5.1   Fractal Dimension

The fractal dimension is defined as a measure of the complexity of objects. When applied to textures, this measure allows quantifying the complexity of the organisation of its pixels (how much the space is filled in). Box counting is one of the frequently techniques used for estimating the fractal dimension of objects and images (Dougherty & Henebry, 2001; Backes & Bruno, 2006).

In this stage, fractal dimension was calculated for the groups SMN, PP and HS. The multiscale approach was achieved by overlaying a grid on the ROIs evaluated. The aim was to obtain the number of squares necessary to cover the image. For an mammographic image (ROI) I as the input, the number of squares that contain structure of interest (SMN, PP or HS) presents in I, $N_r(I)$ depends on the size of the box r (see equation 3). The relation defined in equation 3 allows estimating the fractal dimension D based on equation 4.

$$N_r(I) = \mu r^{-D},\tag{3}$$

$$D = -lim_{r\to 0}\frac{ln(N_r(I))}{ln(r)}.\tag{4}$$

However, equation 4 imposes the calculation of a limit. One solution is to adapt this calculation to a discrete space, in which box counting $N_r(I)$ is performed for different values of r. As consequence, it is necessary to define a set S with the possible sizes of sides r used in the diverse iterations of the method, based on the dimensions of the structure under analysis (Backes & Bruno, 2006), equation 5. The approximation of a straight line is obtained from the regression (log-log graph) of $N_r(I)$ (number of boxes occupied) by r (size of side of this box). It is possible to define $D=-\alpha$ as the fractal dimension of I.

$$\forall r_i \in S \begin{cases} r_0 = max(height, width) \\ r_{i+1} = r_i/2 \end{cases} \tag{5}$$

The Box-Counting method was applied as a texture descriptor for evaluation of ROIs. This technique is an appropriate method of fractal dimension evaluation for images with or without self-similarity. In this study, a luminance of a pixel represents its height. This modification implies dividing the image into cubes with side r, instead of boxes of side r, as a consequence produces a new $N_r(I)$, depending on the number of cubes that contain part of the image. The log-log graphs represent the texture signatures of the groups SMN, PP and HS. The approach used in the transformation reduced the dimensionality of the information examined for a one-dimensional function. This reduction allowed quantifying the behaviour of textures.

2.5.2   Lacunarity

Lacunarity characterises the way the pixels are distributed and organised in a given region of the image. Lacunarity is complementary to the fractal dimension, shapes with the same fractal dimension may have different lacunarity values. One of the most popular methods for estimating lacunarity is the gliding-box method (Brink, 1996; Backes & Bruno, 2006; Neta *et al.*, 2008), which was used in the present study.

The process begins with a box of side r positioned in the upper left corner of the image and a count of the number of points in the image is performed. This process is repeated for all the lines and columns of the image, producing a frequency distribution of the lesion present in image. The number of boxes with side r containing structures of interest (SMN, PP or HS) M of the ROI is designated by $n(M,r)$, with the total number of boxes counted designated by $N(r)$. This frequency distribution is then converted into a probability distribution $F(M,r)$, equation 6. The first (A^1) and second (B^2) moments of this distribution are determined in equations 7 and 8. Lacunarity (L) for a box of size r is defined in equation 9, (Brink, 1996; Backes & Bruno, 2006).

$$F(M,r) = \frac{n(M,r)}{N(r)}, \tag{6}$$

$$A^{(1)} = \sum MF(M,r), \tag{7}$$

$$B^{(2)} = \sum M^2 F(M,r), \tag{8}$$

$$L(r) = \frac{B^{(2)}}{\left(A^{(1)}\right)^2}. \tag{9}$$

In this stage, we also used the multiscale approach similar to fractal dimension. The value of $N(r)$ was evaluated for different values of the parameter r, where: for r the value (r_0) was considered the value of the largest dimension of image, i.e., $r_0=max(height, width)$; and in other iterations, the size of r was successively reduced by half, i.e., $r_i+1=r_i/2$, (Backes & Bruno, 2006). This procedure also follows a limit $(lim_{r\to0})$ which represents multiscale approach. The approximation of a straight line was obtained by regression (log-log graph) of $L(r)$ by r. This allowed determination of $L=-\theta$ as the multiscale lacunarity of structure of interest (SMN, PP or HS). Luminance of a pixel was considered as the height of the pixel in the image in order to implement multiscale lacunarity as a texture descriptor for each ROI. The use of this operation was possible to divide the image into cubes of side r. This resulted in new values of $n(M,r)$ and $N(r)$ according to the total numbered cube. Thus, log-log graphs were used to represent the texture signatures of the groups SMN, PP and HS.

2.6   Performance evaluation

After image processing operations and texture signatures, performance evaluation measures were performed using Receiver Operating Characteristic (ROC) curves. This approach was adopted to describe the relationship between the success and failure rates of the groups, indicate the performance rate of descriptors and identify the most appropriate cut-off points (Dua et al., 2009).

Radiologists have used ROC curve to identify an optimal cut-off point in the stage of clinical test (Erkel & Pattynama, 1998). Patients with the disease have generally values above the cut-off point. On the other hand, values below the optimal cut-off point are generally present in most normal patients. Obviously there will be cases where individuals who truly have the disease present values below the cut-off (false negatives) while normal individuals may possibly have values above the cut-off points (false positives). Diagnostic test is applied in the study group and in the group called "gold-standard" to determine the optimal cut-off point. The ratio of true positive tests and total number of cases known to have the disease (determined by the gold standard) is the true positive rate, also known as sensitivity. The ratio of true negative tests and the total number of cases that are known to be normal, also according to the gold standard is the true negative rate, known as specificity. The expectation is that with the help of the ROC curve one could find a cut-off point that will somehow minimize the number of false positives and false negatives. Minimize false positives and false negatives is the same as maximising sensitivity and specificity (Obuchowski, 2005; Fan et al., 2006).

A ROC curve is constructed considering the true positive rate (sensitivity) plotted against the false positive rate (100 minus specificity). For each point of the ROC curve, a pair of sensitivity / (100-specificity) corresponds to a particular cut-off point (threshold value). This process is adopted for different cut-off points and a test with 100% sensitivity and 100% specificity is considered a perfect discrimination. In this case, the curve is represented in the upper left corner. Thus, the higher the overall accuracy of the test, the more the ROC curve obtained approaches the upper left corner. Therefore, the area under the ROC curve (AUC) is associated to the accuracy of the clinical test. For example, an AUC value of 1.0 indicates that the test is theoretically perfect and an AUC value of 0.5 indicates that there is no discriminative value in the test, which is represented by a straight line which extends diagonally from the lower left to the upper right corner. There are several scales to interpret the value of AUC. An AUC value less than 0.75 is not clinically useful (Obuchowski, 2005; Fan et al., 2006). Examples of ROC curves are shown in Figure 5.

Therefore, the performance evaluation measures are useful to enable an appropriate evaluation of the groups studied, which are: SMN versus PP, SMN versus HS and PP versus HS. The performance of the proposed approach was measured by AUC, precision, sensitivity and specificity (Dua et al., 2009; Fawcett, 2006). Thus, each image was evaluated using the metrics: True positives (TP), true negatives (TN), false positives (FP), and false negatives (FN).

The performance evaluation methods were defined by:

- Precision (PR) is the proportion of positive test results that are true positives (equation (10));

- Sensitivity (SE), measures the proportion of actual positives which are correctly identified (equation (11)); and,

- Specificity (SP), measures the proportion of negatives which are correctly identified (equation (12)).

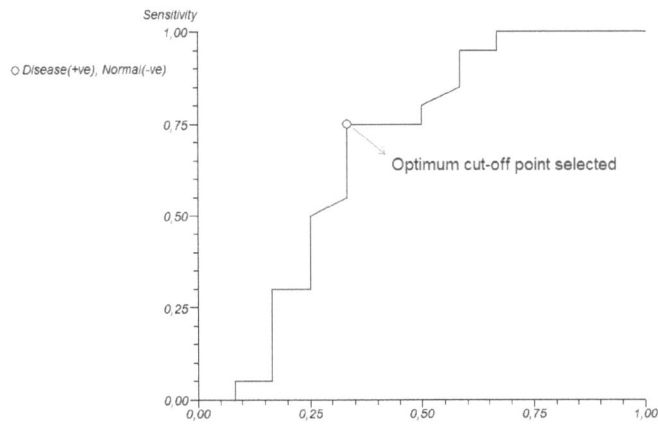

(a)

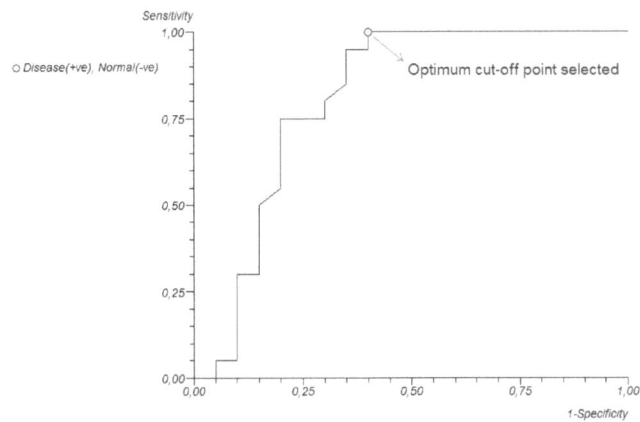

(b)

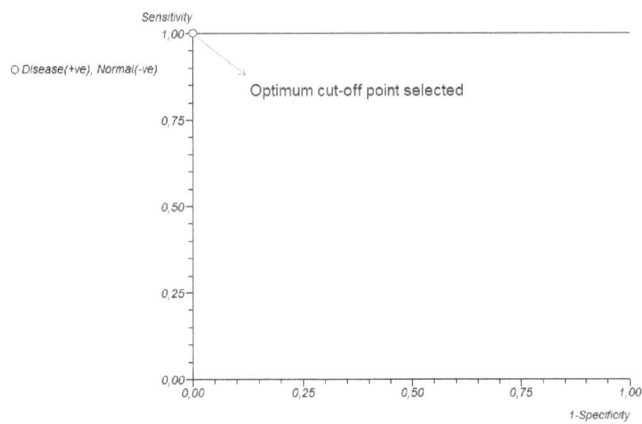

(c)

Figure 5: Examples of ROC curves, considering area under ROC curve with low discriminative value (AUC=0.67) is shown in (a), high discriminative value (AUC=0.8) is shown in (b) and perfect discrimination (AUC=1.0) is shown in (d).

$$Precision = \frac{TP}{TP+FP}, \tag{10}$$

$$Sensitivity = \frac{TP}{TP+FN}, \tag{11}$$

$$Specificity = \frac{TN}{FP+TN}. \tag{12}$$

3   Results

The multilevel thresholding method was applied in images of the group MN and exemplification of the results obtained with ROIs of the CC and MLO views are shown in Figure 6.

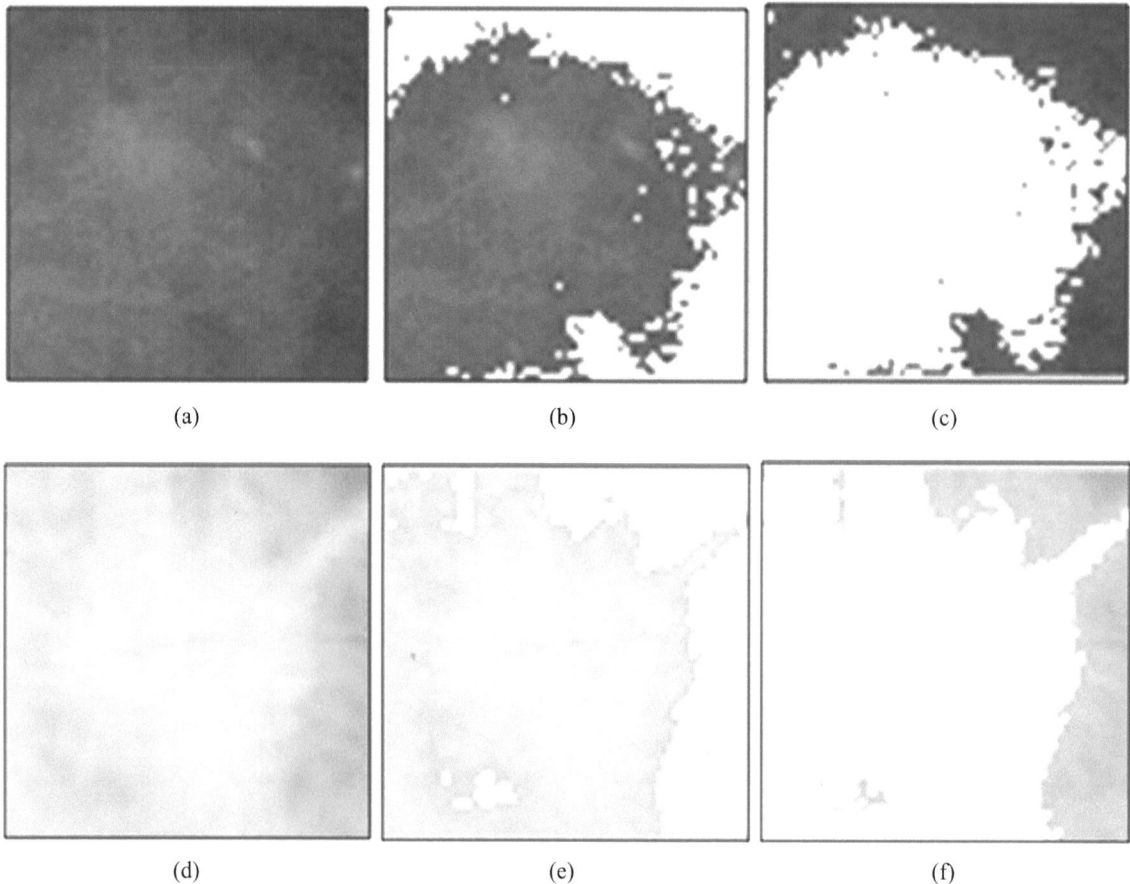

(a)   (b)   (c)

(d)   (e)   (f)

Figure 6: Examples of ROIs used in the proposed approach. The group MN is illustrated in (a) and (d) with ROIs of 64 × 64 pixels in CC and MLO views, respectively. The ROIs of the group MN were segmented with the proposed method (in subsection 2.4), the results are shown in (b) and (e), exemplifying the group SMN, and results of the group PP are presented in (c) and (f).

Texture signatures of the groups SMN versus PP are presented in Figures 7 and 8. Figures show that the group PP presents a behaviour different of the group SMN both observed with the fractal and lacunarity.

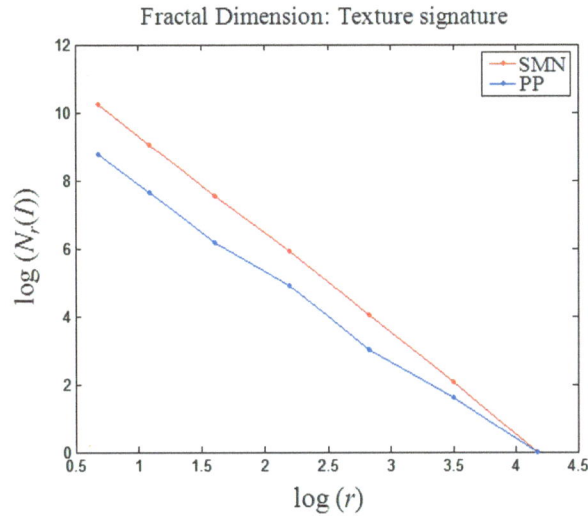

Figure 7: Texture signatures calculated for ROIs shown in Figure 6(e), group SMN, and Figure 6(f), group PP. These signatures were represented in log-log graphs considering the fractal dimension descriptor. The *x* axis indicates the size of the cube and the *y* axis considers the total cubes calculated.

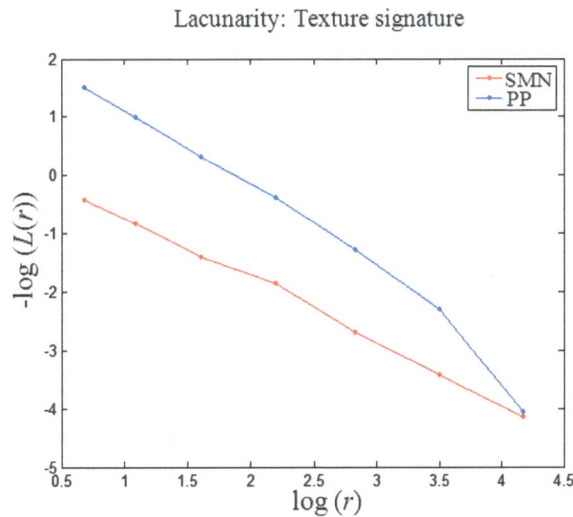

Figure 8: Texture signatures calculated for ROIs shown in Figure 6(e), group SMN, and Figure 6(f), group PP. These signatures were represented in log-log graphs considering the lacunarity descriptor. The *x* axis indicates the size of the cube and the *y* axis considers the lacunarity values.

The ROC curves were generated considering fractal dimension (Figure 9) and lacunarity (Figure 10), both for SMN versus HS, SMN versus PP and PP versus HS. The results obtained with the use of ROC curves are shown in Tables 1 and 2. These tables present area under ROC curve (AUC), with confidence intervals (CI 95%), cut-off points, precision (PR), sensitivity (SE) and specificity (SP).

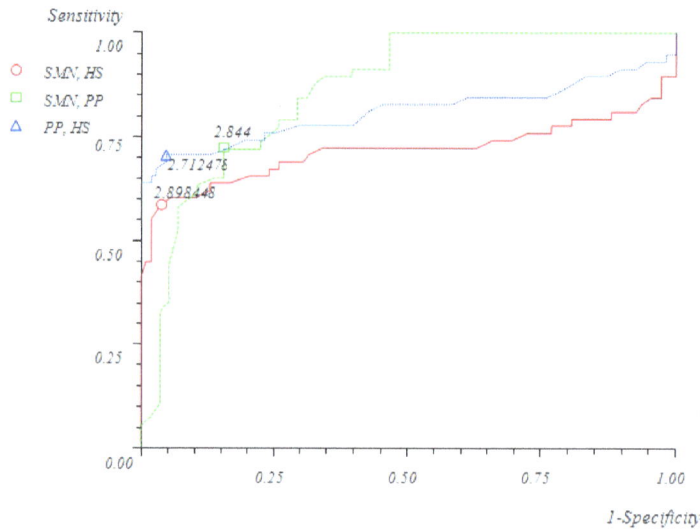

Figure 9: ROC curves considering the fractal dimension values as descriptor: SMN versus HS, SMN versus PP and PP versus HS.

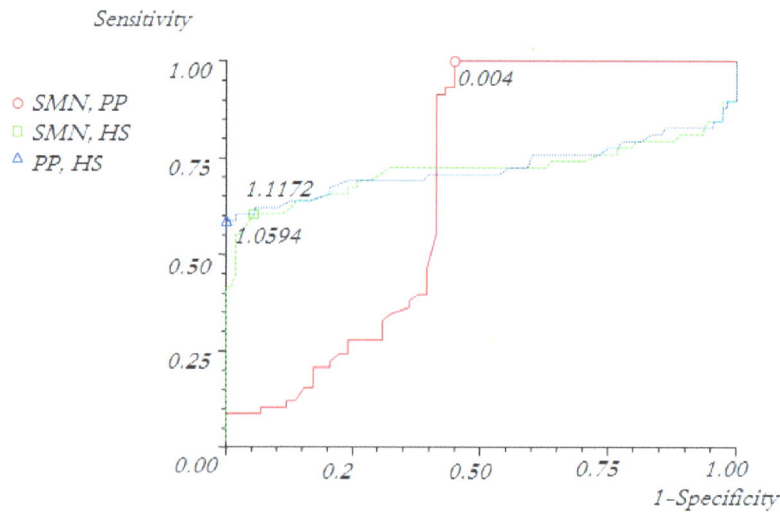

Figure 10: ROC curves considering the lacunarity values as descriptor: SMN versus PP, SMN versus PP and PP versus HS using the lacunarity.

4   Discussion and Conclusion

The stage of identification of threshold values in histograms is relatively simple when the objects present in an image have intensities very distinct with no overlap. Images with irregular intensities can provide histograms with several candidate valleys in the process of definition of a threshold value, the problem focused here. Determination of the valleys allows obtaining the threshold values that separate the most important regions to evaluate a ROI.

Groups	AUC	CI	Cut-off point	PR	SE	SP
SMN versus HS	0.7169	0.6289 - 0.8049	2.8984	0.8947	0.5862	0.9629
SMN versus PP	0.8635	0.7886 - 0.9385	2.844	0.8235	0.7241	0.8448
PP versus HS	0.8109	0.7337 - 0.8882	2.7124	0.8913	0.7068	0.9537

Table 1: Evaluation results with the fractal dimension descriptor considering the groups compared and shown in Figure 9

Groups	AUC	CI	Cut-off point	PR	SE	SP
SMN versus HS	0.7169	0.6289 - 0.8049	1.1172	0.8536	0.6034	0.9444
SMN versus PP	0.6768	0.5750 - 0.7786	0.004	0.6904	1	0.5517
PP versus HS	0.7234	0.6361 - 0.8108	1.0594	1	0.5862	1

Table 2: Evaluation results with the lacunarity descriptor considering the groups compared and shown in Figure 10

Thus, the proposed segmentation algorithm enabled the identification of candidate regions with deeper valleys. In our experiments, this process may have the presence of flat valleys which can be treated as noise present in the histogram of each ROI evaluated. Then, a valley was defined as candidate using the following parameters: comparison with user input values, class sizes and the percentage of slope (region characterised by deeper valleys). The appropriate threshold values for segmentation were obtained from the combination of parameters, which can be considered a disadvantage of the method. However, we suggests that further studies should be performed to determine a more robust method for automation of stage of obtaining of the appropriate combination for the input parameters. Even so, the proposed segmentation method was efficient for the context explored. The method allowed differentiation of structures of interest (Figure 6) with appropriate information to implement the feature extraction stage. This affirmation is based on the evaluation of the different behaviours of the texture signatures (Figures 7 and 8), as well as using the ROC curves (Figures 9 and 10). In our study, different one-dimensional patterns, as shown in Figures 7 and 8, were important features to use of proposed segmentation method. Therefore, we have not used preprocessing filters to modify the features of the histograms in experiments with these images.

In our study, we show that the ROIs contain regions defined as partial pixels (PP) with different patterns of malignant nodule. The results shown in the ROC curves for the groups SMN versus PP and PP versus HS demonstrated tissues with different patterns for descriptor fractal dimension (Figures 9). The group PP has distinctions (AUC) of 81.09% of the group HS and 86.35% of SMN, Table 1. The experiments performed with groups SMN versus PP and SMN versus HS provided significant values to the sensitivity (above 70 %), specificity (above 82 %) and AUC (values above 84 %). The comparison of the groups SMN versus HS provided AUC rate of 71.69 % and a sensitivity rate of 58%. These values show differences, but are not clinically relevant.

Even so, the attribute possible to obtain an important value of specificity (96%), considering that this metric relates to the ability of the test to identify negative results. The results presented allow the inference that the group PP had tissue in degenerative process, with different features of masses and healthy tissues. These values demonstrate the ability of the descriptor to distinguish and quantify the structures investigated.

These procedures confirms the study presented by Mancanttini et al. (Mencattini *et al.*, 2010). The proposed approach also shows the levels of cut-off points needed to determine the rates in comparison among groups presented in Table 1. These information are useful for studies about CAD with decisions based on ROIs defined on the square or rectangular windows (Mencattini *et al.*, 2010). The quantification allows consider the groups focused here in the decision protocols and can providing more accurate results. Furthermore, fractal signature can be features vectors in the decision protocols of CAD and investigating possible patterns exist for each scale of observation.

Considering the lacunarity descriptors, the groups SMN versus PP and PP versus HS demonstrated tissues with distinctions of 67.68% and 72.34%, respectively (Table 2). These values allow the inference that the lacunarity does not show the tissues in transition (PP).

The results obtained in this study allow to define the fractal dimension descriptor as the most suitable to demonstrate a possible behaviour of the structures that constitute the groups SMN, PP and HS. For this, the average fractal dimension was calculated and results are shown in Figure 11. This study demonstrates that fractal dimensions lower are associated with breast cancer (group SMN). Furthermore, fractal dimension allows verify different behaviours between of the groups PP versus HS and SMN. This can indicate tissues in transition. In addition, the fractal dimension was used as a multiscale texture descriptor and this approach demonstrates that breast cancer causes tissues with radiological more uniform and less dense. The distinctions of behaviours also provided important information about the tissues: SMN, PP and HS. This approach shows the differences presented previously.

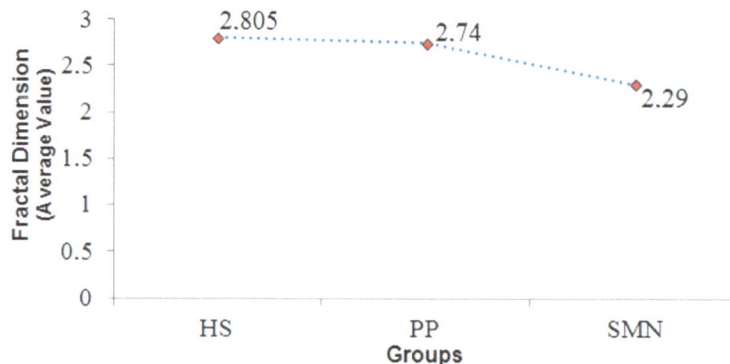

Figure 11: Results of the average values obtained with descriptors fractal dimensions to quantify the behaviour of the groups HS, PP and SMN.

The results obtained by multilevel thresholding method, fractal descriptors, texture signatures and ROC curves shown inter-group differences, mainly considering the groups SMN versus PP and PP versus HS. The AUC values were relevant, with the advantage of quantifying the behaviour of regions with partial pixels. The information presented are important, mainly when CAD system is development with decisions based on ROIs defined on the square or rectangular windows. Furthermore, the contributions mentioned are meaningful and useful for future work to support association signatures of textures in CC and MLO views.

Acknowledgement

This study was supported by UNESP/PROPe (Pro-Reitoria de Pesquisa).

References

Abutableb, A. S. (1989). *Automatic thresholding of gray-level pictures using two-dimensional entropy. Comput. Vision Graph. Image Process., 47(1), 22–32.*

Astley, S. & Gilbert, F. (2004). *Computer-aided detection in mammography. Clinical Radiology, 59(5), 390 – 399.*

Ayres, F. & Rangayyan, R. (2005). *Characterization of architectural distortion in mammograms. Engineering in Medicine and Biology Magazine, IEEE, 24(1), 59 –67.*

Backes, A. R. & Bruno, O. M. (2006). *Segmentacao de texturas por an?lise de complexidade. INFOCOMP Journal of Computer Science, (pp. 87–95).*

Backes, A. R., Casanova, D., & Bruno, O. M. (2012). *Color texture analysis based on fractal descriptors. Pattern Recognition, 45(5), 1984 – 1992.*

Baish, J. M. & Jain, R. K. (2000). *Fractals and cancer. Cancer Res, 60, 3683–3688.*

Borys, P., Krasowska, M., Grzywna, Z. J., Djamgoz, M. B., & Mycielska, M. E. (2008). *Lacunarity as a novel measure of cancer cells behavior. Biosystems, 94(3), 276 – 281.*

Brink, A. D. (1996). *Using spatial information as an aid to maximum entropy image threshold selection. Pattern Recognition Letters, (pp. 29–36).*

Chaudhuri, B. B. & Sarkar, N. (1995). *Texture segmentation using fractal dimension. IEEE Transactions on Pattern Analysis and Machine Intelligence, (pp. 72–76).*

Cheng, H., Cai, X., Chen, X., Hu, L., & Lou, X. (2003). *Computer-aided detection and classification of microcalcifications in mammograms: a survey. Pattern Recognition, 36(12), 2967–2991.*

Coelho, R. C. & Costa, L. d. F. (1995). *The box-counting fractal dimension: Does it provide an accurate subsidy for experimental shape characterization? if so, how to use it? In Symp. on Comp. Graphics and Image Processing (pp. 183–191).*

Dantas, R. D., Nascimento, M. Z., Jacomini, R. S., Pereira, D. C., & RAMOS, R. P. (2012). *Fusion of two-view information: Svd based modeling for computerized classification of breast lesions on mammograms. In N. Uchiyama & M. Z. do Nascimento (Eds.), Mammography - Recent Advances (pp. 261–278).: Intech.*

do Nascimento, M. Z., Frere, A. F., & Germano, F. (2008). *An automatic correction method for the heel effect in digitized mammography images. Journal of Digital Imaging, 21(2), 177 – 187.*

Dougherty, G. & Henebry, G. M. (2001). *A new method for gray-level picture thresholding using the entropy of the histogram. Medical engineering and physics, (23), 369–380.*

Du, G. & Yeo, T. S. (2002). *A novel lacunarity estimation method applied to sar image segmentation. IEEE Transactions on Geoscience and Remote Sensing, 40(12), 2687–2691.*

Dua, S., Singh, H., & Thompson, H. W. (2009). *Associative classification of mammograms using weighted rules. Expert Syst. Appl., 36(5), 9250–9259.*

Dua, S., Singh, H., & Thompson, H. W. (2010). *Associative classification of mammograms using weighted rules. Expert Syst Appl, (pp. 9250–9259).*

Duncan, J. & Ayache, N. (2000). *Medical image analysis: Progress over two decades and the challenges ahead. Pattern Analysis and Machine Intelligence, IEEE Transactions on, 22(1), 85–106.*

Emerson, C. W., Lam, N. N., & Quattrochi, D. A. (1999). *Multi-scale fractal analysis of image texture and patterns. . Photogrammetric Engineering and Remote Sensing, 65(1), 51?62.*

Erkel, A. R. V. & Pattynama, P. M. T. (1998). *Receiver operating characteristic (roc) analysis: Basic principles and applications in radiology. European Journal of Radiology, 27, 88–94.*

Fan, J., Upadhye, S., & AWorster (2006). *Understanding receiver operating characteristic (roc) curves. Canadian Journal of Emergency Medicine, 8(1), 19–20.*

Fawcett, T. (2006). *An introduction to roc analysis. Pattern Recogn. Lett., 27(8), 861–874.*

Gennaro, G. & di Maggio, C. (2006). *Dose comparison between screen/film and full-field digital mammography. European radiology, 16(11), 2559–2566.*

Goldberger, A. L., Rigney, D. R., & West, B. (1990). *Chaos and fractals in human physiology. Sci Am, 262, 42?49.*

Gonzalez, G. C. & Woods, R. E. (2008). *Digital Image Processing, Third Edition. Prentice Hall.*

Gorgel, P., Sertbas, A., Kilic, N., Osman, N., & Osman, O. (2009). *Mammographic mass classification using wavelet based support vector machine. Journal of Eletrical Electronics Engineering, (pp. 867 – 875).*

Gupta, S., Chyn, P. F., & Markey, M. K. (2006). *Breast cancer cadx based on bi-rads descriptors from two mammographic views. Med Phys, 33(6), 1810–7.*

H Li, M L Giger, O. I. O. L. N. L. (2007). *Fractal analysis of mammographic parenchymal patterns in breast cancer risk assessmen. Academic Radiology, (pp. 513–521).*

Hukkinen, K. & Pamilo, M. (2005). *Does computer-aided detection assist in the early detection of breast cancer? Acta Radiologica, 46(2), 135–139.*

Kallergi, M. (2004). *Computer-aided diagnosis of mammographic microcalcification clusters. Medical physics, 31, 314.*

Kaplan, L. (1999). *Extended fractal analysis for texture classification and segmentation. Image Processing, IEEE Transactions on, 8(11), 1572 –1585.*

Kapur, J. N., Sahoo, P. K., & Wong, A. K. C. (1985). *A new method for gray-level picture thresholding using the entropy of the histogram. Computer Vision, Graphics, and Image Processing, 29(3), 273–285.*

M. Ivanovici, N. R. (2011). *Fractal dimension of color fractal images. IEEE Transactions on Image Processing, (pp. 227–235).*

Mancardi, D., Varetto, G., Bucci, E., Maniero, F., & Guiot, C. (2008). *Fractal parameters and vascular networks: facts & artifacts. Theoretical Biology and Medical Modelling, 5(12), 1–8.*

Mandelbrot, B. (1995). *Les Objets fractals : forme, hasard et dimension, survol du langage fractal. Flammarion, 4 edition.*

Mencattini, A., Rabottino, G., Salmeri, M., Lojacono, R., & Colini, E. (2008a). *Breast mass segmentation in mammographic images by an effective region growing algorithm. In Advanced Concepts for Intelligent Vision Systems (pp. 948–957).: Springer.*

Mencattini, A., Salmeri, M., Lojacono, R., Frigerio, M., & Caselli, F. (2008b). *Mammographic images enhancement and denoising for breast cancer detection using dyadic wavelet processing. Instrumentation and Measurement, IEEE Transactions on, 57(7), 1422 –1430.*

Mencattini, A., Salmeri, M., Rabottino, G., & Salicone, S. (2010). *Metrological characterization of a cadx system for the classification of breast masses in mammograms. Instrumentation and Measurement, IEEE Transactions on, 59(11), 2792 –2799.*

Neta, S. R. A., Dutra, L. V., & Erthall, G. J. (2008). Limiariza?§?£o autom??tica em histogramas multimodais. In 7th Brazilian Conference on Dynamics, Control and Applications (pp. 7–9).

Neves, L. A., Oliveira, F. R., Peres, F. A., Moreira, R. D., Moriel, A. R., de Godoy, M. F., & Junior, L. O. M. (2011). Maximum entropy, fractal dimension and lacunarity in quantification of cellular rejection in myocardial biopsy of patients submitted to heart transplantation. Journal of Physics: Conference Series, 285(1), 012032.

Obuchowski, N. A. (2005). Fundamentals of clinical research for radiologists: roc analysis. American Journal of Roentgenology, 184, 364□372.

Otsu, N. A. (1979). A threshold selection method from gray-level histograms. IEEE Transactions on Systems, Man, and Cybernetics, (pp. 62–66).

Plotnick, R. E., Gradner, R. H., Hargrove, W. W., Prestegaard, K., & Perlmutter, M. (1996). Lacunarity analysis: a general technique for the analysis of spatial patterns. Physical Review E, (pp. 5461–5468).

Plotze, R. O., Falvo, M., P?dua, J. G., Bernacci, L. C., Vieira, M. L. C., Oliveira, G. C. X., & Bruno, O. M. (2005). Leaf shape analysis using the multiscale minkowski fractal dimension, a new morphometric method: a study with passiflora (passifloraceae). Canadian Jornal of Botany, 83, 287?301.

Pruess, S. (2007). Some remarks on the numerical estimation of fractal dimension. New-York: Fractals in the Earth Sciences, C.C. Barton and P.R. La Pointe, Plenum Press (Eds).

Qian, W., Sun, X., Song, D., & Clark, R. A. (2001). Digital mammography: Wavelet transform and kalman-filtering neural network in mass segmentation and detection. Academic Radiology, 8(11), 1074 – 1082.

Ramos, R. P., Nascimento, M. Z., & Pereira, D. C. (2012). Texture extraction: An evaluation of ridgelet, wavelet and co-occurrence based methods applied to mammograms. Expert Systems with Applications, 39, 11036 –11047.

Sahoo, P., Soltani, S., & Wong, A. (1988). A survey of thresholding techniques. Computer Vision, Graphics, and Image Processing, 41(2), 233 – 260.

Stojic, T., Reljin, I., & B, R. (2006). Adaptation of multifractal analysis to segmentation of microcalcications in digital mammograms. Physica A, (pp. 494–508).

Verma, B., McLeod, P., & Klevansky, A. (2010). Classification of benign and malignant patterns in digital mammograms for the diagnosis of breast cancer. Expert Systems with Applications, 37(4), 3344 – 3351.

Wei, J., Chan, H.-P., Zhou, C., Wu, Y.-T., Sahiner, B., Hadjiiski, L. M., Roubidoux, M. A., & Helvie, M. A. (2011). Computer-aided detection of breast masses: Four-view strategy for screening mammography. Medical Physics, 38(4), 1867–1876.

Advances in Raman-based Optical Biopsy

Herculano da Silva Martinho

Centro de Ciencias Naturais e Humanas - CCNH
Universidade Federal do ABC - UFABC, Santo Andre-SP, Brazil

1   Introduction

Among several diseases cancer has become the most devastating worldwide (Boyle & Levin, 2008). When detected at its early stages it is well known that the treatment could be very successful. The number of global cancer deaths is projected to increase 45% from 2007 to 2030 (from 7.9 million to 11.5 million deaths), influenced in part by an increasing and aging global population. New cases of cancer in the same period are estimated to jump from 11.3 million in 2007 to 15.5 million in 2030 (Boyle & Levin, 2008). In most developed countries, cancer is the second largest cause of death after cardiovascular disease, and epidemiological evidence points to this trend emerging in the less developed world. Already more than half of all cancer cases occur in developing countries. Cancer prevention is an essential component of all cancer control plans because 40% of all cancer detects can be prevented (Boyle & Levin, 2008). The research for new diagnostic methods and techniques is a very active field. New approaches to obtain early diagnosis of cancer are essential for the cure of patients.

1.1   Current Diagnostic Methods

New developments in medical imaging technologies such as ultrasonography, computer tomography, and magnetic resonance imaging, have improved the quality, selectivity, sensitivity, and quickness of the cancer diagnosis. However, the gold standard method for discriminating normal and altered tissues is still the histopathological analysis performed on a biopsied tissue. Considerable time and cost are required to obtain the biopsy, and the specialized knowledge of a pathologist is needed for diagnosis. In order to overcome these problems and costs, various attempts to achieve a minimally invasive clinical discrimination of cancers have been made, such as those using biomarkers (see Chapter 4 of ref. (Boyle & Levin, 2008)).

The currently available screening and diagnostic methods have their shortcomings that make fast, effective and efficient detection of cancer in the general population impossible, most importantly in developing countries. These limitations are due to the fact that all methods are based on subjective interpretations of morphological abnormalities. For example, the cytological analysis of the cervix, which is the elementary principle of the Pap smear and colposcopy for cervical cancer diagnosis, has a high false negative rate of ~ 50% (Nanda et al., 2000). This fact is inherent to the subjective histological grading of pathologies.

It is common atypical cells be associated with inflammatory infiltrates and the slice be misinterpreted by the pathologist as simple inflammation instead of a malignancy or vice-versa. Data from the World Cancer Report 2008 (see Chapter 4 of ref.: (Boyle & Levin, 2008)) revealed that tests with the best overall serum biomarker (prostate specific antigen) presented 90% sensitivity (S_e) and 25% specificity (S_p). The same resource indicated that S_e and S_p for the Pap smear test that detects cervical intra epithelial cancer fall in the $47-62\%$ and $60-95\%$ ranges, respectively. Oral cytology is one of the most accurate conventional methods with a sensitivity of $S_e = 92\%$ and $S_p = 94\%$.

1.2   Optical Biopsy

Recently, there has been developed new diagnosis tools based on photonic technology. One of these tools is the **optical biopsy**. Optical biopsy refers to techniques where the light-tissue interaction is analyzed and information concerning the state of the tissue is obtained both *"in vivo"* or *"ex vivo"*. Optical spectroscopy techniques such as infrared absorption, fluorescence, and Raman scattering could be also employed. (Holmstrup et al., 2007) described many molecular interaction features in cells and tissues that cannot be accessed by conventional histopathology, that can be probed by optical techniques.

It is important to introduce a general comparison of the S_e and S_p for several optical biopsy methods and conventional histopathological methods as well.

(Backhaus *et al.*, 2010) developed a simple and rapid method for the detection of breast cancer with infrared spectroscopy. With cluster analysis (a method of unsupervised learning) they were able to achieve a S_e = 98% and a S_p = 95%.(Griebe *et al.*, 2007) analyzed biological markers which play an evolving role in the diagnosis of Alzheimer disease. The Fourier-Transform Infrared (FT-IR) spectroscopy data showed S_e = 88.5% and S_p = 80%.

Another example of a new tool for use in optical diagnosis is elastic scattering spectroscopy, which is a point-contact technique where one collects broadband optical spectra sensitive to absorption and scattering within the tissue. Using this technique,(Austwick *et al.*, 2010) obtained a S_e = 69% for detection of clinically relevant metastases and a S_p = 96%. (Canpolat *et al.*, 2012) investigated the potential application of elastic light single-scattering spectroscopy as an adjunctive tool for noninvasive, in vivo, real-time differentiation of malignant and benign skin lesions and to detect positive surgical margins of excised biopsy samples.The *in vivo* spectroscopic measurements and analysis performed on 28 lesions in 23 patients discriminated malignant and benign lesions with a S_e and S_p of 87% and 85%, respectively.

Due to their high sensitivity in the detection of tiny biochemical and molecular variations in tissues the optical biopsy techniques based on Raman spectroscopy are of special interest. They will be exploited in more details in the following sections.

2   Raman-based Optical Biopsy

2.1   The Raman Effect

From the light matter interaction point of view, tissues behave like any bulk medium in which light propagation produces absorption, scattering, refraction, and reflection processes. Since a tissue is a highly scattering turbid medium, the most pronounced effect is scattering. The turbidity or apparent non-transparency of a tissue is caused by multiple scattering from a very heterogeneous structure consisting of macromolecules, cell organelles, and a pool of water (see section 6.3 of (Prasad, 2003)).

When one illuminates a given molecule with a large amount of photons with frequency v_i and energy hv_i ($h = 6.626068 \times 10^{-34}$ J.s is the constant of Planck) the more usual or statistically probable scattering process is the elastic where the scattered photons emerge with the same energy of the incident ones. This is Rayleigh or elastic scattering. However, a small fraction of the photons (typically 1 in 10^5) is inelastically scattered and emerges with energy hv_s different from the incident. The Raman effect corresponds to this inelastic scattering of light and was first described in 1928 by Chandrasekhara Venkata Raman (Raman, 1928) Raman received the Nobel Prize 2 years later for this discovery (Singh & Riess, 1998). The inelastically scattered photons could have their energies higher or lower respect to the incident. The corresponding processes are labeled anti-Stokes and Stokes, respectively. Figure 1 represents a simplified picture of the Raman effect compared to the usual absorption/emission process. In the last the incident photons impinging the molecule induce transitions between the electronic states. The scattered photons will have energies will fit to the energy difference of available states. In the former, the transitions occur among vibrational states and virtual electronic states in the continuum. The incident photon generates a electron-hole pair. The electron may interacts with the quantum of vibration (phonon) destroying it (anti-Stokes process) or creating one (Stokes process). After electron-hole recombination there will be the emission of the inelastic photon. The difference in the energy (or Raman shift) will be the phonon energy. Each molecule presents a characteristic set of vibrational modes or phonons. Thus, the Raman spectroscopy can be used to optically

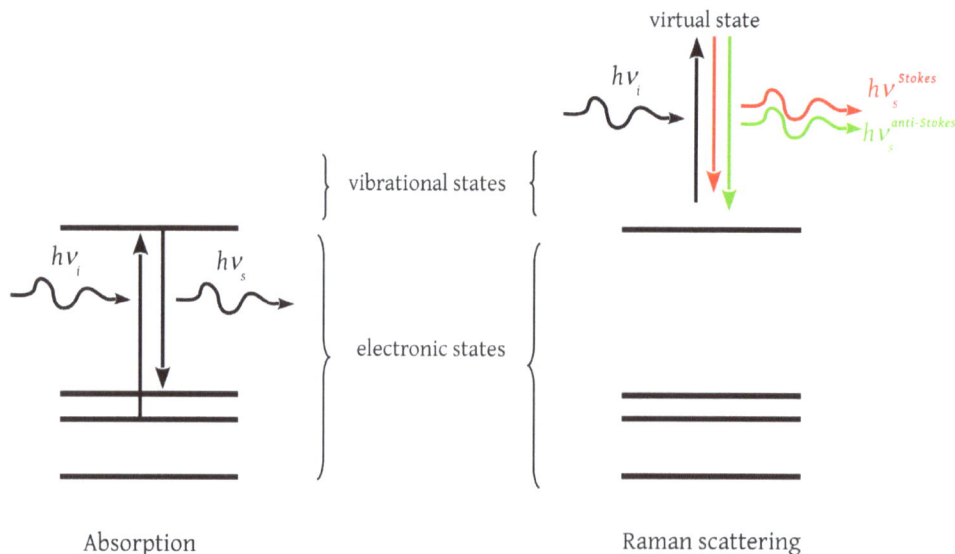

Figure 1: Simplified Jablonsky diagram for the absorption/emission (left) and Raman scattering (right) processes.

probe molecular changes in a given material.

It is important to notice that close to room temperature or temperatures above, the Stokes process is more probable. Thus the Stokes spectra is more intense and the standard choice for displaying Raman data. However, the anti-Stokes spectra has some special characteristics which enable very promising imaging capabilities. The coherent anti-Stokes Raman spectroscopy (CARS) is a very powerful imaging technique subjected to intense developments recently. To the reader interested in this subject it is recommended the reviews by (Evans & Xie, 2008) and (Hashimoto *et al.*, 2012).

When the photon energy fits some set of electronic energy states the Absorption/Emission and Raman process occur simultaneously. However, the corresponding auto-fluorescence process is several orders of magnitude more intense than the Raman scattering. The strongest luminescent emission obscures the tiny Raman bands.

2.2   Raman Spectroscopy and Diagnosis

Recently Raman spectroscopy has become a very important tool for biological samples analysis, including cancer diagnosis (Andrade *et al.*, 2007; Bitar *et al.*, 2006; da Silva Martinho *et al.*, 2008; de Carvalho *et al.*, 2010; Lieber & Kabeer, 2010; Mahadevan-Jansen *et al.*, 2008; Martinho *et al.*, 2008), tropical diseases (Webster *et al.*, 2008), mineralized tissues (Carden & Morris, 2000), and cell studies (Wang *et al.*, 2012; Movasaghi *et al.*, 2012; Verrier *et al.*, 2011; Guze *et al.*, 2011).

The Raman technique offers certain advantages over others optical spectroscopic techniques, such as luminescence spectroscopy, polarized light scattering spectroscopy, optical coherence tomography and confocal reflectance microscopy. These advantages include high spatial ($\lesssim 1\ \mu$m for micro-Raman setups) and spectral ($\lesssim 0.1\ $cm^{-1}) resolutions, the possibility of using less harmful near-infrared (NIR) radiation, less laborious preparation of samples since it is not necessary to introduce exogenous labels and *"in situ"* analysis could be performed, high chemical sensitivity, minimal influence of water bands, and the possibility of *"in vitro"* or *"in vivo"* data acquisition (de Carvalho *et al.*, 2010).

Usually the spectral region between 500 and $1,800$ cm^{-1} (labeled as *fingerprint region*) has the most relevant biochemical information concerning biological tissues (Naumann, 2001). The frequencies of many vibrational bands of amino acids, nucleic acids, proteins, lipids, glucose and other carbohydrates fall in this region (Naumann, 2000). The fingerprint window was extensively studied by Fourier transform-Raman (FT-Raman) using $1,064$ nm laser excitation and NIR (785 and 830 nm laser excitation) Raman techniques: (Naumann, 2001; Naumann, 2000; Martinho *et al.*, 2008).

(Frank *et al.*, 1994) was pioneering using a compact, portable 785 nm Raman-based setup in a clinical setting. In a subsequent work (Frank *et al.*, 1995) used the same setup to obtain Raman spectra of normal, benign (fibro-adenoma), and malignant tissues (infiltrating duct carcinoma not otherwise specified - NOS). They noticed that the band at $1,439$ cm^{-1} in the normal tissue shifted to $1,450$ cm^{-1} in the infiltrating duct carcinoma NOS and they had attributed this change to increased protein concentration in malignant samples. Using the area ratio of 1654/1439 cm^{-1} bands, they easily differentiate infiltrating duct carcinoma from normal tissue. However, they were unable to statistically differentiate among infiltrating duct carcinoma and fibro-adenoma.

The FT-Raman spectra of biological samples are almost auto-fluorescence free, minimizing the need for pre-processing the data (Martinho *et al.*, 2008). (Alfano *et al.*, 1991) were the first to employ FT-Raman spectroscopy in the study of human breast tissues. They studied 14 breast tissues being 3 normal, 4 benign, and 7 malignant, do not regarding the several subtypes of these carcinomas. They observed spectral differences between malignant, benign and normal tissues but they were unable to associate these differences to biochemical changes.

Spectral contamination by auto-fluorescence and difficulties to discriminate malignant and benign lesions or those with similar pathologic grade were features observed at these foremost studies which still persist up to day. As pointed out by (Austwick *et al.*, 2010) several technological obstacles still restrict the wide clinical application of Raman spectroscopy as an optical biopsy technique.

3   Technological Challenges

3.1   The Auto-fluorescence Problem

The auto-luminescence (or simply fluorescence or luminescence) originates on the optical activity of a set of chromophores present in the tissue. Various electronic transitions could be responsible for the absorption and respective auto-luminescence emission. Following (Atkins & De Paula, 2009) are listed the processes important the most in the visible region.

- $d-d$ transition, which involve the excitation of an electron from one d orbital of the transition metal atom to another d level. They are encountered in an organometallic biomolecule involving a transition metal complex with organic ligands. The hemoglobin involving Fe or a porphyrin involving Mn or Zn are the classical examples.

- $\pi-\pi^*$ transition, which involve the promotion of an electron from a bonding π orbital to an antibonding π^* orbital. They are associated with double bonds or a conjugated structural unit. One example of this kind of transition is provided by the absorption in the 11-cis-retinal chromophore in eye. Other important example is a porphyrin such as the heme group in hemoglobin. The absorption spectra of porphyrins exhibit an intense $\pi-\pi^*$ transition in blue region at 400 nm which is called the *Soret band*. In addition, there are a series of weaker $\pi-\pi^*$ transitions in the region, 450-650 nm which are called

Q bands.

- $n - \pi^*$ transition, which involves the excitation of an electron from a non-bonding orbital to an empty π^* orbital. An example is the excitation of an electron of the electron pair in the outer nonbonding orbital of oxygen in a $>C = O$ group to the π^* molecular orbital of the $C = O$ double bond.

- Charge transfer transition, which involves the excitation of an electron from the highest occupied orbital centered on one atom (or a group) to the lowest unoccupied orbital centered on another atom or a group. Complexes of cysteine, methionine, and organometallics usually display charge transfer bands in their absorption spectra.

The auto-luminescence emitted is several orders of magnitude intense than the Raman effect and interferes with the Raman spectra when the excitation light falls in the visible region. (de Veld *et al.*, 2005).

The spectroscopic instrumentation (detectors, gratings, lasers, etc.) and technology available today have better performance in the visible spectral region (400 – 700 nm). However, Raman excitation in this range is not suitable for biological samples studies due to the strong auto-luminescence arising from samples. The strong luminescence signal masks the majority of Raman bands and decreases the signal to noise (S/N) ratio of the measurements affecting directly the sensitivity and specificity values. This limitation is one of the major obstacles to the wider use of Raman spectroscopy for medical optical diagnosis.

This auto-fluorescence problem can also be minimized by using excitation sources close to the infrared. (Lieber & Kabeer, 2010) demonstrated the application of Raman spectroscopy and its auto-fluorescence free background for pediatric Wilms' tumor diagnosis. The fluorescence free background spectra were able to discriminate normal kidney from Wilms' tumor with $S_e = 81\%$ and $S_p = 100\%$. The Raman spectra obtained $S_e = 93\%$ and $S_p = 100\%$. Nd:YAG lasers at 1,064 nm could also be used. Reasonable S/N ratio spectra with this excitation are obtained only with the FT-Raman technique, but due to the poor efficiency of CCD detectors in the infrared region, linear semiconductors detectors (InGaAs or Ge) must be used. But in this case the multiplexing advantage of the dispersive setup is totally or partially lost. The FT technique demands higher acquisition times than the dispersive one (typically a factor of 1,000) with poor spectral resolution and sensitivity.

Another option is employ ultraviolet (UV) radiation, where it is usually possible to obtain high quality spectra due to the elimination of luminescence and increase in the Raman intensity (Pajcini *et al.*, 1997; Asghari-Khiavi *et al.*, 2009). Nevertheless, the availability of UV instrumentation is limited, expensive, and can cause various types of damage to tissues, specially for *"in vivo"* applications.

Some methods have been developed in order to reduce luminescence and extract the vibrational information from the scattered Raman signal. We would cite the are polarization modulation (Angel *et al.*, 1984), time-resolved picosecond excitation pulse and gating (Matousek *et al.*, 2001), shifted-excitation Raman difference spectroscopy (SERDS) (Shreve *et al.*, 1992), and computational algorithms for automated background subtraction (see, e.g. (Krishna *et al.*, 2012)).

Polarization modulation is based on the fact that the emitted luminescence does not conserve the polarization state of the exciting source. Thus, polarization sensitive detection will almost certainly eliminate the cross-polarized luminescence component of the Raman spectra. However, as the parallel-polarized fluorescence is normally non-negligible, this method has been ineffective in achieving this goal. Time-resolved Raman utilizes the fact that luminescence has a relatively longer life time ($\sim 10 - 1,000$ ps) compared to Raman (~ 10 fs). Thus, by using pulsed lasers and limiting signal collection to just the time of the short pulse, can prevent the luminescence emission. This technique, however, involves sophisticated instrumentation and is not effective when the fluorescence lifetime is comparable to the excitation pulse duration (Zhao *et al.*, 2002). Moreover, the spectral resolution decreases due to finite pulse of the laser.

3.2 The SERDS Method: A Way to Correctly Manage Auto-luminescence Contamination on Raman Spectra

The characteristics of Raman, absorption/emission (auto-fluorescence) processes were commented on section 2.1. However, it is important to stress some fundamental differences between them. The first relates to the energy shift of the scattered and emitted photons compared to the incident ones. The **Raman shift is independent** of the excitation energy $h\nu_i$. Thus, is it possible (in principle) to detect the Raman effect exciting the sample with photons with any energy since the Raman bands will appear as side-bands around the excitation line (see Fig.2). Luminescence as any electronic transition could be excited once $h\nu_i$ greater than a minimum value. Obviously the selection rules will be diverse in each case. The broad luminescence peak does not display appreciable chance in both intensity or maximum position for small laser excitation energy/wavelength variations. On the other hand, the Raman bands will follow the wavelength excitation $\Delta\lambda$ as shown on Fig.2. Altogether, one could take advantage of these characteristics and eliminates the negative interference of the auto-luminescence on the Raman spectrum since a tunable laser source is available. Once subtracted two slightly shifted Raman spectra a derivative-like luminescence free signal could be obtained, as observed on Fig. 3. This is the basis of the Shifted Excitation Raman Difference Spectroscopy (SERDS) method.

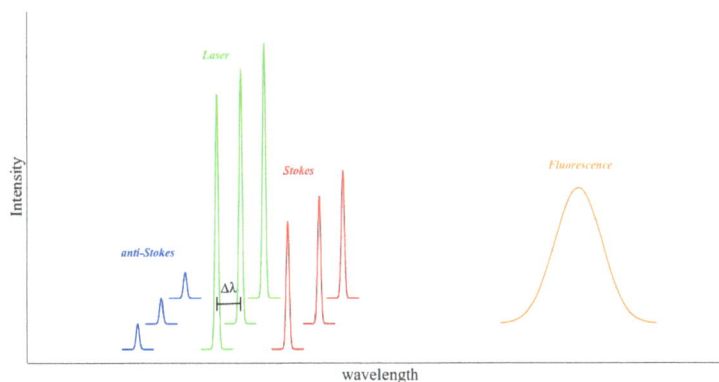

Figure 2: Schematic representation of the Raman spectra compared to the auto-luminescence emission. Both Stokes and anti-Stokes Raman bands shift their position responding to laser wavelength change $\Delta\lambda$.

(Shreve *et al.*, 1992) were the first to propose the SERDS method. It is based on fact that the luminescence spectrum is nearly insensitive to small energy excitation changes in contrast to that of the Raman bands. Thus, subtracting two Raman spectra, each one excited by slightly shifted laser lines could enable the elimination of the luminescence. Shreve et al. observed very good fluorescence removal using this method to measure the Raman spectra of a dye diluted in alcohol. A variation of this method was proposed by (Mosier-Boss *et al.*, 1995). In their proposal there was no shift of the excitation laser line, but a slight movement on the angle of the spectrometer diffraction grating to get two spatially shifted spectra. It was shown (Zhao *et al.*, 2002) that this is a poor method to remove the luminescence. (Bell *et al.*, 1998) proposed a similar method of subtracting spectra taken at several different, closely spaced spectrometer positions ex-

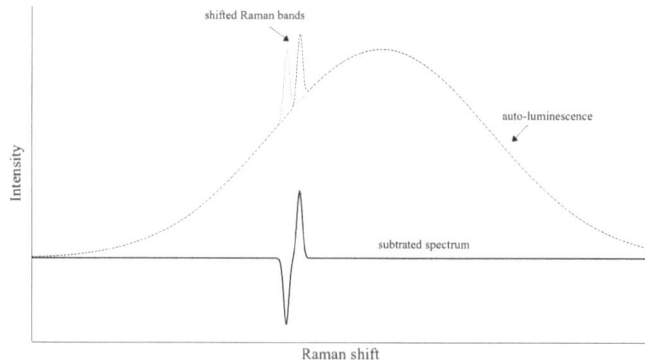

Figure 3: Illustration of how the shifted Raman spectra could be used to eliminate the auto-fluorescence.

cited with the same laser energy. The fluorescence-free Raman spectra were obtained by iterative fitting the bands to double Lorentzian functions. They obtained promising results using a dye in cyclohexane as the sample. However, it was pointed out that the main disadvantage of the method is the need for further complex data processing to obtain a recognizable Raman spectra.

(Zhao *et al.*, 2002) and (Osticioli *et al.*, 2007) used a mathematical method based on Fourier transform to automatically process the SERDS spectrum and obtain the pure Raman signal. The procedure applied to isopropanol, acetamide-phenol powder, cinnabar pigment, and sulfur was reasonably successful to reconstruct the Raman bands. However, noise and spurious bands were observed. As pointed out by the authors the ability for good spectral reproduction strongly depends on the noise level in the raw spectra (Osticioli *et al.*, 2007). A similar limitation could be considered for the automated background subtraction (Mosier-Boss *et al.*, 1995); (Beier & Berger, 2009); (McCain *et al.*, 2008); (Zhang & Ben-Amotz, 2000); (Brennan *et al.*, 1997) methods. In addition, it is desirable to develop a correct reconstruction procedure to know the spectra of the specific interfering fluorophore.

3.2.1 Basic SERDS Theory

The total signal (S_R) measured when exciting a sample with light at wavelength λ is

$$S_R(\lambda) = \{L(\lambda) + R(\lambda)\}M(\lambda) + B(\lambda) \tag{1}$$

where $L(\lambda)$, $R(\lambda)$, $M(\lambda)$, and $B(\lambda)$ are the luminescence signal, Raman signal, optical response of the system, and background, respectively. For excitation at two slightly different wavelengths (λ_1 and λ_2) the above equation becomes:

$$S_R(\lambda_1) = \{L(\lambda_1) + R(\lambda_1)\}M(\lambda_1) + B(\lambda_1) \tag{2}$$

$$S_R(\lambda_2) = \{L(\lambda_2) + R(\lambda_2)\}M(\lambda_2) + B(\lambda_2) \tag{3}$$

since L, B, and M are almost λ-independent.

The difference $\delta S \equiv S_R(\lambda_2) - S_R(\lambda_1)$ is the subtracted derivative-like signal. It will be

$$\delta S = \{R(\lambda_2) - R(\lambda_1)\} = \delta R(\lambda)M(\lambda) \tag{4}$$

The pure Raman signal could be recovered integrating eq.4

$$R(\lambda) = \int M^{-1} \delta S d\lambda \qquad (5)$$

where M^{-1} does not vary appreciably in the interval of interest for Raman measurements. Singularities, oscillatory, or fast decreasingly behavior of the quantum response of detectors or diffraction gratings could induce some artifacts when integrating the above expression. M could be obtained, e.g., by measuring the emission of a tungsten lamp and comparing it with the emissivity of a black-body at same temperature.

3.2.2 Raman Spectroscopy Instrumentation

Two different optical setups for dispersive Raman experiments were employed for *in vitro* and *in vivo* macro-Raman applications. Figure 4 shows the schematic view of the SERDS system for macro-Raman measurements. A tunable Lithrow-configuration diode laser ($\lambda = 785$ or 830 nm - Sacher Lasertechnik) was used as the excitation source. The wavelength was mechanically adjusted using a home-made gear which enabled reproducible λ-shifts in 0.5 nm steps. For *in vitro* experiments (Fig.4a), the laser was guided by optics and the Raman signal collected using a telescope. The laser spot diameter on the sample was 200 while typical acquisition time was 2 seconds. A notch filter (Semrock) was used to reject the Rayleigh scattering. The Raman signal was detected by a spectrometer (PiActon SpectraPro model 2500i) equipped with a N_2 cooled CCD detector (Princeton Instruments Spec-10). For *in vivo* applications it is desirable to take advantage of the remote probing characteristic of the optical fiber probes. The *in vivo* setup one (Fig. 4b) used an optical probe (EMVISION LLC) for both exciting the sample and collecting the Raman signal. In this case a laser at 785 nm was used as excitation source. To eliminate both the signals produced in the fibers and the elastically scattered light that enters into the collection fibers, a set of a long-pass and notch filter were glued on the distal side. A SMA connector made the coupling between spectrometer and optical fiber. In all cases the slit of the spectrometer was set to 100. A home-made holder was employed to kept the proximal portion of the optical fiber 2 mm above the skin.

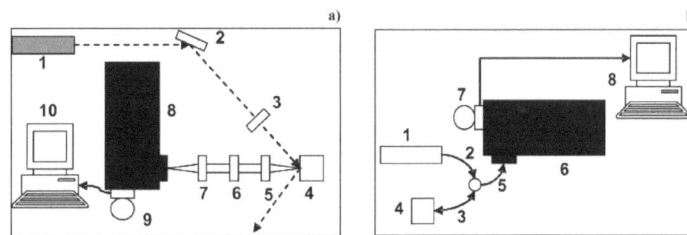

Figure 4: a) Schematic view of the SERDS system for macro-Raman in vitro measurements. (1) laser; (2) mirror; (3) convergent lens; (4) sample holder; (5) and (7) telescope; (6) notch filter; (8) spectrometer; (9) CCD camera; (10) computer. b) Schematic view of the SERDS system for *in vivo* measurements. (1) laser; (2) optical probe laser-guide ; (3) optical probe excitation; (4) sample environment; (5) optical probe collecting; (6) spectrometer; (7) CCD camera; (8)computer.

The tested parameters were: (i) the grating grooves (300, 600, and $1,200$ gr/mm) of the spectrometer holographic gratings; (ii) the laser line shifts $\lambda = 0.5$; 1.5; 2.5; and 3.5 nm and (iii) laser excitation powers between 10 and 110 mW.

For comparative purposes, the FT-Raman spectra were also taken in each case. An FT-Raman spectrometer (Bruker RFS 100/S) with a Nd:YAG laser at 1064 nm as excitation source was used.

3.2.3 *In vitro* Results

A non-carious third molar tooth was used to test the *in vitro* setup. It was sliced in a disc form with 4 mm of thickness and had been already characterized in a previous study (da Silva Tagliaferro *et al*., 2009).

Figure 5 shows the Raman spectra of human tooth taken with 300 (Fig. 5a); 600 (Fig. 5b); and 1,200 (Fig. 5c) gr/mm with different excitation laser output powers (P = 15, 45, 80, and 110 mW) at 830 nm. The light power delivered was almost the same since the absorption in the mirrors (Fig. 4a) is minimal. All spectra were normalized to 1. The prominent band at 950 cm^{-1} is the PO_4 vibration of hydroxy-apatite (da Silva Tagliaferro *et al*., 2009). The spectral window/resolution were 1,850/1.6; 960/0.8; 420/0.3 cm^{-1} for 300;600; and 1,200 gr/mm gratings, respectively. The 300 gr/mm (Fig. 5a) grating presented the most intense peaks, with the largest spectral window, but with the smallest spectral resolution if compared to the others. The 1,200 gr/mm grating (Fig. 5b) presented the best spectral resolution but the less intense peaks and the smallest spectral window. The 600 gr/mm grating presented intermediated characteristics between the 300 and the 1,200 gr/mm gratings.

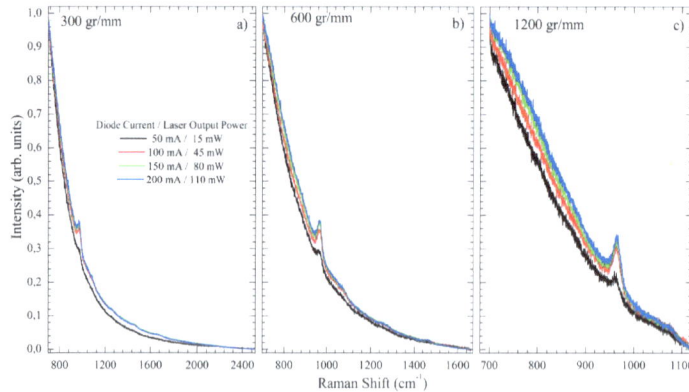

Figure 5: Raman spectrum of a human tooth with 300 (a); 600 (b); and 1,200 (c) gr/mm gratings in function of outputs power 15, 45, 80 and 110 mW.

The spectral difference δS is shown on Fig.6 for several conditions. Panels I, II, and III show the spectra obtained with 300, 600, and 1,200 gr/mm gratings, respectively. The powers employed were P = 15 mW (a), 45 mW (b), 80 mW (c) and 110 mW (d) and δ = 0.5; 1.5,2.5 and 3.5 nm. With $P < 15$ mW (Fig. 6a Panels I-III) the height of the derivative-like Raman band at 960 cm^{-1} was less than two times the noise level. This ratio is greater than 10 for other powers. The signal to noise ratio (S/N) became constant (~ 0.013) at $P = 80$ mW (Fig. 6c) for all gratings. This indicates that better spectra were acquired with $P > 80$ mW. Higher $\Delta\lambda$ distorted the linear form of the inflection signal among the maximum and minimum peaks. For example, for 300, 600, and 1,200 gr/mm gratings this distortion started at $\Delta\lambda$ = 3.5, 2.5 and 1.5 nm, respectively.

Figure 7 shows the inverse of the normalized optical response $M^{-1}(\lambda)$ for 300 (a), 600 (b), and 1,200 (c) gr/mm gratings. The 300 gr/mm (Fig. 7a) grating presented a very flat signal between 1,000 and 2,200 cm^{-1}. The 600 gr/mm grating showed a quite smooth behavior between 780 and 1,450 cm^{-1} while

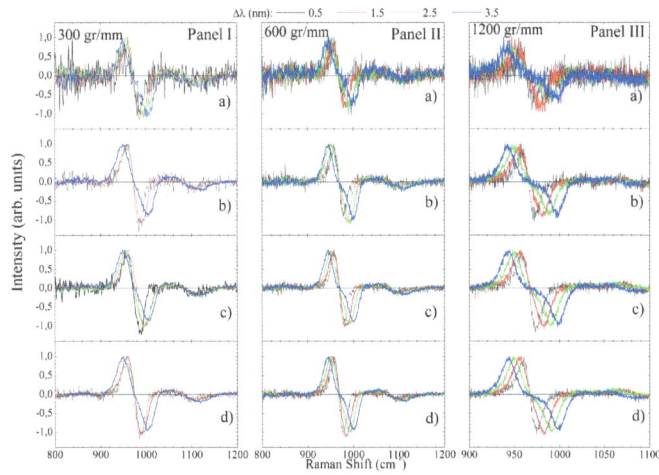

Figure 6: δS of human tooth comparing obtained with 300 (Panel I); 600 (Panel II); and 1200 (Panel III) gr/mm gratings. It was tested different output powers (15 (a); 45(b); 80(c); and 110 (d) mW) and wavelength displacements ($\Delta\lambda = 0.5$; 1.5; 2.5; and 3.5 nm) from the principal laser line.

presenting nonlinearities at borders. The $1,200$ gr/mm grating showed a exponentially decreasing response modulated by several bumps and peaks.

The integrated spectra of Fig.6 after correction to M^{-1} are shown in Fig. 8. At first glance it is clear the broadening effect at higher $\Delta\lambda$s. It was observed bands at 800; 871; 882; 961; $1,040$; and $1,071$ cm^{-1} for the 300 gr/mm grating with $\Delta\lambda = 0.5$ nm (Fig. 8 a). As the expected bands would be at 816; 856; 880; 961; $1,005$; $1,030$; $1,045$; and $1,071$ cm^{-1} (da Silva Tagliaferro et al., 2009), those seen at 800 and 871 cm^{-1} were spurious signal. Moreover, the expected bands at 816; 856; $1,005$; $1,030$ cm^{-1} were not observed. Increasing the λ-shift to $\Delta\lambda = 1.5$ nm the band at 800 cm^{-1} disappear; those at 871 and 882 cm^{-1} superimposed into a single band at 867 cm^{-1}; the band at 961 cm^{-1} shifted to 966 cm^{-1} while presented an increasing broadening; and those at $1,040$ and $1,071$ cm^{-1} collapsed into a broad band centered at $1,075$ cm^{-1}. These spectral features were broadened for $\Delta\lambda = 2.5$ and 3.5 nm. An additional band at $1,060$ cm^{-1} was seen in the $\Delta\lambda = 3.5$ nm spectra.

Figure 8b) presents the data for the 600 gr/mm grating. For $\Delta\lambda = 0.5$ nm bands at 816; 823; 856; 880; 961; $1,045$; and $1,071$ cm^{-1} were observed. Those at $1,045$ and $1,071$ cm^{-1} were more resolved than in the previous case while just one spurious band at 823 cm^{-1} was observed. It was observed similar artifacts as discussed in Fig. 8a) with $\Delta\lambda = 1.53.5$ nm for the 600 gr/mm grating. Figure 8c) shows the spectra for the $1,200$ gr/mm grating. Above the noise level the 914; 850; 880; 961 and $1,081$ cm^{-1} bands were observed for $\Delta\lambda = 0.5$ nm. Only two bands (880 and 961 cm^{-1}) correspond to the expected ones. For $\Delta\lambda = 1.5$ nm, the $1,081$ cm^{-1} band shifted to $1,084$ cm^{-1}. Its frequency decreases to $1,065$ cm^{-1} for $\Delta\lambda = 2.5$ and 3.5 nm.

Another important parameter to discuss is the root mean square signal to noise ratio ($S/N(RMS)$). For comparison we will discuss the S/N ratio only for $\Delta\lambda = 0.5$ nm data. It was found $S/N(RMS) = 0.373$; 0.434; and 0.371 for 300, 600, and $1,200$ gr/mm, respectively. Thus, the best S/N ratio was found with the 600 gr/mm grating. It also had good spectral resolution (0.8 cm^{-1}) while displaying spectral window width ~ 960 cm^{-1} and relatively smooth behavior between 780 and $1,450$ cm^{-1}. Nevertheless, it was concluded that the best set of parameters was $\Delta\lambda = 0.5$ nm and the 600 gr/mm grating.

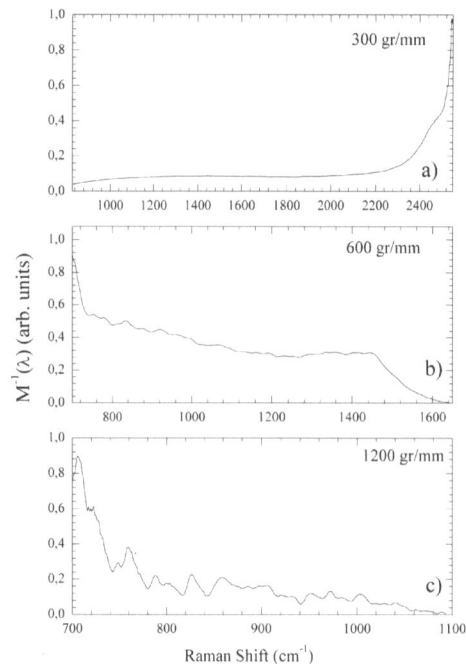

Figure 7: The inverse of the optical response (M^{-1}) for 300 (a); 600 (b); and $1,200$ (c) gr/mm gratings.

Figure 9 shows the SERDS spectra for human tooth using the best set of parameters ($\Delta\lambda = 0.5$ nm; 600 gr/mm; 110 mW) and following the steps commented before to acquire the pure Raman signal. Figure 9a) displays the two shifted spectra while Fig. 9b) and c) shows the subtracted signal and the integrated one, respectively. The fluorescence removal is evident when comparing Fig. 9a) and c). It is also shown in Fig. 9c) the FT-Raman spectra of the same tooth. The spectra were almost the same.

3.2.4 *In vivo* Measurements

The *in vivo* setup was tested on human skin of two voluntary students. They were informed about the objectives of the research as well as its ethical aspects and signed a consent form.

Figure 10 shows the SERDS procedure to take human skin spectra with an optical fiber probe. It was employed similar analysis of in vitro case and it was concluded that the best set of parameters were $\Delta\lambda = 0.5$ nm; 600 gr/mm grating; and 70 mW laser power. Figures 10a), b) and c) displays the two shifted spectra (in wavelength units), the subtracted signal, and the integrated one, respectively. The SERDS and FT-Raman spectra are compared in Fig. 10c). The overall spectral features are present on the SERDS spectra. However, some relevant differences could be identified when subtracting FT-Raman and SERDS spectra (Fig. 10d). Bands between 750 and $1,200$ cm^{-1} appeared less intense in the SERDS spectra when compared to the FT-Raman one. Otherwise, the $1,200 - 1,580$ cm^{-1} ones appeared more intense in the SERDS spectra.

We argue that the main cause of these differences relies on the etaloning effect that occurs on back-illuminated CCD detectors working in the near infrared. The coating of the CCD surface with anti-reflecting material could minimize this effect but does not completely suppress it. Reflections between parallel front and back surfaces cause CCD act as partial etalon. The effect is an oscillatory modulation of the detected signal. The two arrows on Fig. 10 a) indicates two bands probably due to etaloning modulation. The

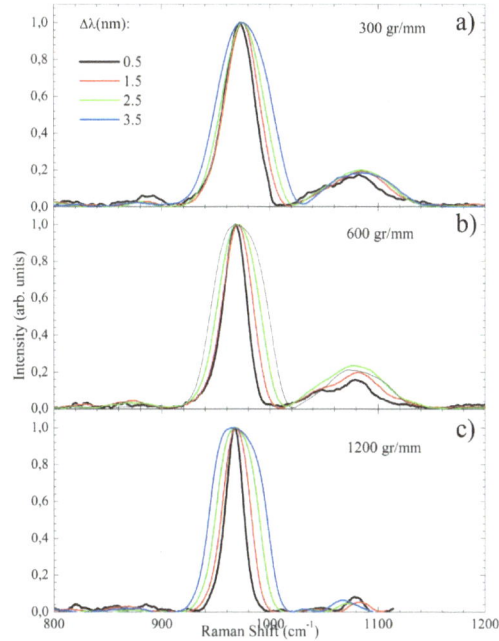

Figure 8: SERDS spectrum of human tooth for 300 (a); 600 (b); and 1,200 (c) gr/mm gratings and $\Delta\lambda = 0.5$; 1.5; 2.5 and 3.5 nm.

three factors determine the shape and intensity of the etaloning effect are the thickness of the CCD, d, the wavelength of the light, and the light absorption by the CCD material expressed as the finesse constant, Q (Saleh & Teich, 1991). The resulting etaloning intensity will follows the equation (Saleh & Teich, 1991)

$$E(\lambda) = \frac{I_{max}}{1 + (\frac{2Q}{\pi})^2 \sin^2 (\frac{2\pi d}{\lambda})} \qquad (6)$$

Thus, the total signal in eq. 5 need be modified to $S_R(\lambda) = [L(\lambda) + R(\lambda)]M(\lambda)E(\lambda) + B(\lambda)$. As just stayed before, at very close wavelength shift one could consider L and M as λ-independent. As consequence the M^{-1}-corrected differential of S_R will be

$$M^{-1}dS_R = R(\lambda)\frac{dE(\lambda)}{d\lambda}d\lambda + E(\lambda)\frac{dR(\lambda)}{d\lambda}d\lambda \qquad (7)$$

and to completely recover the pure Raman signal $R(\lambda)$ one will need solve this differential equation. As first approximation one could also consider E almost constant and the derivative of $E(\lambda)$ respect to λ as zero. Thus, eq.7 simplifies to

$$M^{-1}dS_R = E(\lambda)\frac{dR(\lambda)}{d\lambda}d\lambda \qquad (8)$$

and eq.5 will be re-written as

$$R(\lambda) = \int M^{-1}\delta S d\lambda \qquad (9)$$

which implies consider the etaloning effect as a correction factor after the integration of the subtracted signal. The etaloning parameters in our case were estimated analyzing the subtracted FT-Raman and SERDS signal (Fig. 10 d). It is clear the modulation of the overall signal by an envelope due to the oscillatory function.

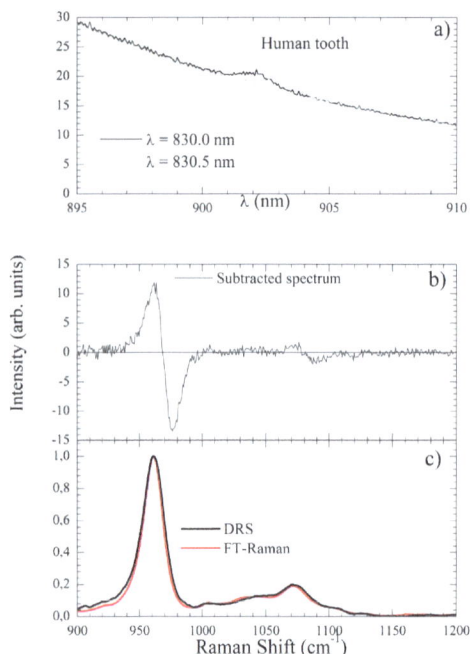

Figure 9: a) Two spectra obtained for a human tooth at λ_1 = 830.0 nm and λ_2 = 830.5 nm. b) Subtracted spectrum (δS). c) SERDS spectrum compared to the FT Raman one.

The fitting of the signal envelope is shown as a dashed line on Fig.10d). The obtained parameters were I_{max} = 1.33; Q = 1.31; and d = 4 nm.

The dashed line in Fig.10c) is the SERDS spectra corrected by the above-estimated etaloning signal. It could be observed that the relative intensities were more realistic when compared to the FT-Raman signal. However differences still persist and we argue that they will be fixed once $R(\lambda)$ be obtained directly from eq. 7 without approximations. It is possible numerically solve this equation is a bit complex procedure and is beyond the scope of the present work.

This discussion indicated that SERDS could be used to eliminate undesired luminescence background in a very systematic and reproducible way. It is reported successful background removal from different kinds of human biological tissues as tooth and skin. It was found that each sample had a specific set of parameters (grooving of the grating, laser power, and $\Delta\lambda$) that maximizes the luminescence elimination and minimizes the spectra distortion. It was found $\Delta\lambda$ = 0.5 cm^{-1} as the best wavelength variation in all experiments. The grating and laser power depends on the specific case. The etaloning effect could represent an important source of interference mainly when the overall scattered signal is high (as in the human skin case). One way to overcome this problem is perform a preliminary characterization of the etaloning signal present in the detector conjugated to some previous knowledge about the expected Raman bands.

3.3   Biological Variability and Misclassification Sources: Inflammatory Infiltrates

It has been recognized that the sensitivity of Raman spectroscopy to subtle biochemical differences must be considered in order to successfully implementation it in a clinical setting for diagnosing even for tissues histopathologically normal (Vargis *et al.*, 2011). Other several restriction to the wide application of Raman-based optical biopsy relies on the misleading or confusing discrimination that arises from pre-altered, pre-

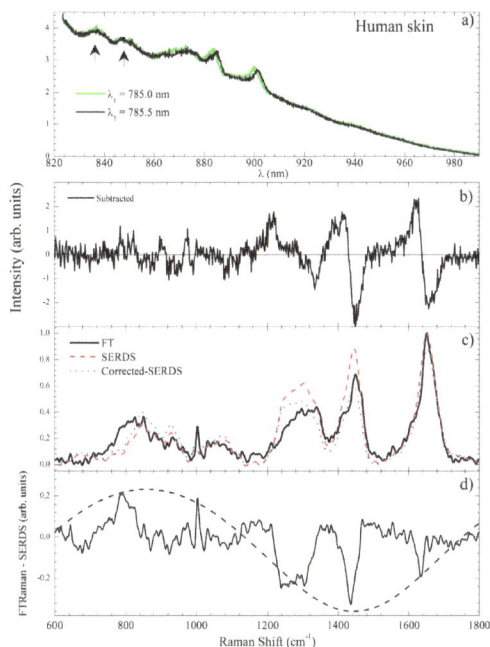

Figure 10: a) Two human skin spectra obtained at $\lambda_1 = 785.0$ nm and $\lambda_2 = 785.5$ nm. b) Subtracted spectrum. c) FT-Raman (solid line), SERDS (dashed line) and corrected-SERDS (dotted line) spectra. d) SERDS subtracted FT-Raman spectra. The dashed line is a fitting to eq. (6) as discussed in text.

malignant, and/or inflammatory tissues. In fact, the development of a malignancy is related to an inflammatory process that occurs simultaneously and generally surrounding the neoplastic process. The available screening and diagnosis methods have some shortcomings that make impossible fast, effective and efficient supervision of cancer in the general population, mainly in development countries. These limitations are due to the fact that all methods are based on subjective interpretations of morphological abnormalities. This fact is inherent to the subjective histological grading of pathologies. It is common atypical cells be associated within inflammatory infiltrates and the slice be misinterpreted by the pathologist as simple inflammation instead of a malignancy or neoplastic or vice-versa. This high false negative rate of histopathological findings had implications on optical biopsy studies. Thus the correct identification of inflammatory infiltrates contribution to the optical biopsy signal is of great relevance to boost advances in the field. In the following it will be discussed some selected works of our research group concerning this topic.

3.3.1 Breast Cancer

(Bitar *et al.*, 2006) analyzed the Raman spectra covering the spectral region of 500 to $2,100$ cm^{-1} of several human breast tissues in order to obtain a differentiation between normal tissues and 8 subtypes of breast pathologies, including fibrocystic condition, duct carcinoma-in-situ, duct carcinoma-in-situ with necrosis, infiltrating duct carcinoma-NOS, inflammatory infiltrating duct carcinoma, medullary infiltrating duct carcinoma, colloid infiltrating duct carcinoma, and invasive lobular carcinoma. Almost, differentiation between normal and pathological breast tissues is well established in literature, the complete differentiation including subtypes of cancer is of special interest for clinical applications of Raman spectroscopy. In this

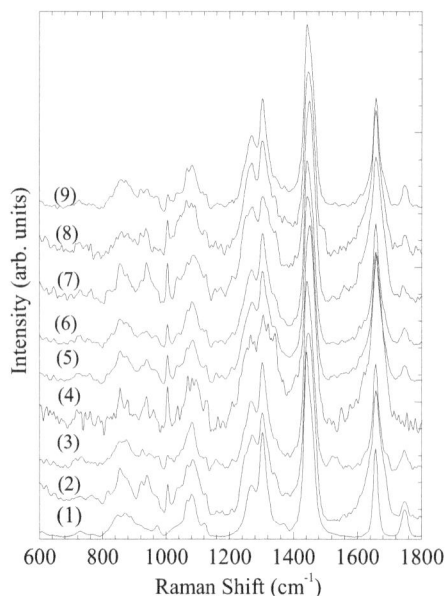

Figure 11: Normalized average Raman spectrum of (1) normal; (2) fibrocystic condition; (3) duct carcinoma-in-situ; (4) duct carcinoma-in-situ with necrosis; (5) infiltrating duct carcinoma; (6) infiltrating duct carcinoma inflammatory; (7) infiltrating duct carcinoma medullar; (8) infiltrating duct carcinoma colloid and (9) infiltrating lobular carcinoma groups. The spectra were vertically translated for clarity.

study it was analyzed the Raman spectra of normal and tumoral breast tissues, including several subtypes of cancers, searching for specific spectral features that could differentiate normal from pathological tissues. The collected samples were histopathologically classified into 9 groups according to their morphological features. Through the qualitative analysis of the Raman spectra (see Fig. 11) and assignment of the relevant bands from the literature, it was possible built spectral models and differentiates among normal breast, fibrocystic condition, duct carcinoma-in-situ, duct carcinoma-in-situ with necrosis, infiltrating duct carcinoma NOS, colloid infiltrating duct carcinoma and invasive lobular carcinoma. These differences were established through the comparative study between the spectral differences and the histopathological diagnosis. Furthermore, it was able to establish the biochemical basis for each spectrum, relating the observed peaks to specific biomolecules that have special role in the carcinogenesis process. It was noticed that we are not able to differentiate inflammatory and medullary duct carcinomas from infiltrating duct carcinoma NOS. The results were summarized in the Fig.12.

3.3.2   Cervical Cancer

Cervical cancer is the second most common cancer among women worldwide and it is generally more common in developing countries. (Martinho *et al.*, 2008) Each year, 471 thousand new cases are reported and approximately 230 thousand of woman had found the death due to this kind of cancer. (Martinho *et al.*, 2008) The main causing agent is the sexually transmitted papilloma human virus (HPV). Cervical malignancy is usually preceded by cervical intra epithelial neoplasia (CIN) of grades I, II, and III before becoming invasive. It is widely known that a large amount of deaths by this pathology (estimated as ~ 90%) would be avoided with early diagnosis. This emphasizes the search for effective screening methods for

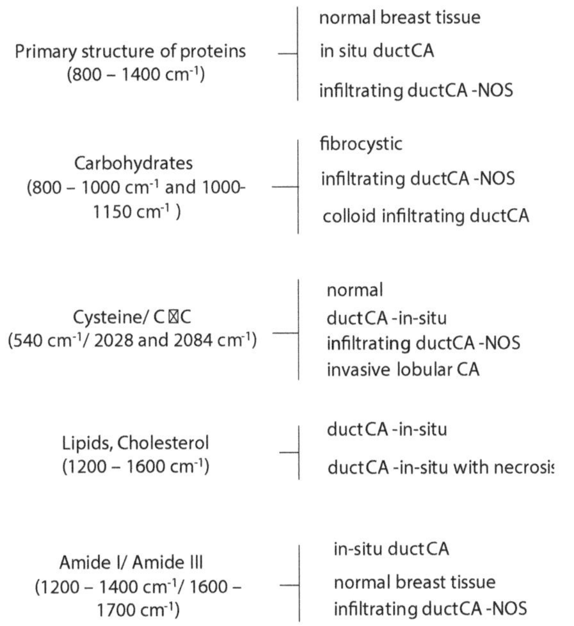

Figure 12: Summary of the several breast cancers classes and their corresponding main Raman spectral differences. At left we present the main bimolecular vibration enabling one to discriminate the specific kind of tissue indicated in the right.

cervix neoplasia.

The available screening and diagnosis methods (mainly Pap smear and colposcopy) have some shortcomings that make impossible fast, effective and efficient supervision of cancer in the general population, mainly in development countries. These limitations are due to the fact that all methods are based on subjective interpretations of morphological abnormalities. The cytological analysis of cervix, which is the elementary principle of Pap smear and colposcopy, for example, had a high false negative rate of ~ 50%. (Martinho *et al.*, 2008) This fact is inherent to the subjective histological grading of this pathology. It is common atypical cells be associated to inflammatory infiltrates and the slice be misinterpreted by the pathologist as simple cervix inflammation (cervicitis) instead of a malignancy or neoplasia or vice-versa. This high false negative rate would limit the accuracy of screenings at very initial stages of the cervical cancer which prevents an adequate treatment at this stage. As consequence a large number of patients will need a surgical procedure to remove the cancer that otherwise would be detected and treated at beginning.

The Raman-based optical diagnosis of normal cervix, inflammatory cervix (cervicitis), and cervical intra epithelial neoplasia (CINI) was investigated on samples of 63 patients. (Martinho *et al.*, 2008) The main alterations were found in the 857 cm^{-1} (*CCH* deformation aromatic); 925 cm^{-1} (*C – C* stretching); ~ 1247 cm^{-1} (*CN* stretch, *NH* bending of Amide III); 1370 cm^{-1} (*CH$_2$* bending); and 1525 cm^{-1} (*C = C/C = N* stretching) vibrational bands in accordance with previously reported on literature comparing normal and malignant cervix tissues.

3.3.3 Statistical Analysis

A typical spectra could be composed of couple of thousand of experimental points or variables. Thus, minering the relevant pieces of information among several groups which could be composed of hundreds of patientes is a hard task. In this sense, compressing methods are valuable tools for analyis of the multidi-mensional spectroscopic data (Kemsley, 1996). The Principal Components Analysis (PCA) is one of these methods.(Dunteman, 1989)

The main goal of PCA is to reduce the dimensionality of a data set whilst retaining as much as possible of the information present in the original data. This goal is achieved by a linear transformation to a new set of variables, the principal component (PC) scores. They are uncorrelated, and ordered such that the first few retain most of the variation present in all of the original variables. The PCs can accurately characterize all of the spectral changes in a set of spectral data. The first principal component (PC1) accounts for the maximum variance in the data, the second principal component (PC2) for the next greatest variance, and so on, until additional principal components describe only noise. These last principal components are discarded. Using a simple tridimentional analogy one could think the PC construction as shadow projection of some object. In Fig. 13 a cylinder is illuminated from three different positions. Projections on specific planes retain only sets of partial characteristics of the object (the PCs). Usually a minimum set of PCs is necessary to classify the subpopulations of a experimental data set and the separation could be seen by visual inspection of the scattering plot. The scattering plot comprises bi or tridimentional graphs were 2 ou 3 specific PCs are plotted for all groups (see, e.g., Fig.14).

A linear combination of the PCs can then be used to model the measured spectra. PCA has already been used in conjunction with a range of discriminant analysis techniques to tackle classification problems (Kemsley, 1996). Because of the way in which principal components are generated, the fits of the principal components to all of the spectra in the data set will be excellent. The fit coefficients in this linear model are often called scores.

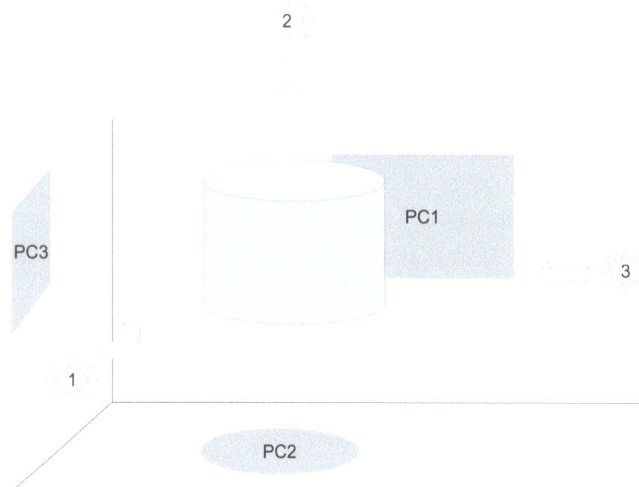

Figure 13: Projection of a object shadow along three different directions illustrating the principal components construction.

The principal component scores can, e.g., then be correlated with the concentrations of specific biochemicals compounds in a least-squares step known as regression. The regression model could be used to classify the spectra in groups which were previously established. For diagnostic purposes, these groups refer to the normal and pathologic kinds of tissues previously screened and classified using an standardized methodology, e.g., histopathological analysis of selected slices. The simplest regression modeling is the binary logistic where it is assumed a division on two groups (e.g., normal and altered for tissues) (Bewick et al., 2005). The probability of a tissue spectrum belongs to the altered group is p and the odds for the altered group is modeled as a linear combination of a set of PCs

$$ln(\frac{p}{1-p}) = \sum_i \alpha_i PC_i \tag{10}$$

For the cervix tissue, PCA analysis applied to the spectral data indicated that the full discrimination among normal and neoplastic tissues by Raman optical biopsy is seriously affected by the presence of inflammatory infiltrates which increases the false positive rate. This fact is especially relevant once cervicitis is a very common state (non-cancerous) of the cervix of sexually active woman. The results suggest that for the correct Raman-based diagnosis of normal cervix from cervical intra epithelial neoplasia it is necessary to use an auxiliary way to discriminate the contribution from the inflammatory infiltrates. The results of our work (Martinho et al., 2008) indicated that the full discrimination among normal and neoplastic CIN I tissues of cervix by Raman optical biopsy was seriously compromised by the presence of inflammatory infiltrates. Fig. 14 shows the scattering plot for PC2, PC3, and PC4. It is clear the mixing among normal and CIN I tissue signal due to the presence of cervicitis. However, once considering only two classes of tissues, normal and altered, a better separation could be found. The data was modeled to

$$ln(\frac{p}{1-p}) = 0.6667 - 13.98PC_3 + 29.25PC_4 \tag{11}$$

The scaled scattering plot of ($29.25PC_4$(versus ($0.6667 - 13.98PC_3$) is shown on Fig.:15.

In fact, both the crude biochemical analysis obtained by direct spectral comparison among normal, cervicitis, and CIN I samples; the clustering procedure; and the LR diagnosis model results indicated that the cervicitis samples were always misclassified as CIN I (see Fig. 15). This fact increases the false positive rate of a Raman-based diagnosis. This is especially relevant since cervix inflammation is very common (non-cancerous) disease of cervix.

Thus, the results suggest that for a safe and useful optical diagnosis of cervix it is mandatory find out a cervicitis-marker-like signal that could be found, e.g., by coupling an auxiliary technique (fluorescence, dichroism, etc) to the Raman-based one.

3.3.4   Inflammatory Fibrous Hyperplasia

FT-Raman Spectroscopy was applied to identify biochemical alterations existing between inflammatory fibrous hyperplasia (IFH) and normal tissues of buccal mucosa. (de Carvalho et al., 2010) The IFH is a good prototype for study inflammatory process. One important implication of this study is related to the cancer lesion border. In fact, the cancerous - normal border line is characterized by the presence of inflammation and its correct discrimination would increase the accuracy in delimiting the lesion frontier. Seventy spectra of IFH from 14 patients were compared to 30 spectra of normal tissue from 6 patients. The statistical analysis was performed with Principal Components Analysis and Soft Independent Modeling Class Analogy methodologies in order to find out the set of spectral bands which enabled the best discrimination among normal and IFH tissues. Bands close to 574; 1,100; 1,250 − 1,350; and 1,500 cm^{-1} (mainly amino acids

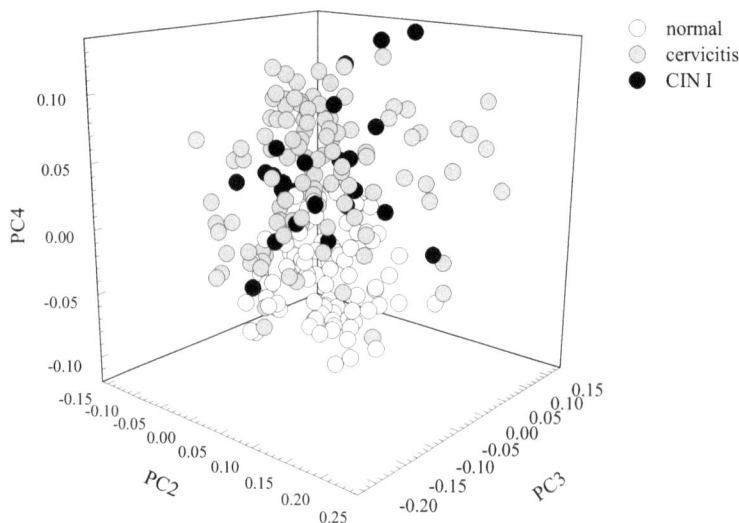

Figure 14: Scattering plot of PC2-PC4 for the normal (open circle), CIN I (solid cyan circle), and cervicitis (solid black circle).

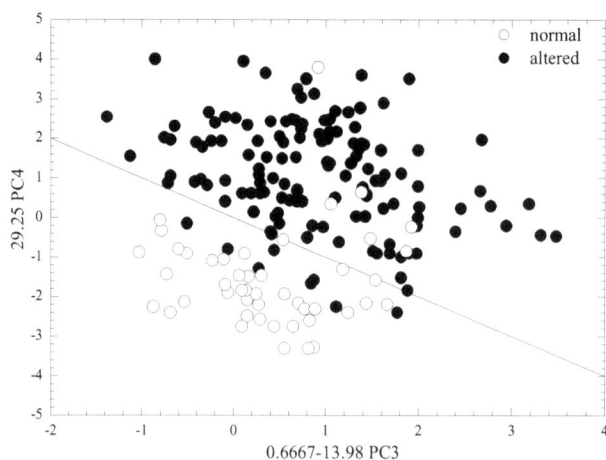

Figure 15: Scattering plot for the best fitted LR model. The solid line is a diagnosis line based on eq.11 with $p = 0.50$.

and collagen bands) presented the main intra-group variations which are due to the acanthosis process in the IFH epithelium. The $1,200$ (C-C aromatic/DNA), $1,350$ (CH$_2$ Bending/Collagen 1) and $1,730$ cm^{-1} (Collagen III) regions presented the main inter-group variations. This finding was interpreted as originated on extracellular matrix degeneration process occurring in the inflammatory tissues.

After studying several spectral ranges with help of the PCA-based Soft independent modelling by class analogy (SIMCA) method(Wold & Sjostrom, 1977) it was concluded that the best discrimination capability (sensibility of 95% and specificity of 100%) was found using the $530 - 580$ cm^{-1} wavenumber (see Fig. 16). The bands in this region are related to vibrational modes of Collagen amino acids Cistine,

Cysteine, and Proline and their relevant contribution to the classification probably relies on the extracellular matrix degeneration process occurring in the inflammatory tissues. Thus only exploring this narrow spectral window it is possible to discriminate normal and inflammatory tissues. This is very useful information for accurate cancer border lesion determination. The existence of this narrow spectral window enabling normal and inflammatory diagnosis had also useful implications for an *in vivo* dispersive Raman setup for clinical applications. (de Carvalho *et al.*, 2010)

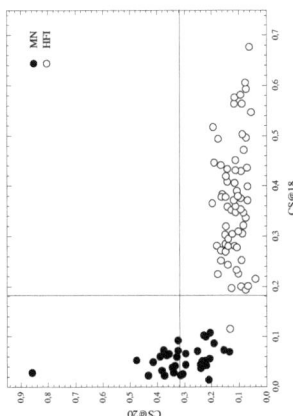

Figure 16: Three-dimensional projection of the samples obtained by the SIMCA method.

4   News Perspectives

In the effort to find out the experimental setup or Raman-configuration furnishing the best discriminative power among pathological and normal tissues one interesting alternative has becoming analyze those bands which are away from the laser line in the high wavenumber region ($2,800 - 3,600$ cm^{-1}) that are related to $O-H$, CH, CH_2, CH_3, and NH vibrations due to lipids, proteins, carbohydrates, among other species present. This region is far from laser line, which prevents almost all undesirable effects just commented in the previous sections. For example, (Mo *et al.*, 2009) studied the high-wavenumber Raman spectroscopy spectral region and concluded that the diagnostic algorithms based on principal components and linear discriminant analysis together with the leave-one-patient-out cross-validation method furnished S_e = 93.5% and S_p = 97.8% for dysplasia tissue identification. (Lin *et al.*, 2012) reported the implementation of a miniaturized fiber-optic Raman probe for trans nasal image-guided high wavenumber Raman spectroscopy to differentiate tumor from normal laryngeal tissue at endoscopy. The diagnostic S_e = 90.3% and S_p = 90.9% for laryngeal cancer identification was reported.

Our group shown that exploring this spectral region could also shine light on the question relative to the confounding or misleading effect of the inflammatory infiltrates. In a recent work (de Carvalho *et al.*, 2011) we have investigated the vibrational spectra of normal (NM) and oral inflammatory fibrous hyperplasia (IFH) tissues of buccal mucosa in the high-wavenumber region using a 1,064 nm laser source. IFH is a good inflammatory tissue prototype. The epithelium of the oral mucosa shows changes induced by the inflammatory process located in the lamina propria. The alterations of IFH are observed in the epithelium and connective tissue. Usually, the IFH in the oral mucosa is caused by some previous trauma, for example due to the habitual biting of the mucosa. Thus, an inflammatory response is started at this site, which leads to increased tissue damage caused by this inflammation that ceases when the inflammatory factor is also interrupted.

Figure 17 shows the Box Plot for the NM (Fig. 17a) and IFH (Fig. 17b) baseline corrected spectral data. The black lines correspond to the average spectrum while the vertical gray ones are the regions between the first and third quartiles.It is important to note that the $2,800 - 3,050$ cm^{-1} region (CH_2 and CH_3 vibrations) showed greater intra-group variation for normal mucosa. However, the IFH spectra showed the highest intra-group variation in the $3,050 - 3,600$ cm^{-1} region (CH, OH, and NH vibrations). The relative area $\frac{A_{2,800-3,050}}{A_{3,050-3,600}} \sim$ for NM while it decreases to ~ 1.5 for IFH. The two above-cited regions present subtle spectral structures consisting of a set of superposed nearly overlapping bands that are related to CH, CH_2, CH_3, OH, and NH vibrations on different molecules, respectively. A simple classification model based on the relative areas of the above cited regions resulted in concordant pairs of 95.3%. Considering the standard errors in the model parameters, it was found that $87\% < S_e < 100\%$ and $73\% < S_p < 93\%$, respectively. In addition, it has been found that the Raman scattering cross-sections in the NH, OH, and CH stretching region are more intense than in the mid-IR/Raman (fingerprint) region.

More subtle information could be extracted from these results. In fact, there are a set of overlapping bands originating from specific locations, which are not equally contributing to the diagnosis. One interesting example is the structured water around proteins. Water and other biomolecules inside the cells have different properties than the water outside (Gniadecka et al., 2003; Bohr & Olsen, 2011). The viscosity of the intracellular water, for example, is higher and its ability to spread is smaller, as observed by nuclear magnetic resonance (NMR) (Gniadecka et al., 2003). As water molecules occupy specific sites and form localized clusters with structures that are determined by their hydrogen-bonding capabilities they are able to influence the vast majority of physical and chemical properties of the tissues, thus the water may be self-structured differently in normal and inflammatory tissues (de Carvalho et al., 2011). (Cybulski & Sadlej, 2007) observed that spectra in the OH-stretching vibrations region are related to local structures and interactions of the hydrogen-bonds networks, so each cluster has a characteristic Raman spectrum. Since water is one important constituent, which has vibrational bands falling in this spectral window, we argue

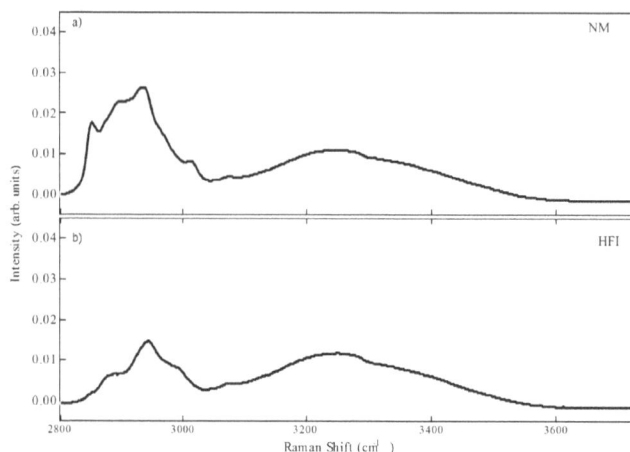

Figure 17: a) Box Plot of IFH and b) Box Plot of NM, The black line is related to the average of the spectrum obtained and the region shaded in gray refers to the variation found in groups.

that this is could be origin of the discriminative power of the high-wavenumber region closely related to the hydropic degeneration process in IFH.

Simultaneous fingerprint and high-wavenumber Raman measurements are also possible and some groups have reporting important progress using this methodology (see, e.g, (Duraipandian *et al.*, 2012)). Other promising trend in the optical biopsy field relies to the combination of two or more techniques in order to achieve improvements on S_e and S_p. (Cicchi *et al.*, 2012) tested an experimental setup which combines fluorescence spectroscopy and Raman spectroscopy in a multidimensional approach. The preliminary results on fresh human skin biopsies clinically diagnosed as malignant melanoma, melanocytic nevus, or healthy skin, found an optimal correlation with the subsequent histological exam. (Patil *et al.*, 2011) reported the development of a clinical instrument combining optical coherence tomography (OCT) and Raman spectroscopy (RS-OCT). It is based on pioneer setup described by (Patil *et al.*, 2008). They demonstrated the capability to identify structurally ambiguous features within an OCT image with Raman spectroscopy both in a phantom, *ex vivo* and *in vivo* tissues.

References

Alfano, R. R., Liu, C. H., Sha, W. L., Zhu, H. R., Akins, D. L., Cleary, J., Prudente, R., & Cellmer, E. (1991). *Human breast tissues studied by ir fourier transform raman spectroscopy. Lasers in the life sciences, 4(1), 23–28.*

Andrade, P. O., Bitar, R. A., Yassoyama, K., Martinho, H., Santo, A. M. E., Bruno, P. M., & Martin, A. A. (2007). *Study of normal colorectal tissue by ft-raman spectroscopy. Anal. and Bioanal. Chem., 387, 1643.*

Angel, S. M., DeArmond, M. K., Hanck, K. W., & Wertz, D. W. (1984). *Computer-controlled instrument for the recovery of a resonance raman spectrum in the presence of strong luminescence. Analytical Chemistry, 56(14), 3000–3001.*

Asghari-Khiavi, M., Mechler, A., Bambery, K. R., McNaughton, D., & Wood, B. R. (2009). *A resonance raman spectroscopic investigation into the effects of fixation and dehydration on heme environment of hemoglobin. Journal of Raman Spectroscopy, 40(11), 1668–1674.*

Atkins, P. & De Paula, J. (2009). *Elements of physical chemistry. WH Freeman.*

Austwick, M. R., Clark, B., Mosse, C. A., Johnson, K., Chicken, D. W., Somasundaram, S. K., Calabro, K. W., Zhu, Y., Falzon, M., & Kocjan, G. (2010). *Scanning elastic scattering spectroscopy detects metastatic breast cancer in sentinel lymph nodes. J Biomed Opt, 15, 047001–.*

Backhaus, J., Mueller, R., Formanski, N., Szlama, N., Meerpohl, H. G., Eidt, M., & Bugert, P. (2010). *Diagnosis of breast cancer with infrared spectroscopy from serum samples. Vib Spectrosc, 52, 173–177.*

Beier, B. D. & Berger, A. J. (2009). *Method for automated background subtraction from raman spectra containing known contaminants. Analyst, 134(6), 1198–1202.*

Bell, S. E. J., Bourguignon, E. S. O., & Dennis, A. (1998). *Analysis of luminescent samples using subtracted shifted raman spectroscopy. ANALYST-LONDON-SOCIETY OF PUBLIC ANALYSTS THEN ROYAL SOCIETY OF CHEMISTRY-, 123, 1729–1734.*

Bewick, V., Cheek, L., Ball, J., et al. (2005). *Statistics review 14: Logistic regression. Crit Care, 9(1), 112–118.*

Bitar, R. A., da Silva Martinho, H., Tierra-Criollo, C. J., Ramalho, L. N. Z., Netto, M. M., & Martin, A. A. (2006). *Biochemical analysis of human breast tissues using fourier-transform raman spectroscopy. J. Biom. Opt., 11(5), 054001–054001.*

Bohr, J. & Olsen, K. (2011). *The close-packed triple helix as a possible new structural motif for collagen. Theoretical Chemistry Accounts: Theory, Computation, and Modeling (Theoretica Chimica Acta), 130(4), 1095–1103.*

Boyle, P. & Levin, B. (2008). World Cancer Report 2008. Lyon: IARC Press.

Brennan, J. F., Wang, Y., Dasari, R. R., & Feld, M. S. (1997). Near-infrared raman spectrometer systems for human tissue studies. Applied spectroscopy, 51(2), 201–208.

Canpolat, M., Akman-Karakaş, A., Gökhan-Ocak, G. A., Başsorgun, I. C., Çiftçioğlu, M. A., & Alpsoy, E. (2012). Diagnosis and demarcation of skin malignancy using elastic light single-scattering spectroscopy: A pilot study. Dermatologic Surgery, 38(2), 215–223.

Carden, A. & Morris, M. (2000). Application of vibrational spectroscopy to the study of mineralized tissues (review). J. Biom. Opt., 5, 259.

Cicchi, R., Cosci, A., Rossari, S., Giorgi, V. D., Kapsokalyvas, D., Massi, D., & Pavone, F. S. (2012). Double optical fibre-probe device for the diagnosis of melanocytic lesions. In Proceedings of SPIE, volume 8427 (pp. 842714).

Cybulski, H. & Sadlej, J. (2007). On the calculations of the vibrational raman spectra of small water clusters. Chemical Physics, 342(1), 163–172.

da Silva Martinho, H., Yassoyama, M. C. B. M., de Oliveira Andrade, P., Bitar, R. A., do Espírito Santo, A. M., Arisawa, E. A., A A Martin, A., et al. (2008). Role of cervicitis in the raman-based optical diagnosis of cervical intraepithelial neoplasia. Journal of biomedical optics, 13, 054029.

da Silva Tagliaferro, E. P., Rodrigues, L. K. A., Soares, L. E. S., Martin, A. A., & dos Santos, M. N. (2009). Physical and compositional changes on demineralized primary enamel induced by co2 laser. Photomedicine and Laser Surgery, 27(4), 585–590.

de Carvalho, L., Bitar, R., Arisawa, E., Brandão, A., Honório, K., Cabral, L., Martin, A., Martinho, H., & Almeida, J. (2010). Spectral region optimization for raman-based optical biopsy of inflammatory lesions. Photomedicine and Laser Surgery, 28(S1), 111–117.

de Carvalho, L. F. C. S., Sato, E. T., J D Almeida, J., & da H S Martinho (2011). Diagnosis of inflammatory lesions by high-wavenumber ft-raman spectroscopy. Theoretical Chemistry Accounts: Theory, Computation, and Modeling (Theoretica Chimica Acta), 130(4), 1221–1229.

de Veld, D., Bakker, S. T., Skurichina, M., Witjes, M., der Wal, J. V., Roodenburg, J. L., & HJ, H. J. S. (2005). Autofluorescence and raman microspectroscopy of tissue sections of oral lesions. Las Med Sci, 19, 203–209.

Dunteman, G. H. (1989). Principal components analysis, volume 69. SAGE Publications, Incorporated.

Duraipandian, S., Zheng, W., Ng, J., Low, J. J. H., Ilancheran, A., & Huang, Z. (2012). Simultaneous fingerprint and high-wavenumber confocal raman spectroscopy enhances early detection of cervical precancer in vivo. Analytical Chemistry, 84(14), 5913–5919.

Evans, C. & Xie, X. (2008). Coherent anti-stokes raman scattering microscopy: chemical imaging for biology and medicine. Annu. Rev. Anal. Chem., 1, 883–909.

Frank, C. J., McCreery, R. L., & Redd, D. C. B. (1995). Raman spectroscopy of normal and diseased human breast tissues. Analytical chemistry, 67(5), 777–783.

Frank, C. J., Redd, D. C. B., Gansler, T. S., & McCreery, R. L. (1994). Characterization of human breast biopsy specimens with near-ir raman spectroscopy. Analytical Chemistry, 66(3), 319–326.

Gniadecka, M., Nielsen, O. F., & Wulf, H. C. (2003). Water content and structure in malignant and benign skin tumours. Journal of Molecular Structure, 661, 405–410.

Griebe, M., Daffertshofer, M., Stroick, M., Syren, M., Ahmad-Nejad, P., Neumaier, M., Backhaus, J., Hennerici, M. G., & Fatar, M. (2007). Infrared spectroscopy: a new diagnostic tool in alzheimer disease. Neurosci Lett, 420, 29–33.

Guze, K., Short, M., Zeng, H., Lerman, M., & Sonis, S. (2011). Comparison of molecular images as defined by raman spectra between normal mucosa and squamous cell carcinoma in the oral cavity. Journal of Raman Spectroscopy, 42(6), 1232–1239.

Hashimoto, M., Minamikawa, T., & Araki, T. (2012). Coherent anti-stokes raman scattering microscopy for high speed non-staining biomolecular imaging. Current pharmaceutical biotechnology.

Holmstrup, P., Vedtofte, P., Reibel, J., & Stoltze, K. (2007). Oral premalignant lesions: is a biopsy reliable? Journal of oral pathology & medicine, 36(5), 262–266.

Kemsley, E. (1996). Discriminant analysis of high-dimensional data: a comparison of principal components analysis and partial least squares data reduction methods. Chemometrics and Intelligent Laboratory Systems, 33(1), 47 – 61.

Krishna, H., Majumder, S. K., & Gupta, P. K. (2012). Range-independent background subtraction algorithm for recovery of raman spectra of biological tissue. Journal of Raman Spectroscopy.

Lieber, C. A. & Kabeer, M. H. (2010). Characterization of pediatric wilms' tumor using raman and fluorescence spectroscopies. J Pediat Surg, 45, 549–554.

Lin, K., Cheng, D. L. P., & Huang, Z. (2012). Optical diagnosis of laryngeal cancer using high wavenumber raman spectroscopy. Biosensors and Bioelectronics, 35, 213–217.

Mahadevan-Jansen, A., Mitchell, M. F., Ramanujamf, N., Malpica, A., Thomsen, S., Utzinger, U., & Richards-Kortumt, R. (2008). Near-infrared raman spectroscopy for in vitro detection of cervical precancers. Photochemistry and photobiology, 68(1), 123–132.

Martinho, H. S., Yassoyama, M. C. B. M., de Oliveira, P. A., Bitar, R. A., Santo, A. M. E., Arisawa, E. A. L., & Martin, A. A. (2008). Role of cervicitis in the raman-based optical diagnosis of cervical intraepithelial neoplasia. J Biomed Opt, 13, 054029–.

Matousek, P., Towrie, M., Ma, C., Kwok, W. M., Phillips, D., Toner, W. T., & Parker, A. W. (2001). Fluorescence suppression in resonance raman spectroscopy using a high-performance picosecond kerr gate. Journal of Raman Spectroscopy, 32(12), 983–988.

McCain, S., Willett, R., & Brady, D. (2008). Multi-excitation raman spectroscopy technique for fluorescence rejection. Optics Express, 16(15), 10975–10991.

Mo, J., Zheng, W., Low, J. J. H., Ilancheran, J. N. A., & Huang, Z. (2009). High wavenumber raman spectroscopy for in vivo detection of cervical dysplasia. Anal Chem, 81, 8908–8915.

Mosier-Boss, P. A., Lieberman, S. H., & Newbery, R. (1995). Fluorescence rejection in raman spectroscopy by shifted-spectra, edge detection, and fft filtering techniques. Applied spectroscopy, 49(5), 630–638.

Movasaghi, Z., Rehman, S., & ur Rehman, I. (2012). Raman spectroscopy can detect and monitor cancer at cellular level: Analysis of resistant and sensitive subtypes of testicular cancer cell lines. Applied Spectroscopy Reviews, 47(7), 571–581.

Nanda, K., McCrory, D. C., Myers, E. R., Bastian, L. A., V, V. H., Hickey, J. D., & Matchar, D. B. (2000). Accuracy of the papanicolaou test in screening for and follow-up of cervical cytologic abnormalities. Ann Int Med, 132, 810–919.

Naumann, D. (2000). Infrared spectroscopy in microbiology. Chichester: John Wiley and Sons.

Naumann, D. (2001). Ft-infrared and ft-raman spectroscopy in biomedical research. Appl Spectrosc Rev, 36, 239–298.

Osticioli, I., Zoppi, A., & Castellucci, E. M. (2007). Shift-excitation raman difference spectroscopy–difference deconvolution method for the luminescence background rejection from raman spectra of solid samples. Applied spectroscopy, 61(8), 839–844.

Pajcini, V., Munro, C. H., Bormett, R. W., Witkowski, R. E., & Asher, S. A. (1997). Uv raman microspectroscopy: Spectral and spatial selectivity with sensitivity and simplicity. Applied Spectroscopy, 51(1), 81–86.

Patil, C., Bosschaart, N., Keller, M., van Leeuwen, T., & Mahadevan-Jansen, A. (2008). Combined raman spectroscopy and optical coherence tomography device for tissue characterization. Optics letters, 33(10), 1135–1137.

Patil, C. A., Kirshnamoorthi, H., Ellis, D. L., van Leeuwen, T. G., & Mahadevan-Jansen, A. (2011). A clinical instrument for combined raman spectroscopy-optical coherence tomography of skin cancers. Lasers in Surgery and Medicine, 43(2), 143–151.

Prasad, P. N. (2003). Introduction to biophotonics. New Jersey: John Wiley and Sons.

Raman, C. (1928). A new radiation. Indian Journal of physics, 2, 387–398.

Saleh, B. & Teich, M. (1991). Fundamentals of Photonics. New York: John Wiley and Sons.

Shreve, A. P., Cherepy, N. J., & Mathies, R. A. (1992). Effective rejection of fluorescence interference in raman spectroscopy using a shifted excitation difference technique. Applied spectroscopy, 46(4), 707–711.

Singh, R. & Riess, F. (1998). Raman and the story of nobel prize. Curr Sci, 75, 965–971.

Vargis, E., Byrd, T., Logan, Q., Khabele, D., & Mahadevan-Jansen, A. (2011). Sensitivity of raman spectroscopy to normal patient variability. Journal of Biomedical Optics, 16(11), 117004–117004.

Verrier, S., Zoladek, A., & Notingher, I. (2011). Raman micro-spectroscopy as a non-invasive cell viability test. Methods in molecular biology (Clifton, NJ), 740, 179.

Wang, H., Tsai, T., Zhao, J., Lee, A., Lo, B., Yu, M., Lui, H., McLean, D., & Zeng, H. (2012). Differentiation of hacat cell and melanocyte from their malignant counterparts using micro-raman spectroscopy guided by confocal imaging. Photodermatology, Photoimmunology & Photomedicine, 28(3), 147–152.

Webster, G. T., Tilley, L., Deed, S., McNaughton, D., & Wood, B. R. (2008). Resonance raman spectroscopy can detect structural changes in haemozoin (malaria pigment) following incubation with chloroquine in infected erythrocytes. FEBS Letters, 582, 1087.

Wold, S. & Sjostrom, M. (1977). Simca: a method for analyzing chemical data in terms of similarity and analogy. Chemometrics: theory and application, 52, 243–282.

Zhang, D. & Ben-Amotz, D. (2000). Enhanced chemical classification of raman images in the presence of strong fluorescence interference. Applied Spectroscopy, 54(9), 1379–1383.

Zhao, J., Carrabba, M. M., & Allen, F. S. (2002). Automated fluorescence rejection using shifted excitation raman difference spectroscopy. Applied spectroscopy, 56(7), 834–845.

www.ingramcontent.com/pod-product-compliance
Lightning Source LLC
Chambersburg PA
CBHW050816220326
41598CB00006B/228

* 9 7 8 1 9 2 2 2 2 7 4 9 2 *